T5-COA-557

Review copy
not for sale

Clinical Aspects of IgG Subclasses and Therapeutic Implications

Monographs in Allergy

Vol. 23

Series Editors
P. Dukor, Basel; *L. Å. Hanson,* Göteborg; *P. Kallós,* Helsingborg;
F. Shakib, Derby; *Z. Trnka,* Basel; *B.H. Waksman,* New York, N.Y.

KARGER

Basel · München · Paris · London · New York · New Delhi · Singapore · Tokyo · Sydney

2nd Workshop on Clinical Aspects of IgG Subclasses and Therapeutic Implications, Interlaken, May 4 and 5, 1987

Clinical Aspects of IgG Subclasses and Therapeutic Implications

Volume Editors
F. Skvaril, Bern
A. Morell, Bern
B. Perret, Bern

41 figures and 65 tables, 1988

KARGER

Basel · München · Paris · London · New York · New Delhi · Singapore · Tokyo · Sydney

Monographs in Allergy

Cover illustration
Modified according to Morell, A.; Skvaril, F.; Hitzig, W.; Barandun, S.: IgG Subclasses: Development of Serum Concentrations in 'Normal' Infants and Children. J. Pediatr. *80:* 960–964 (1972).

Library of Congress Cataloging-in-Publication Data
Workshop on Clinical Aspects of IgG Subclasses and Therapeutic Implications (2nd: 1987: Interlaken, Switzerland)
Clinical aspects of IgG subclasses and therapeutic implications.
(Monographs in allergy; vol. 23)
Includes bibliographies and index.
1. Immunoglobulin G – Physiological effect – Congresses. 2. Immunoglobulin allotypes – Congresses. 3. Immunopathology-Congresses. 4. Immunotherapy-Congresses. I. Skvaril, F. II. Morell, A. (Andreas) III. Perret, B. (Beat), 1944 – . IV. Title. V. Series.
[DNLM: 1. IgG-immunology-congresses. 2. IgG-therapeutic use-congresses. W1 M0567E v. 23/QW 601 W926 1987c]
QR186.8.G2W67 1987 616.07'93 87-33888
ISBN 3-8055-4671-8

Bibliographic Indices.
This publication is listed in bibliographic services, including Current Contents® and Index Medicus.

Drug Dosage
The authors and the publisher have exerted every effort to ensure that drug selection and dosage set forth in this text are in accord with current recommendations and practice at the time of publication. However, in view of ongoing research, changes in government regulations, and the constant flow of information relating to drug therapy and drug reactions, the reader is urged to check the package insert for each drug for any change in indications and dosage and for added warnings and precautions. This is particularly important when the recommended agent is a new and/or infrequently employed drug.

All rights reserved
No part of this publication may be translated into other languages, reproduced or utilized in any form or by any means, electronic or mechanical, including photocopying, recording, microcopying, or by any information storage and retrieval system, without permission in writing from the publisher.

© Copyright 1988 by S. Karger AG, P.O. Box, CH-4009 Basel (Switzerland)
Printed in Switzerland by gdz (Genossenschaftsdruckerei Zürich)
ISBN 3-8055-4671-8

Contents

Foreword IX

Introductory Presentation

Schur, P.H. (Boston, Mass.): IgG Subclasses. A Historical Perspective 1

IgG Subclasses and Antibody Activities

Djurup, R. (Copenhagen): Immunochemical Quantitation of IgG Subclass Proteins and IgG Subclass Antibodies: Status and Perspectives 12

Hammarström, L. (Huddinge and Stockholm); *Insel, R.A.* (Rochester, N.Y.); *Persson, M.A.A.; Smith, C.I.E.* (Huddinge and Stockholm): The IgG1 Subclass Preference of Selected, Naturally Occuring Antipolysaccharide Antibodies 18

Linde, A.; Sundqvist, V.-A.; Mathiesen, T.; Wahren, B. (Stockholm): IgG Subclasses to Subviral Components. 27

Urbanek, R. (Freiburg i. Br.): IgG Subclasses and Subclass Distribution in Allergic Disorders 33

Yount, W.J.; Cohen, P.; Eisenberg, R.A. (Chapel Hill, N.C): Distribution of IgG Subclasses among Human Autoantibodies to Sm, RNP, dsDNA, SS-B and IgG Rheumatoid Factor 41

Oxelius, V.-A. (Lund): Restrictive Murine Monoclonal IgG Subclass Antisera Revealing Antigenic Variants of Human IgG Subclasses 57

Ferrante, A.; Beard, L.J. (Adelaide): IgG Subclass Assays with Polyclonal Antisera and Monoclonal Antibodies 61

Jefferies, R.; Walker, M.R. (Birmingham): The Biological Significance of Specific Antibody IgG Subclass Profiles 73

Radl, J. (Rijswijk); *Jol-van der Zijde, C.M.; Tol, M.J.D, van; Vossen, J.M.* (Leiden): IgG Subclass Representation within Homogenous Immunoglobulins in Immunodeficiency Diseases 78

Clinical Aspects of IgG Subclasses

Reimer, C.B.; Black, C.M.; Holman, R.C.; Wells, T.W.; Ramirez, R.M.; Sa-Ferreira, J.A.; Nicholson, J.K.A.; McDougal, J.S. (Atlanta, Ga.): Hypergammaglobulinemia Associated with Human Immunodeficiency Virus Infection 83
Geha, R.S. (Boston, Mass.): IgG Antibody Response to Polysaccharides in Children with Recurrent Infections 97
Mac Lennan, I.C.M.; Chandramukhi, A.; Lane, P.J.L.; Oldfield, S. (Birmingham): The Cellular Basis of Selective Defects in IgG Subclass Responses 103
Preud'homme, J.L.; Aucouturier, P.; Barra, A.; Duarte, F. (Poitiers); *Intrator, L.; Cordonnier, C.; Vernant, J.P.* (Creteil); *Schulz, D.; Noël, L.H.; Lesavre, P.* (Paris): Serum IgG Subclasses in Secondary Immunodeficiencies 113
Insel, R.A.; Anderson, P.W. (Rochester, N.Y.): IgG Subclass Distribution of Antibody Induced by Immunization with the Isolated and Protein-Conjugated Polysaccharide of *H. influenzae* b and G2m(n) Distribution of Serum IgG2 in Man 128
Christensen, K.K.; Christensen, P. (Lund): IgG Subclasses and Neonatal Infections with Group B Streptococci 138
Quinti, I.; Papetti, C.; Hunolstein, C., von; Orefici, G.; Aiuti, F. (Rome): IgG Subclasses to Group B Streptococci in Normals, Colonized Woman and IgG2 Subclass-Deficient Patients 148
Chandra, R.K. (St. John's, Newfoundland): Concentrations and Production of IgG Subclasses in Preterm and Small-for-Gestation Low Birth Weight Infants 156

IVIG Replacement Therapy in IgG Subclass Deficiency States

Björkander, J. (Göteborg); *Oxelius, V.-A.* (Lund); *Söderström, R.; Hanson, L.Å.* (Göteborg): Immunoglobulin Treatment of Patients with Selective IgG Subclass and IgA Deficiency States 160
Smith, T.F.; Muldoon, M.F.; Bain, R.P.; Wells, E.L. (Atlanta, Ga.); *Tiller, T.L.* (Greensville, S.C.); *Kutner, M.H.* (Atlanta, Ga.); *Schiffman, G.* (Brooklyn, N.Y.); *Pandey, J.P.* (Charleston, S.C.): Clinical Results of a Prospective, Double-Blind, Placebo-Controlled Trial of Intravenous γ-Globulin in Children with Chronic Chest Symptoms 168
Gelfand, E.W.; Reid, B.; Roifman, C.M. (Denver, Colo. and Toronto, Ont.): Intravenous Immune Serum Globulin Replacement in Hypogammaglobulinemia. A Comparison of High-versus Low-Dose Therapy 177
Heiner, D.C.; Lee, S.I.; Kim, K.; Schoettler, J. (Torrance, Calif.): Replacement Therapy in IgG4-Deficient Patients 187
Beard, L.J.; Ferrante, A. (Adelaide): IgG Replacement Therapy in IgG Subclass-Deficient Children 194
Plebani, A. (Pavia); *Duse, M.; Tiberti, S.* (Brescia); *Avanzini, M.A.; Monafo, V.* (Pavia); *Menegati, E.; Ugazio, A.G.* (Brescia); *Burgio, G.R.* (Pavia): Intra-

Contents

venous γ-Globulin Therapy and Serum IgG Subclass Levels in Intractable
Childhood Epilepsy 204
Emanuel, D. (New York, N.Y.): Issues Concerning the Use of Intravenous Immunoglobulins for the Immunoprophylaxis of Cytomegalovirus Infections in Allogeneic Bone Marrow Transplant Recipients 216
Fischer, S.H.; Ochs, H.D.; Wedgwood, R.J. (Seattle, Wash.); *Skvaril, F.; Morell, A.* (Bern); *Hill, H.R.* (Salt Lake City, Utah); *Schiffman, G.* (Brooklyn, N.Y.); *Corey, L.* (Seattle, Wash.): Survival of Antigen-Specific Antibody Following Administration of Intravenous Immunoglobulin in Patients with Primary Immunodeficiency Diseases 225

New Biological Aspects of IgG Subclasses

Söderström, T.; Söderström, R.; Andersson, R.; Lindberg, J.; Hanson, L.Å. (Göteborg): Factors Influencing IgG Subclass Levels in Serum and Mucosal Secretions 236
Ambrosino, D.M. (Boston, Mass.); *Morell, A.; Vassalli, G.* (Bern); *Lange, G.D., de* (Amsterdam); *Skvaril, F.* (Bern); *Siber, G.R.* (Jamaica Plain, Mass.): Correlations of G2m(n) and Km(1) Allotypes with Subclass- and Light-Chain-Specific Antibody 244
Granoff, D.M.; Sheetz, K.E.; Nahm, M.H.; Madassery, J.V.; Shackelford, P.G. (St. Louis, Mo.): Further Immunologic Evaluation of Children Who Develop Haemophilus Disease Despite Previous Vaccination with Type b Polysaccharide Vaccine 256
Shackelford, P.G.; Granoff, D.M. (St. Louis, Mo.): IgG Subclass Composition of the Antibody Response of Healthy Adults, and Normal or IgG2-Deficient Children to Immunization with *H. influenzae* type b Polysaccharide Vaccine or Hib PS-Protein conjugate Vaccines 269
Rijkers, G.T.; Roord, J.J.; Struyvé, M.C. (Utrecht); *Poolman, J.T.* (Bilthoven); *Zegers, B.J.M.* (Utrecht): Development of IgG Antipolyribosylribitolphosphate Antibodies in the Course of *H. influenzae* Type b Meningitis in Infants below 2 Years of Age 282

Subject Index 289

Foreword

In recent years, knowledge on IgG subclasses in health and in various disease states has been rapidly growing. Many investigators have analyzed the influence of age, genetic makeup and other biological factors on the subclass serum concentrations. Moreover, the subclass composition of IgG antibodies against a host of microbial and other antigens was established. The clinical significance of partial as well as complete deficiencies of any of the four IgG subclasses was impressively documented. Evidence is now emerging that the underlying defect may be an incapacity to respond to certain groups of antigens which are known to induce subclass-restricted antibodies. The most prominent example are IgG antibodies to bacterial capsular polysaccharides.

Not long ago, a selection of important studies of the leading investigators in this field was published in volumes 19 and 20 of this series. In view of the great interest which is currently focussed on clinical aspects and therapeutic implications of IgG subclasses, as well as in view of the many new exciting findings, we felt that the state of the art should again be documented. Therefore, a second workshop was held at Interlaken on May 4 and 5, 1987. It was made possible by the generous support from the Central Laboratory of the Swiss Red Cross Blood Transfusion Service, Berne. The present volume includes the presentation and discussions of this meeting. We wish to thank all the authors, discussants and chairmen who devoted their time and effort to contribute to this work.

F. Skvaril
A. Morell

Introductory Presentation

IgG Subclasses
A Historical Perspective[1]

Peter H. Schur

Departments of Rheumatology/Immunology and the Clinical Immunology Laboratory, Brigham and Women's Hospital, Harvard Medical School, Boston, Mass., USA

History is usually thought of as what happened in the past, and how it possibly relates to the present. Historians often perceive themselves as clairvoyants trying to predict the future, based on recognized patterns of the past. Trained as a scientist, however, I am basically curious, and often wonder, how did it all begin?

Phase 1

In the beginning (that is in the 1930s) there was but one γ-globulin, until Kabat [1], Tiselius [2], and Pedersen [3] showed that it could be divided into 7S and 19S fractions. By the 1950s, immunological techniques demonstrated three immunological classes, IgG, IgA, and IgM. Critical in these advancements were the techniques of electrophoresis (developed by Tiselius [2] in the 1930s and 1940s), ultracentrifugation (developed in the 1940s by Tiselius, Pedersen, and Svedberg [3]), double diffusion in agar (developed by Ouchterlony [4] in 1953), immunoelectrophoresis (developed in 1958 by Grabar and Williams [5]), and the use of myeloma proteins, which were shown to be structurally similar to normal Ig [6]. Critical to these studies were the use of rabbits to make antisera. The stage was set for a new discovery.

The discovery of the IgG subclasses represents the results of parallel work by a number of groups, working independently but aware of each others' work. The groups were either in New York City, at the NIH, or in Florida. In 1956, Oudin [7], by immunizing different strains

---

[1] Supported in part by a grant from the USPHS, AM 37005.

of rabbits, was the first to demonstrate allotypy of IgG. The same year (1956), Korngold and Lipari [8] reported that rabbits immunized with normal IgG and myeloma proteins made antibodies which demonstrated antigenic differences (by double diffusion in agar) between the myeloma proteins.

Korngold [9] was able to describe three IgG, and became the first investigator to note IgG subclasses. In retrospect, he probably recognized κ and λ and possibly one IgG subclass. In 1959, Edelman [10] demonstrated that IgG had both heavy (H) and light (L) chains, and in 1962 showed that L chains were the same as Bence-Jones proteins [11]. Meanwhile, Dray and Young [12] confirmed Oudin's observations of allotypy of IgG in rabbits and in 1958 decided to look for allotypy in human Ig. Unable to immunize humans with Ig plus Freund's adjuvant, he picked the closest species to man, primates (Rhesus monkeys) – and appeared to be the first to use primates to make antisera. The antisera did not detect antigenic differences between individuals, but by immunoelectrophoresis detected three IgG [13, 14]. By absorbing with myeloma proteins (obtained from Fahey) the antiserum would give but one line on immunoprecipitation with normal serum. Dray presented the data at the Rockefeller University and compared results with those of Edelman and Kunkel. Edelman had an antiserum which detected two different IgG, of the same mobility, which (antiserum) subsequently recognized κ and λ. In 1962 and 1963, Fahey and Solomon [15], Mannik and Kunkel [16], and Migita and Putnam [17] reported on two types of light chains (called by different names but basically Type I and II), and correspondingly two types of IgG, IgA, and IgM. These observations were made with both normal immunoglobulins and myeloma proteins.

1962. Meanwhile, Harboe [18] became one of the first Scandinavians to reciprocate Kunkel's sabbatical in Tiselius's laboratory and worked under Kunkel at the Rockefeller University. Harboe [18] extended the basic observations of Grubb [19] and noted that IgG myeloma proteins could be either a+b– or Gm a–b+ [20]. The differences were thought to reflect heterogeneity of genetic characters among normal IgG in a given individual. Allen, Kunkel and Kabat [21] then collaborated to study the structure and function of isolated antibodies and also found differences in their Gm characteristics. In the same year (1962), Hess and Butler [22] demonstrated that monkeys could make antibodies with Gm specificity when immunized with normal IgG and IgG myeloma proteins. They also concluded that these observations suggested differences among IgG molecules.

1963. In this year, Benacerraf et al. [23] demonstrated that guinea pig IgG could be separated electrophoretically into slow and fast moieties, which differed in complement-fixing and skin-sensitizing properties – demonstrating again that there was more than one IgG, not based on light chain specificities, and the first to demonstrate that animals could have more than one type of IgG.

1964. Much of all of this work came to fruition in the recognition of four IgG subclasses although, as I have noted, subdivision of IgG had in fact been noted for a number of years, albeit less than four.

The group working under Putnam was interested in immunoglobulin structure. Stimulated by the recent discovery of heavy chain diseases [24, 25], they obtained the heavy chain Crawford (CR) (IgG1) from Franklin and Zucker (ZU) (IgG3) from Osserman. Rabbit antisera were made to both and could differentiate CR from ZU. These differences could also be defined in normal IgG. More myeloma proteins were obtained which could be defined as either corresponding to CR, ZU. These results were discussed with Osserman prior to the FASEB meeting in 1964, and were discussed with Terry, Fahey, Grey, and Kunkel after their FASEB presentations. The results were published on July 10, 1964 (submitted on March 26, 1964) [26]. What was never published were the results with another antiserum which reacted with all non-CR, non-ZU (that is non-IgG1, IgG3), proteins, except for one IgG myeloma protein. Thus, in retrospect this additional antiserum recognized IgG2, while no antiserum recognized the last myeloma protein, which was presumably a IgG4.

1964. Takatsuki and Osserman analyzed five of their heavy chain proteins and one from Franklin. They were able to observe, as did Ballieux et al. [26], that antisera to these proteins defined two types of IgG called C (after Crawford the IgG1) and Z (after Zucker the IgG3). Then they analyzed 20 myeloma proteins. Eighteen were IgG1 und two IgG3. In retrospect, surprisingly, no IgG2 were found. Their paper was published on July 21, 1964 (having been submitted on April 9, 1964) [27].

1964. Terry and Fahey, stimulated by the work of Dray and Benacerraf, were trying to define Ig subclasses in both mice and humans. Solomon, affiliated with their laboratory at the time, found a myeloma protein that was neither IgG, IgA, or IgM. Only years later was it found to be a IgD. They immunized monkeys and rabbits with normal γ-globulin and myeloma proteins. The antisera recognized three IgG in normal sera by immunoelectrophoresis. The three types corresponded to those described earlier by Dray. The immunoprecipitation lines were decreased or absent in patients with agammaglobulinemia or hypogammaglobulinemia. Terry and Fahey were therefore the first to describe a deficiency in the IgG subclasses! They also recognized antithyroglobulin antibodies in all three IgG subclasses – and were again the first to recognize antibodies in the IgG subclasses. Their paper was presented at the 1964 FASEB meeting [28] and published on October 26, 1964 (having been submitted on July 8, 1964 [29]. Subsequently they took isolated myeloma proteins that were either slow or fast on electrophoresis, or of different carbohydrate content, and those proteins and their Fc pieces (often isolated with great difficulty) were used to immunize monkeys and rabbits. The antisera recognized differences among the myeloma proteins.

1964. Grey came to Kunkel's laboratory in 1963 and began to utilize the many anti-immunoglobulin antisera available in the laboratory. Thanks to the diligent efforts of Solomon (Ne-Newman), Yount (Vi-Vilkes), Mannik (Ge-Gerolman) and myself, many myeloma proteins were available for study. Grey and Kunkel [30] began to recognize antigenic differences between myeloma proteins that could not be accounted for by κ/λ differences. The antisera were made specific by absorption with myeloma proteins until four subclasses to IgG could be defined. Thus, they were the first group to recognize four subclasses of IgG. The availability of many myeloma proteins no doubt facilitated this finding. The study was presented at the 1964 FASEB meeting [30] and was published on August 1, 1964 (having been submitted on April 24, 1964) [31].

Shortly after, four IgG subclasses were recognized; Terry and Fahey [32] confirmed these findings. At one point, a fifth IgG was reported by Spiegelberg in an abstract at the FASEB meetings, but was subsequently recognized to be a IgG2n+.

Phase 2

Phase 2 of this historical perspective was essentially deciding what to do with the knowledge that IgG is divided into four subclasses. Is there any special significance to four from either the biological, historical, or other point of view? From the point of view of mythology, the numbers 3 and 7 have greater significance. Nevertheless, the number 4 has its own status: there are 4 limbs, 4 chambers of the heart, 4 corners of the earth, 4 seasons (and 4 languages in Switzerland). What was done in this phase was a reflection of the particular interests of the investigator. For instance, Fahey reaffirmed his Cleveland connection and collaborated with Steinberg, while the Kunkel group gravitated to their Scandinavian connections and collaborated with Grubb. Both groups (and others) demonstrated the association of particular allotypic markers (Gm) with the IgG subclasses [6, 32–39]. In fact initial credit should be given to Prendergast who observed the association during one of the Thursday afternoon Kunkel laboratory meetings when others were presenting their data. Most of the investigators in the field at this point were immunochemists who studied subjects such as structural and antigenic differences, including enzyme sensitivity, the number of disulfide bonds and free sulfhydryl groups, electrophoretic mobility, peptide differences, and ultimately amino acid sequences [38–41, and reviewed in ref. 42]. Others used the antisera to determine the concentration of IgG subclasses in normal individuals [reviewed in ref. 42–44], which naturally led to the determination of IgG subclass levels in disease [reviewed in ref. 42–45]. Having started with myeloma proteins it was natural to look at the frequency of myeloma proteins among the subclasses and compare it to the percentage in normals – they are similar but significantly not quite the same [reviewed in ref. 42]. Others with a pediatric or a genetic background often look for things that are missing and discovered individuals who were deficient in an IgG subclass [reviewed in ref. 42–44] and, influenced no doubt by the findings in agammaglobulinemia, noted recurrent infections in most of these individuals. Later on, IgG subclass levels were determined in patients with other immune diseases [reviewed in ref. 43, 44]. Others more biologically oriented began to look at the IgG subclass composition of antibodies, of cell surface immunoglobulin, of immunoglobulins in immune deposits, and in particular their biological properties (namely PCA, complement fixation) [46, 47, reviewed in ref.

Table I. IgG subclass publications

Year	Total number	DNA mapping	Genetics	Structure	Biology	Antibodies	Measure	Monoclonals	Immunodeficiencies	Treatment	IgG4
1960	1			1							
1961	1			1							
1962	1			1							
1964	12		2	8	1	1					
1965	7		2	4		1					
1966	11		5	4	1	1					
1967	13		5	5	1		2				
1968	14		2	3		3			1		1
1969	17		4	7	1	2			3		
1970	40		5	14	7	2	3		6		3
1971	23		1	14	5		3				
1972	24		3	5	7	5	2				1
1973	18		2	5	3	5	2				1
1974	19		2	7	2	2	3		1		1
1975	19			6	1	4	4		2		1
1976	22		3	6	3	4	4		1	1	
1977	17		2	4	2	1	3			1	4
1978	19	1	1	4	1	7	4				2
1979	25			4	2	4	9		3	1	2
1980	26		1	2	3	8	2		1	1	3
1981	32	2	2	2	4	4	6		3	2	5
1982	34	5	1	1	1	4	6	4	2		8
1983	58	1		3	8	14	4	4	8		16
1984	59	1	2		9	17	14	4	2		8
1985	56	3		1	5	27	8	3	3	1	5
1986	96	1	4	2	5	19	20	5	22	4	9

42–45]. Of particular interest to many was IgG4, which is the IgG subclass found in least concentration in normals, was antigenically more different from the other IgG subclasses, does not fix complement, but yet was found – often in relatively large amounts – in pathological lesions. These studies have raised the possibility that IgG4 is the non-IgE reagin, and involved in histamine release and allergic disease reactions [reviewed in ref. 43–45]. We have clearly not heard the last word from the proponents and detractors of this theory. Hopefully, constructive criticism of each other's works will lead to more critical analysis of the issues.

Phase 3

The Present. To date, there have been approximately 664 papers written on the subject of IgG subclasses (table I). I have divided the papers into 10 groups. One can discern trends of increasing and decreasing numbers of papers per year, in particular areas, presumably reflecting both interests and advances in technology (namely monoclonal antisera, solid-phase immunoassays, enzyme-linked immunosorbent assay). Clearly the steady increase in the number of papers per year, the PhD theses, involvement by industry, monographs, and of course international meetings (in lovely settings) speak to an expanding important field. Examination of table I for trends suggests that the interest in structure and genetics seems to have peaked and then waned, while the number of papers on biological properties of the IgG subclasses has remained relatively steady. On the other hand, the typing of antibodies (to every conceivable foreign and autoantigen) has increased as of late, reflecting the parallel increase in availability of the monoclonal antisera and the improved technology to utilize them in sensitive assays. There also appears to be increased interest in immunodeficiencies, and their treatment, while the special interest in IgG4 seems to have peaked. Lastly, the interest in the DNA control, and regulation of the IgG subclasses, and its role in defining immunodeficiencies on a genomic basis, seems perhaps to be generating much interest.

The present workshop reflects current interests in defining the use and specificity of reagents, the IgG subclass nature of antibodies, especially to polysaccharides, defining immunodeficiencies, and seeking paths to their therapy.

Phase 4

The Future. As noted in the beginning of this paper, a historian often acts as a clairvoyant, using the past to predict the future. I venture into this area with care and dread, knowing of many past predictions in many areas that failed – namely world peace, a cure for cancer, and even for the common cold! The only prediction I make with confidence is that where will be more and more papers published on the subject. Neverthless, I feel compelled to try and predict specifically what will be investigated in the near future and hope that these thoughts will serve as a stimulus to the participants of this meeting as well as to a younger generation of scientists.

I predict that the further use of monoclonal antibodies will define further subdivisions of the IgG subclasses. These subdivisions will then be studied in respect to: their structure, function, and genetic associations; serum levels in normals (of all ages) and in diseases; serum levels in patients with immunodeficiencies (and what it clinically correlates with) and how these deficiencies can be replaced; their distribution in antibodies and pathological deposits; and the role of IgG4 in allergy.

I also predict that the techniques of molecular biology will be used to initially define the immunodeficiency on a genomic basis, and will note many (different forms) of deletions and mutations, many of which (but not necessarily all) result in different forms of immunodeficiency. An international workshop will sort them and define a nomenclature to classify them. Ultimately, these tools of molecular biology will be used as genetic engineering tools to correct a defect – where clinically indicated. Molecular biological tools will also be used to help explain why the immune response to some antigens results in predominately an IgG1 response (anti-Sm), IgG2 (polysaccharides) and IgG4 (allergens, clotting factors). Once we know which antibody class/subclass/subdivision provides us with maximal protection from pathogens/allergens, this knowledge will be useful in designing better vaccines. Molecular biological tools will also tell us why individual clones of B cells become malignant and make monoclonal Ig – and also facilitate ways of turning this system off. Ideally IgG subclasses will be turned on to make effective antibodies that may prevent cancer, the common cold, and other diseases. Then we can all retire – or begin research on some other problem.

Acknowledgements

I am grateful to the following colleagues for sharing some of their reminiscences and unpublished anecdotes regarding the early discovery of the IgG subclasses: Drs. J.

Allen, G. Bernier, S. Dray, J. Fahey, S. Litwin, R. Prendergast, A. Solomon, and H. Spiegelberg.

References

1 Kabat, E.A.: Getting started 50 years ago – experiences, perspectives, and problems of the first 21 years. A. Rev. Immunol. *1:* 1–32 (1983).
2 Tiselius, A.: Electrophorectic analysis and the constitution of native fluids. Harvey Lect. *35:* 37–70 (1939–40).
3 Pedersen, K.O.: Ultracentrifugal studies on serum and serum fractions (Almqvist & Wiksell, Uppsala 1945).
4 Ouchterlony, O.: Diffusion in gel methods for immunological analysis. Prog. Allergy, vol. 5, pp. 1–78 (Karger, Basel 1958).
5 Grabar, P.; Williams, C.A., Jr.: Méthode immuno-électrophorétique d'analyse de mélanges de substances antigéniques. Biochim. biophys. Acta *17:* 67–74 (1955).
6 Kunkel, H.G.: Myeloma proteins and antibodies. Harvey Lect. *59:* 219–242 (1965).
7 Oudin, J.: 'L'allotypie' de certains antigènes protéidiques du sérum. C.r. hebd. Séance. Acad. Sci., Paris *242:* 2606–2608 (1956).
8 Korngold, L.; Lipari, R.: Multiple-myeloma proteins. III. Antigenic relationship of Bence-Jones proteins to normal gamma-globulin and multiple-myeloma serum proteins. Cancer *9:* 262–272 (1956).
9 Korngold, L.: Abnormal plasma components and their significance in disease. Ann. N.Y. Acad. Sci. *94:* 110–130 (1961).
10 Edelman, G.M.: Dissociation of gamma-globulin. J. Am. chem. Soc. *81:* 3155–3156 (1959).
11 Edelman, G.M.; Poulik, M.D.: Studies on structural units of the gamma-globulins. J. exp. Med. *113:* 861–884 (1962).
12 Dray, S.: Young, G.O.: Differences in the antigenic components of sera of individual rabbits as shown by induced isoprecipitins. J. Immun. *81:* 142–149 (1958).
13 Dray, S.: Three gamma-globulins in normal human serum revealed by monkey precipitins. Science *132:* 1313–1314 (1960).
14 Lichter, E.A.; Dray, S.: Immunoelectrophoretic characterization of human serum proteins with primate antisera. J. Immun. *92:* 91–99 (1964).
15 Fahey, J.L.; Solomon, A.: Two types of gamma myeloma proteins, B2A myeloma proteins, gamma-1-globulins-macroglobulins and Bence Jones proteins identified by two groups of common antigenic determinants. J. clin. Invest. *42:* 811–822 (1963).
16 Mannik, M.; Kunkel, H.G.: Classification of myeloma proteins, Bence Jones proteins, and macroglobulins into two groups on the basis of common antigenic determinants. J. exp. Med. *116:* 859–877 (1962).
17 Migita, S.; Putnam, F.W.: Antigenic relationships of Bence Jones proteins, myeloma proteins, and normal human gamma-globulin. J. Exp. Med. *117:* 81–104 (1963).
18 Harboe, M.: A new hemagglutinating substance in the Gm system, anti-Gm. Acta path. microbiol. scand. *47:* 191–198 (1959).

19 Grubb, R.: Agglutination of erythrocytes coated with 'incomplete' anti-Rh by certain rheumatoid arthritic sera and some other sera. The existence of human serum groups. Acta path. Microbiol. scand. *39:* 195–197 (1956).
20 Harboe, M.; Osterland, C.K.; Mannik, M.: Kunkel, H.G.: Genetic characters of human gamma-globulins in myeloma proteins. J. exp. Med. *116:* 719–738 (1962).
21 Allen, J.C.; Kunkel, H.G.; Kabat, E.A.: Studies on human antibodies. II. Distribution of genetic factors. J. exp. Med. *119:* 453–465 (1964).
22 Hess, M.; Butler, C.: Anti-Gm specifities in sera of rhesus monkeys immunized with human gamma-globulin. Vox Sang. *7:* 93–95 (1962).
23 Benacerraf, B.: Ovary, Z.; Bloch, K.J.; Franklin, E.C.: Properties in guinea pig 7S antibodies. I. Electrophoretic separation of two types of guinea pig 7S antibodies. J. expl. Med. *117:* 937–949 (1963).
24 Franklin, E.C.; Meltzer, M.; Guggenheim, F.; Lowenstein, J.: An unusual micro globulin in the serum and urine of a patient. Fed. Proc. *22:* 264 (1963).
25 Osserman, E.F.; Takatsuki, K.: Plasma cell myeloma: globulin synthesis and structure. Medicine *42:* 357–384 (1963).
26 Ballieux, R.E.; Bernier, G.M.; Tominaga, K.; Putnam, F.W.: Gamma globulin antigenic types defined by heavy chain determinants. Science *145:* 168–170 (1964).
27 Takatsuki, K.; Osserman, E.F.: Structural differences between two types of 'Heavy Chain' disease proteins and myeloma globulins of corresponding types. Science *145:* 499–500 (1964).
28 Terry, W.D.; Fahey, J.L.: Heterogeneity of the H chains of human 7S gamma-globulin. Fed. Proc. *23:* 454 (1964).
29 Terry, W.D.; Fahey, J.L.: Subclasses of human gamma-globulin based on differences in the heavy polypeptide chains. Science *146:* 400–401 (1964).
30 Grey, H.M.; Kunkel, H.G.: Subdivision of myeloma proteins. Fed. Proc. *23:* 454 (1964).
31 Grey, H.M.; Kunkel, H.G.: H chain subgroups of myeloma proteins and normal 7S gamma-globulin. J. exp. Med. *120:* 253–266 (1964).
32 Terry, W.D.; Fahey, J.L.; Steinberg, A.G.: Gm and InV factors in subclasses of human IgG. J. exp. Med. *122:* 1087–1102 (1965).
33 Martensson, L.; Kunkel, H.G.: Distribution among the gamma-globulin molecules of different genetically determined antigenic specificities in the Gm system. J. exp. Med. *122:* 799–811 (1965).
34 Kunkel, H.G.; Allen, J.C.; Grey, H.M.; Martensson, L.; Grubb, R.A.: A relationship between the H chain groups of 7S gamma-globulin and the Gm system. Nature *203:* 413–414 (1964).
35 Kunkel, H.G.; Allen, J.C.; Grey, H.M.: Genetic characters and polypeptide chains of various types of gamma globulin. Cold Spring Harb. Symp. quant. Biol. *29:* 443–447 (1964).
36 Natvig, J.B.; Kunkel, H.G.; Litwin, S.D.: Genetic markers of the heavy chain subgroups of human gamma-globulin. Cold Spring Harb. Symp. quant. Biol. *32:* 173–180 (1967).
37 Litwin, S.D.; Kunkel, H.G.: A gamma-globulin genetic factor related to Gm(a) but localized to a different portion of the same heavy chains. Nature *210:* 866 (1966).

38   Meltzer, M.; Franklin, E.C.; Fudenberg, H.; Frangione, B.: Single peptide differences in gamma-globulin of difference genetic (Gm) types. Proc. natn. Acad. Sci. USA *51:* 1007–1014 (1964).
39   Frangione, B.; Franklin, E.C.; Fudenberg, H.H.; Koshland, M.E.: Structural studies of human gamma G-myloma proteins of difference antigenic subroups and genetic specificities. J. exp. med. *124:* 715–732 (1966).
40   Frangione, B.; Franklin, E.C.: Structural studies of human immunoglobulins. Differences in the Fd fragments of the heavy chains of G myeloma proteins. J. exp. Med. *122:* 1–10 (1965).
41   Grey, H.M.; Kunkel, H.G.: Heavy-chain subclasses of human gamma G-globulin. Peptide and immunochemical relationships. Biochemistry *6:* 2326–2334 (1967).
42   Schur, P.H.: Human gamma-G subclasses. Prog. clin. Immunol. *1:* 71–104 (1972).
43   Schur, P.H.: IgG Subclasses – a review. Ann. Allergy *58:* 89–100 (1987).
44   Shakib, F.: Editors of basic and clinical aspects of IgG subclasses. Monogr. Allergy, vol. 19 (Karger, Basel 1986).
45   Hanson, L.Å.; Söderström, T.; Oxelius, V.A. (eds): Immunoglobulin subclass deficiencies. Monogr. Allergy, vol. 20 (Karger, Basel 1986).
46   Yount, W.J.; Dorner, M.M.; Kunkel, H.G.; Kabat, E.A.: Studies on human antibodies. VI. Selective variations in subgroup composition and genetic markers. J. exp. Med. *127:* 633–646 (1968).
47   Ishizaka, T.; Ishizaka, K.; Salmon, S.; Fudenberg, H.H.: Biologic activity of aggregated gamma-globulin. VIII. Aggregated immunoglobulins of different classes. J. Immun. *99:* 82–91 (1967).

Peter H. Schur, MD, Departments of Rheumatology/Immunology and the Clinical Immunology Lab., Brigham and Women's Hospital, Harvard Medical School, Boston, MA 02115 (USA)

IgG Subclasses and Antibody Activities

Immunochemical Quantitation of IgG Subclass Proteins and IgG Subclass Antibodies: Status and Perspectives

R. Djurup

Department of Clinical Chemistry, Bispebjerg Hospital, Copenhagen, Denmark

Within the last few years polyclonal and monoclonal antibodies with good reactivity to and specificity for the 4 human IgG subclasses have become generally available. This has led to the rapid development of a number of different assays for quantitation of human IgG subclass proteins and IgG subclass antibodies. Most of these assays have been developed for research purposes and their performance characteristics and possible suitability for routine clinical laboratory use have not been evaluated to any great detail. In this brief introductory paper I shall put forward some criteria for evaluation of performance characteristics of assays intended for quantitation of IgG subclass proteins or IgG subclass antibodies (Abs) in the routine laboratory.

Quantitation of IgG Subclass Proteins

IgG subclass proteins have been quantified by radial immunodiffusion, rocket immunoelectrophoresis, nephelometry, turbidimetry, agglutination inhibition, competetive radio-immunoassays and enzyme immunoassays. The advantages and disadvantages of most of these methods have recently been reviewed [1]. The turbidimetric method is discussed in [2] and a detailed description of one of the enzyme immunoassays is presented in [3]. Probably, most of these assays may be carried out with both monoclonal and polyclonal antibodies, but a detailed theoretically and statistically sound comparison of the merits of the two types of antibodies in quantitation of polyclonal IgG subclass proteins in sera is still lacking.

Assays for IgG subclass protein quantitation should be evaluated in terms of: (1) subclass reactivity and specificity; (2) sensitivity; (3) imprecision; (4) dynamic range; (5) interference, and (6) practicability, including availability of reagents and instruments, economy and capacity of the analysis.

Evaluation of the subclass-specific antibodies should include testing of the reactivity against a broad panel of highly purified myeloma proteins. The antibody specificity should be tested in exactly the assay in which they are to be used. Thus, Abs working in immunoprecipitation-in-gel techniques do not necessarily work in liquid-phase precipitation assays, as one recent example has shown [4]. It is not sufficient to test the specificity of the Abs against myeloma protein in aqueous buffers as interfering factors in sera may affect the assay specificity [Prassler and Djurup, unpublished observations]. It is therefore necessary also to assess the accuracy and specificity of the assay by addition of known amounts of IgG myeloma proteins of each subclass to normal sera (and ideally to subclass-deficient sera, too) with known IgG subclass levels.

In comparison of different methods or different Abs (e.g. polyclonal versus monoclonal Abs) it is inadequate to compare solely the reactivity against purified myeloma proteins. Thus, this test does not tell much about the relative accuracy or imprecision when the different methods or Abs are applied to quantitation of polyclonal IgG subclass proteins in sera.

A more sound approach would be to compare the test results obtained by quantitation of IgG subclass protein levels in a large number of sera by a two-way analysis of variance or the analogous non-parametric test. Such statistical analysis will reveal whether the two methods or the two types of Abs measure the same substance with the same degree of accuracy – taking into consideration the imprecision of the assays. It may also indicate whether any significant method- or Ab-dependent bias exists.

When the distribution of the subclass protein concentrations for each subclass has been evaluated by a goodness of fit test, some kind of regression or correlation analysis should also be performed. In this context it should be noted that it has not been shown that any of the 4 subclass concentrations is consistently normal or log-normal distributed. Considering the fact that IgG subclass protein levels have now been investigated in a systematic manner for more than 15 years, it is surprising that the distributions of the IgG subclass protein concentrations apparently have not been subjected to rigorous statistical analysis. In a recent interlaboratory study in which we quantified the IgG subclass protein levels in 200 sera from normal adults by radial immunodiffusion [5], we found that only the IgG2 protein concentrations fitted log-normal distributions in both laboratories. The other 3 subclass concentrations were neither consistently normal nor log-normal distributed. This shows that use of the same reagents, the same calibrator, and the same assay technique is not sufficient to obtain the same frequency distributions in different laboratories. The assay protocol probably also needs to be highly standardized. An important task in the next years will therefore be to attempt to define reference reagents, including both antibodies and calibrators, and to propose one or more reference methods for quantitation of IgG subclass proteins in serum. In this context we will have to define exact protocols for carrying out the reference assays and to propose statistical methods for method and antibody comparison studies.

Quantitation of IgG Subclass Antibodies

IgG subclass antibodies have been measured by direct agglutination techniques, the red cell-linked antigen-antiglobulin reaction, radio-immunodiffusion, crossed radio-immunoelectrophoresis, radio-immunoprecipitation, and a variety of solid-phase immunoassays using antibodies labelled with either ^{125}I-iodine (immunoradiometric assays), enzymes (immuno-enzymometric assays also known as ELISA), or fluorescent probes (immunofluorescence assays). As the major part of the recently developed assays has been based on solid-phase immobilized antigens, I shall limit the following discussion to this type of assay. (The advantages and disadvantages of the different methods mentioned above have recently been reviewed [1].)

When evaluating the performance of solid-phase assays for quantitation of IgG subclass antibodies, it is important to consider the following parameters: (1) antigen-specificity; (2) subclass-specificity; (3)

equipotency; (4) imprecision; (5) isotypic competition; (6) calibration of the assay; (7) sensitivity, and (8) practicability, including availability of antigen, subclass-specific antisera and reference sera.

The enthusiasm for the availability of monoclonal Abs with good subclass specificity in assays for specific Abs has been so great that many investigators apparently have neglected testing of antigen specificity and subclass specificity in their assays. Most assays for quantitation of IgG subclass antibodies have been developed from assays for 'total IgG antibodies'. As the antigen specificity of the latter often has been established previously, only little attention has been paid to documentation of the antigen reactivity and specificity of the assays for IgG subclass antibodies. However, the antigen specificity of such assays should be documented for each subclass in question. Thus, specific binding of a dominating subclass may overshadow cross-reactivity of a minor subclass.

Concerning the subclass-reactivity of the assay, it should be recognized that different subclasses may bind to different components of complex antigen mixtures. As an example, IgG2 Abs bind mainly, if not exclusively, to carbohydrate-containing antigens. As pure carbohydrate antigens (Ags) bind poorly to plastic surfaces, it may be difficult to detect IgG2 Abs to such Ags in many types of solid-phase assays. The subclass specificity may be tested in several ways. Probably the most correct way would be to test the subclass specificity with monoisotypic antigen-specific Abs isolated from immune sera or produced by human-human hybridoma technology. However, such reagents are at present not generally available. As an alternative, the subclass specificity may be tested against purified myeloma proteins, immobilized either by simple adsorption, by covalent coupling, or by an anti-immunoglobulin to the plastic surface. As physical adsorption has been found to change the reactivity of some subclass proteins, one of the two latter-mentioned methods is to be preferred.

To compare antibody (Ab) levels in different subclasses, equal amounts of antibodies in different subclasses should give the same (transformed) signal. As mAbs for different subclasses differ somewhat in affinity for their homologous protein, achievement of equipotency requires adjustment of the dilutions of the Abs or separate calibration curves for each subclass. Neither approach is fully satisfactory, and availability of mAbs with equal affinity for their homologous subclass would mean a great advantage.

The imprecision of most assays for IgG subclass Abs is high to very high. In this context it should be noted that variation in the binding characteristics of the plastic devices, antigen purity and composition, and amount of subclass-specific Ab in the ascitic fluid, all may add to the imprecision. Before a subclass Ab assay is taken into routine diagnostic use, the overall long-term imprecision should be established and evaluated, using different batches of plastic devices, antigen (Ag) preparations, and subclass-specific Abs.

The advantage of using non-porous plastic surfaces as basis for IgG and IgG subclass Ab assays is that most of the non-specific binding, which otherwise has been so troublesome in solid-phase assays of this type, is eliminated. The drawback is that the plastic surfaces have only very limited Ag binding capacity. If a major and a minor subclass bind to the same Ag, the binding of the minor subclass may be competitively inhibited by the major one. This may lead to serious underestimation of the minor subclass. Evaluation of subclass-specific assays should therefore include protocols to establish whether such competition occurs.

IgG subclass Ab assays are often calibrated in arbitrary units by use of a single immune serum or by a pool of such sera. Several attempts have been done to obtain 'absolute' estimates (e.g. in ng Ab per ml serum). While such absolute quantitation is attractive and would greatly simplify interlaboratory comparisons, it cannot be considered a realistic goal for assays for Abs to complex Ags and Ag mixtures. Thus, different immune sera contain different mixtures of Abs to individual epitopes and, furthermore, Abs of different affinities to the same epitope. It may therefore give a false impression of exactness to state Ab concentration in absolute units. However, if one measures Abs to homogenous Ags or even better to a single well-defined epitope, quantitation in absolute units may be possible.

Due to the difficulties in absolute calibration of IgG subclass Ab assays, it is at present not possible to compare objectively assay sensitivity.

I should end by suggesting that we in the next years attempt to answer the following questions: (1) Which assays for IgG subclass antibodies do we really need? (2) How do we establish reference reagents (e.g. solid-phase devices, Ag preparations, subclass-specific Abs, calibrator preparations) and reference methods for these assays? (3) How do we best calibrate IgG subclass assays?

References

1 Djurup, R.; Weeke, B.: Methods of detecting IgG subclass proteins and antibodies. Monogr. Allergy, vol. 19, pp. 86–99 (Karger, Basel 1986).
2 Deverill, I.; Jefferis, R.; Ling, N.R.; Reeves, W.G.: Monoclonal antibodies to human IgG: reaction characteristics in the centrifugal analyzer. Clin. Chem. *27:* 2044–2047 (1981).
3 Papadea, C.; Check, I.J.; Reimer, C.B.: Monoclonal antibody-based solid-phase immunoenzymometric assays for quantitating human immunoglobulin G and its subclasses in serum. Clin. Chem. *31:* 1940–1945 (1985).
4 Oxelius, V.-A.: Antigenic variants of human IgG subclasses. Restriction of murine monoclonal IgG subclass antisera. Scand. J. Immunol. *25:* 169–174 (1987).
5 Djurup, R.; Mansa, B.; Søndergaard, I.; Weeke, B.: IgG subclass concentrations in sera from 200 normal adults and IgG subclass determination of 106 myeloma proteins. An interlaboratory study. Scand. J. clin. Lab. Invest. (in press, 1987).

R. Djurup, MD, PhD, Novo BioLabs, Novo Allé 6B 3.59.2,
DK-2880 Bagsværd (Denmark)

The IgG1 Subclass Preference of Selected, Naturally Occurring Antipolysaccharide Antibodies[1]

L. Hammarström[a], R.A. Insel[b], M.A.A. Persson[a], C.I.E. Smith[a, 2]

[a]Department of Clinical Immunology, Karolinska Institute at Huddinge Hospital, Huddinge, and Department of Immunology, Stockholm University, Stockholm, Sweden; [b]Department of Pediatrics, University of Rochester, Rochester, N.Y., USA

Introduction

Antibodies against bacterial antigens arise as a consequence of natural infection or vaccination. Depending on the site of antigenic exposure, the appearing antibodies may be of different classes or subclasses. Gastrointestinal infections may thus result in a predominant IgA response whereas systemic infections mainly induce IgG antibodies.

Since the pioneering days of Yount et al. [1], antibodies against bacterial polysaccharide antigens have been claimed to be mainly or exclusively of the IgG2 subclass [for review see ref. 2]. This suggestion is strengthened by observations of lack of antipolysaccharide antibodies in IgG2-deficient individuals [for review see ref. 3]. In view of the recently suggested IgG1 preference of antibodies against selected polysaccharides [for review see ref. 4], we determined to reexamine the subclass pattern of naturally occurring antibodies against *H. influenzae* and *N. meningitidis* polysaccharide antigens in normal and immunoglobulin-subclass-deficient individuals.

---

[1] This work was supported by the Swedish Medical Research Council, the Sven and Dagmar Salén Foundation, and the Ellen, Walter and Lennart Hesselman Foundation. The skilful technical assistance of Ms. Anette Johnsson is gratefully acknowledged.

[2] We are indebted to Prof. G. Lefranc, Montpellier, France, Dr. B. Zegers, Utrecht, The Netherlands, and Prof. A.O. Carbonara, Torino, Italy, for supplying some of the patient sera used.

Materials and Methods

Sera

Sera from normal healthy adults and immunodeficient individuals were collected and stored frozen until used. The sera from individuals with various forms of IgG subclass gene deletions and from individuals with a suspected regulatory IgG subclass disorder – the respective subclass being below detection level: IgG1 (<0.1 g/l), IgG2 (<0.2 g/l) or IgG4 (<0.02 g/l) have previously been extensively characterized [5, 6]. The US standard anti-*H. influenzae* type b (Hib) capsular polysaccharide antiserum from the FDA Office of Biologics (lot 1983, a pool of sera from adults drawn after immunization with the purified Hib polysaccharide), containing 70 µg/ml of specific antibody and a human IgG2 monoclonal directed against the above polysaccharide (developed by R.A. Insel), served as positive controls.

Antigens

Tyraminated Hib capsular polysaccharide (prepared by Dr. R.A. Insel, Department of Pediatrics, Rochester, N.Y., USA) and meningococcal capsular polysaccharide type A and C (a gift from Prof. A. Lindberg, Department of Bacteriology, Huddinge Hospital, Huddinge, Sweden) were coated in phosphate-buffered saline or bicarbonate buffer at coating concentrations of 2 and 10 µg/ml, respectively.

Enzyme-Linked Immunosorbent Assay

The enzyme-linked immunosorbent assay (ELISA) was performed as described previously in detail [7] using a mixture of polyclonal anti-IgM, anti-IgG and anti-IgA (Dakopatts, Glostrup, Denmark) or monoclonal anti-IgG class (8a4) or subclass (NL-16; anti-IgG1; GOM1; anti-IgG2, ZG4; anti-IgG3 and GB7B; anti-IgG4; the latter purchased from Unipath, Bedford, England) antibodies. An additional monoclonal antibody against IgG2 (HP 6014) was obtained from Dr. C. Reimer, CDC, Atlanta, Ga., USA.

Results

The Antibody Spectrum against H. influenzae Type b Capsular Polysaccharide

It was initially claimed that antibodies against ribosylribitolphosphate were mainly although not exclusively of the IgG2 subclass [8]. Recent data, however, suggests an IgG1 preference both by antibodies induced by the pure polysaccharide [9] and a protein-polysaccharide conjugate [10]. The former notion is supported both by the close correlation between serum IgG2 levels and the response to the polysaccharide [11, 12] and the lack of responsiveness in IgG2-deficient individuals [12–14]. In view of the divergent data, we therefore ex-

Table I. The IgG subclass distribution of naturally occurring antibodies against bacterial capsular polysaccharides[a]

Donor	Defect	H. influenzae type b			N. meningitidis type A			N. meningitidis type C		
		IgG	IgG1	IgG2[b]	IgG	IgG1	IgG2[b]	IgG	IgG1	IgG2[b]
1	IgG1[c]	0.65	0.00	0.00	0.84	0.00	0.00	0.88	0.01	0.02
2	IgG1	0.38	0.00	0.01	1.15	0.00	0.02	1.06	0.00	0.00
3	IgG1,IgG2,IgG4[c]	0.22	0.03	0.00	0.51	0.00	0.00	0.51	0.00	0.00
4	IgG1,IgG2,IgG4[c]	0.10	0.07	0.00	0.40	0.00	0.00	0.38	0.02	0.00
5	IgG2	0.12	0.32	0.01	0.41	0.18	0.00	0.26	0.86	0.00
6	IgG2,IgG4	0.83	1.05	0.00	0.97	1.65	0.00	0.57	1.97	0.02
7	IgG2,IgG4	0.41	0.50	0.00	0.52	0.12	0.00	0.61	0.54	0.00
8	IgG2,IgG4	0.26	0.31	0.00	0.37	0.19	0.00	0.44	0.57	0.00
9	IgG2,IgG4	0.26	0.32	0.00	0.27	0.09	0.00	0.32	0.35	0.00
10	IgG2,IgG4	0.73	0.43	0.00	1.32	0.59	0.00	1.15	1.85	0.00
11	IgG2,IgG4	0.18	0.18	0.00	0.23	0.08	0.00	0.37	0.86	0.00
12	IgG2,IgG4[c]	0.29	0.83	0.00	0.80	1.18	0.00	0.61	1.97	0.00
13	IgG2,IgG4[c]	0.96	1.55	0.00	0.47	0.89	0.00	0.53	1.48	0.00
14	IgG2,IgG4[c]	0.16	0.33	0.02	0.47	0.34	0.00	0.19	0.75	0.00
15	IgG2,IgG4[c]	0.21	0.86	0.00	0.54	0.70	0.00	0.39	1.00	0.00
16	IgG2,IgG4[c]	0.34	0.88	0.00	1.15	2.00	0.00	0.45	1.47	0.00
17[d]	–	0.68	0.60	0.13	0.41	0.32	0.00	0.51	1.14	0.00
18[e]	–	0.29	0.45	0.08	0.22	0.20	0.04	0.52	0.17	0.04
19[f]	–	0.35	0.61	0.15	0.66	0.36	0.08	0.39	0.32	0.10

[a] Results are given as net absorbance after 90 min (IgG) or 60 min (IgG1 and IgG2).
[b] Using GOM1.
[c] Due to gene deletions of the corresponding heavy chain constant region genes.
[d] Pool of 10 sera from normal children 5–10 years of age (age-matched with the IgG1-deficient children).
[e] Reference pool of adult sera obtained after vaccination with purified Hib polysaccharide (diluted 1:7,000. For determination of antimeningococcal antibodies, the reference pool was diluted 1:100.
[f] Mean values for 11 normal healthy blood donors. Range of absorbance for anti-Hib antibodies: 0.17–2.00 for IgG; 0.12–2.00 for IgG1, and 0.02–0.70 for IgG2. Range of absorbance for antimeningococcal antibodies: 0.17–2.00 for IgG; 0.10–0.79 for IgG1, and 0.00–0.56 for IgG2. Range of absorbance for antimeningococcal C antibodies: 0.17–2.00 for IgG; 0.11–0.82 for IgG1, and 0.03–0.47 for IgG2.

amined the subclass profile of naturally occurring antiribosylribitolphosphate antibodies in sera from normal and immunodeficient individuals.

Levels of antibodies in healthy nonimmunized individuals are generally rather low and a majority of healthy adults previously tested showed IgG levels above what has been considered as protective levels (1 µg/ml) [15]. However, a minority of sera from individuals with various forms of IgG subclass deficiencies were found to contain protective antibody levels (data not shown). The reference pool of sera against Hib from adults displayed a high level, measured as net absorbance for IgG1 and a relatively low level of IgG2 (table I). It should be stressed that these data are not quantitative but nevertheless suggest that IgG1 antibodies from the bulk of IgG antiribosylribitolphosphate antibodies in normal adults. As seen in table I, this pattern was found in most normal individuals tested. Similar data were obtained using the HP6014 anti-IgG2 monoclonal (data not shown).

The absorbance values and subclass distribution of sera from immunodeficient individuals are also given in table I. The data imply that background levels of IgG and IgG1 anti-Hib polysaccharide antibodies, comparable to those of normal individuals, are seen in adult IgG2-deficient individuals. Low levels of specific IgG3 antibodies are frequently noted in IgG2-deficient individuals (data not shown). Sera from the two IgG1-deficient individuals tested (both children) showed normal levels of total IgG but markedly low levels of IgG2 antibodies against the polysaccharide.

The Subclass Distribution of Antimeningococcal Polysaccharide Antibodies

Antibodies against meningococcal polysaccharide type A have previously been suggested to display a somewhat unexpected subclass profile since quite substantial amounts of IgG1 (in addition to IgG2) were found in normal donors [16]. Background levels of antimeningococcal antibodies are, in our experience, rather low. The subclass pattern of these antibodies were individually quite variable but suggest a clear IgG1 predominance in nonvaccinated individuals (table I). The levels and subclass distribution of sera from immunodeficient individuals are also given in table I. Similar data were obtained when the antibody pattern against meningococcal polysaccharide type C was tested (table I).

Discussion

In spite of the above results it is clear that a number of polysaccharide antigens do induce mainly IgG2 antibodies in normal adults [for review see ref. 3, 4]. However, it is equally clear that a hitherto unexpected number of polysaccharide antigens induce mainly if not exclusively IgG1 antibodies. The latter group includes, in addition to ribosylribitolphosphate and meningococcal polysaccharides, Klebsiella capsular polysaccharides of selected serotypes [17], and Salmonella lipopolysaccharide [18].

Phosphorylcholine, another carbohydrate antigen, has previously also been suggested to induce mainly IgG2 antibodies in man [19]. However, this view has recently been challenged since antibody levels are only moderately lowered in IgG2-deficient individuals [20] and in normal adults, the naturally occurring antibodies are in fact mainly of the IgG1 subclass [21]. Even though sera containing low levels of antibodies contain mainly IgG1 antibodies, high-titered sera may contain proportionally more IgG2 antibodies against polysaccharides which has previously been suggested in the response to dextran [1, 22], levan [1; and unpublished results] and possibly also meningococcal polysaccharides. High-titered sera also appear to express a different antibody repertoire, i.e. a different set of V genes, as compared to low-titered sera [23].

Antibodies of the IgG2 subclass exhibit a poor capacity to activate complement and do not bind effectively to Fc receptors on phagocytic cells and yet these antibodies appear to constitute the bulk of IgG antibodies against selected polysaccharides. It has previously been suggested that different heavy chain constant region genes preferentially associate with particular sets or families of V genes and, since the affinity of antibodies has been shown to correlate with a number of important biological properties, it is possible that the IgG2 constant region gene primarily interacts with a selected set of V genes, possibly coding for high-affinity antipolysaccharide antibodies. This hypothesis receives support both from experimental animal data [24, 25] (where certain idiotypes are shown to be expressed only in particular immunoglobulin classes) and data on human antibodies [26–29] where affinity/avidity differences between the various subclasses have been suggested both with regard to protein [27, 29] and polysaccharide antigens [29]. In the latter cases, the highest affinity/avidity was present in the major subclass expressed, i.e. IgG1 and IgG2, respectively. In this context, it is also quite interesting that a slight IgG2 preference for the V_HI gene family has previously been shown [26]. The seemingly strong IgG1 preference of antibodies against the Hib capsular polysaccharide and the suggested equal affinity and equipotent biological effect of IgG1 and IgG2 antibodies against Hib that has previously been reported [30] could seen to be in conflict with our hypothesis. However, the affinity of antibodies against ribosylribitolphosphate may actually differ between the IgG1 and IgG2 subclasses (since a higher affinity of IgG2 antibodies is suggested by its enrichment on affinity columns) [30] and IgG1 and IgG2 fractions obtained have, as the authors point out, not yet been tested in relevant biological protection assays [30]. In this paper, normal amounts (as suggested by absorbance values in ELISA similar to those of controls) of total IgG and IgG1 anti-Hib polysaccharide and antimeningococcal polysaccharide antibodies were found in IgG2-deficient adults. Normal baseline levels of anti-Hib capsular polysaccharide antibodies were also recently observed in IgG2-deficient children [31]. However, a proneness to infections with Hib [31–34] and meningococci [34, 35] in IgG2-deficient individuals has previously been well established. A higher than expected rate of Hib infection has also been noted in G2m-negative individuals [23, 36] (an allotype associated with low serum levels of IgG2). Although the latter point has been disputed [37], the above data suggest that the ability to form even low or moderate levels of IgG2 antibodies may be necessary for the successful elimination of capsulated bacteria. IgG2 antibodies would then be expected to be endowed with unique in vivo properties, possibly as a consequence of a higher mean affinity, i.e. a selective subclass associated utilization of the V gene repertoire [for model see ref. 38]. An alternative hypothesis would suggest that a stepwise acquisition of specificities occurs even within the IgG1 subclass [for model see ref. 38], and that the arrest in maturation of the antibody repertoire takes place at an earlier stage in development than previously anticipated. In the latter case, the IgG2 deficiency would thus merely serve as a marker of a delayed maturation resulting in a lack of a given antibody specificity.

References

1 Yount, W.J.; Dorner, M.M.; Kunkel, H.G.; Kabat, E.A.: Studies on human antibodies. VI. Selective variations in subgroup composition and genetic markers. J. exp. Med. *127:* 633–646 (1968).

2 Hammarström, L.; Smith, C.I.E.: IgG subclasses in bacterial infections. Monogr. Allergy, vol. 19, pp. 122–133 (Karger, Basel 1986).
3 Hanson, L.Å.; Söderström, T.; Oxelius, V. (eds): Immunoglobulin subclass deficiencies. Monogr. Allergy, vol. 20, pp. 1–250 (Karger, Basel 1986).
4 Shakib, F. (ed.): Basic and clinical aspects of IgG subclasses. Monogr. Allergy, vol. 19, pp. 1–317 (Karger, Basel 1986).
5 Hammarström, L.; Carbonara, A.O.; DeMarchi, M.; Lefranc, G.; Lefranc, M.P.; Smith, C.I.E.: Generation of the antibody repertoire in donors with multiple heavy chain constant region genes. Scand. J. Immunol. 25: 189–194 (1987).
6 Hammarström, L.; Carbonara, A.O.; DeMarchi, M.; Lefranc, G.; Smith, C.I.E.; Zegers, B.J.M.: Altered subclass restriction pattern of antigen-specific antibodies in donors with defect expression of IgG or IgA subclass heavy chain constant region genes. Clin. Immunol. Immunopathol. (in press).
7 Persson, M.A.A.; Hammarström, L.; Smith, C.I.E.: Enzyme-linked immunosorbent assay for subclass distribution of human IgG and IgA antigen-specific antibodies. J. immunol. Methods 78: 109–121 (1985).
8 Johnston, R.B.; Anderson, P.; Rosén, S.; Smith, D.H.: Characterization of human antibody to polyribophosphate, the capsular antigen of *Haemophilus influenzae* type b. Clin. Immunol. Immunopathol. 1: 234–240 (1973).
9 Shackelford, P.G.; Granoff, D.M.; Nelson, S.J.; Scott, M.G.; Smith, D.S.; Nahm, M.H.: Subclass distribution of human antibodies to *Haemophilus influenzae* type b capsular polysaccharide. J. Immun. 138: 587–592 (1987).
10 Insel, R.; Anderson, P.W.: Activation of human B cells by polysaccharides. VIth Int. Congr. of Immunology, Toronto 1986, abstr.
11 Siber, G.R.; Schur, P.H.; Aisenberg, A.C.; Weitzman, S.A.; Schiffman, G.: Correlation between serum IgG2 concentrations and the antibody response to bacterial polysaccharide antigens. New Engl. J. Med. 303: 178–182 (1980).
12 Umetsu, D.T.; Ambrosino, D.M.; Quinti, I.; Siber, G.R.; Geha, R.S.: Recurrent sinopulmonary infection and impaired antibody response to bacterial capsular polysaccharide antigen in children with selective IgG-subclass deficiency. New Engl. J. Med. 313: 1247–1251 (1985).
13 Insel, R.A.; Anderson, P.W.: Response to oligosaccharide-protein conjugate vaccine against *Hemophilus influenzae* b in two patients with IgG2 deficiency unresponsive to capsular polysaccharide vaccine. New Engl. J. Med. 315: 499–503 (1986).
14 Söderström, T.; Söderström, R.; Bengtsson, U.; Björkander, J.; Hellstrand, K.; Hanson, L.Å.: Clinical and immunological evaluation of patients low in single or multiple IgG subclasses. Monogr. Allergy, vol. 20, pp. 135–142 (Karger, Basel 1986).
15 Käyhty, H.; Peltova, H.; Karanro, V.; Mäkelä, P.H.: The protective level of serum antibodies to the capsular polysaccharide of *Haemophilus influenzae* type b. J. infect. Dis. 147: 1100–1104 (1983).
16 Seppelä, I.J.T.; Routonen, N.; Sarnesto, A.; Mattila, P.A.; Mäkelä, O.: The percentages of six immunoglobulin isotypes in human antibodies to tetanus toxoid: standardization of isotype-specific second antibodies in solid-phase assay. Eur. J. Immunol. 14: 868–875 (1984).

17 Skvaril, F.; Cryz, S.J.; Fürer, E.: IgA and IgG subclass antibodies in individuals vaccinated with Klebsiella capsular polysaccharide vaccine (Abstract). Symp. on Vaccines and Vaccinations (Institut Pasteur, Paris 1985).
18 Persson, M.A.A.; Ekwall, E.; Hammarström, L.; Lindberg, A.A.; Smith, C.I.E.: IgG and IgA subclass patterns of human antibodies to Shigella flexneri and Salmonella serogroup B and D O antigens. Infect. Immunity 52: 834–839 (1986).
19 Brown, M.; Schiffman. G.; Rittenberg, M.B.: Subpopulations of antibodies to phosphocholine in human serum. J. Immun. 132: 1323–1328 (1984).
20 Cunningham-Rundles, C.: Antibodies to phosphorylcholine in sera of patients with humoral immunodeficiency disease. Monogr. Allergy, vol. 20, pp. 42–49 (1986).
21 Freijd, A.; Johnsson, A.; Rynnel-Dagöö, B.: Age-dependent IgG subclass distribution of phosphocholine antibodies in humans. Clin exp. Immunol. (submitted).
22 Hammarström, L.; Persson, M.A.A.; Smith, C.I.E.: Immunoglobulin subclass distribution of human anti-carbohydrate antibodies: aberrant pattern in IgA deficient donors. Immunology 54: 821–826 (1985).
23 Baker, C.J.; Kasper, D.L.; Edwards, M.S.; Schiffman, G.: Influence of preimmunization antibody levels on the specificity of the immune response to related polysaccharide antigens. New Engl. J. Med. 303: 173–178 (1980).
24 Scott, M.G.; Fleischman, J.B.: Preferential idiotype-isotype associations in antibodies to dinitrophenyl antigens. J. Immun. 128: 2622–2628 (1982).
25 Nishinarita, S.; Claflin, J.L.; Lieberman, R.: IgA isotype-restricted idiotypes associated with T15 Id + PC antibodies. J. Immun. 134: 2544–2549 (1985).
26 Förre, O.; Natvig, J.B.; Kunkel, H.G.: Serological detection of variable region (V_H) subgroups of Ig heavy chains. J. exp. Med. 144: 897–905 (1976).
27 Devey, M.; Bleasdale, K.M.; French, M.A.H.; Harrison, G.: The IgG4 subclass is associated with a low affinity antibody response to tetanus toxoid in man. Immunology 55: 565–568 (1985).
28 Emmrich, F.; Zenke, G.; Eichmann, K.: Isotype restriction of idiotopes associated with human anti-streptococcal A carbohydrate antibodies. Eur. J. Immunol. 16: 542–546 (1986).
29 Persson, M.A.A.; Brown, S.E.; Steward, D.M.W.; Hammarström, L.; Smith, C.I.E.; Howard, C.R.; Wahl, M.; Rynnel-Dagöö, B.; Lefranc, G.; Carbonara, A.O.: IgG subclass associated differences of specific antibodies in humans. Different patterns for protein and polysaccharide antigens (submitted).
30 Weinberg, G.A.; Granoff, D.M.; Nahm, M.H.; Shackelford, P.G.: Functional activity of different IgG subclass antibodies against type b capsular polysaccharide of Haemophilus influenzae. J. Immun. 136: 4232–4236 (1986).
31 Shackelford, P.G.; Polmar, S.H.; Mayus, J.L.; Johnson, W.L.; Corry, J.M.; Nahm, M.H.: Spectrum of IgG2 subclass deficiency in children with recurrent infections: prospective study, J. Pediat. 108: 647–653 (1986).
32 Oxelius, V.: Chronic infections in a family with hereditary deficiency of IgG2 and IgG4. Clin. exp. Immunol. 17: 19–27 (1974).
33 Sjöholm, A.; Hallberg, T.; Oxelius, V.; Hammarström, L.; Smith, C.I.E.; Lindgren, F.: C2 deficiency, moderately low IgG2 concentrations and lack of the G2m(23) allotype marker in a child with repeated bacterial infections. Acta Pediat. scand. 76: 533–538 (1987).

34 Quinti, I.; Paretti, C.; Testi, R.; Bonomo, R.; Aiuti, F.: IgG subclass deficiency in adults: a clinical and immunological study. Monogr. Allergy, vol. 20, pp. 143-148 (Karger, Basel 1986).
35 Bass, J.L.; Nuss, R.; Metha, K.A.; Morganelli, P.; Bennett, L.: Recurrent meningococcemia associated with IgG2-subclass deficiency. New Engl. J. Med. *309:* 430-434 (1983).
36 Ambrosino, D.M.; Schiffman, G.; Gotslich, E.C.; Schur, P.H.; Rosenberg, G.A.; DeLange, G.G.; van Loghem, E.; Siber, G.R.: Correlation between G2m(n) immunoglobulin allotype and human antibody response and susceptibility to polysaccharide encapsulated bacteria. J. clin. Invest. *75:* 1935-1942 (1985).
37 Granoff, D.M.; Shackelford, P.G.; Panden, J.P.; Boies, E.G.: Antibody responses to *Haemophilus influenzae* type b polysaccharide vaccine in relation to Km(1) and G2m(23) immunoglobulin allotypes. J. infect. Dis. *14:* 257-264 (1986).
38 Hammarström, L.; Lefranc, G.; Lefranc, M.P.; Persson, M.A.A.; Smith, C.I.E.: Aberrant pattern of anti-carbohydrate antibodies in immunoglobulin class or subclass-deficient donors. Monogr. Allergy, vol. 20, pp 50-56 (Karger, Basel 1986).

Lennart Hammarström, MD, Department of Clinical Immunology (F79),
Karolinska Institute at Huddinge Hospital, S-141 86 Huddinge (Sweden)

IgG Subclasses to Subviral Components

Annika Linde, Vivi-Anne Sundqvist, Tiit Mathiesen, Britta Wahren

Department of Virology, National Bacteriological Laboratory, Stockholm, Sweden

Immunoassays have recently been developed to determine antiviral IgG subclass reactivity. This was made possible by use of mouse monoclonal antibodies [6] reactive with the four human IgG subclasses. Most published results have been excellently summarized [15]. In general, there is an agreement that IgG1 is the dominant antiviral subclass. Little of antiviral IgG2 has been found so far, but the role of IgG2 in antiviral defense is still not entirely settled [19]. Discrepant results have also been presented concerning virus-specific IgG3. Most investigators have found antiviral IgG3 antibodies in connection with current viral disease [3, 5, 7–10, 18]. After infections with nonlatent viruses, such as rotavirus, rubella virus or respiratory syncytial virus (RSV), the specific IgG3 activity has been found to decrease considerably or disappear 3–6 months after infection [3, 5, 8, 9]. In contrast, at least 50% of serum samples from healthy individuals who previously experienced herpes simplex virus (HSV), cytomegalovirus (CMV), or Epstein-Barr virus (EBV) infections, contain virus-specific IgG3. The herpes viruses give rise to latent infections. Clinical reactivations are also frequent. The disappearance of IgG3 after infection with viruses without latency, and the presence of IgG3 to latent viruses in healthy individuals, indicates that the presence of viral antigen is a prerequisite for maintenance of a specific IgG3 response. Virus-specific IgG4 has been found only infrequently. Exceptions are IgG4 reactivities found against HSV [11, 18] in healthy seropositive individuals and against hepatitis B virus surface antigen [16] after vaccination. Repeated antigenic stimulation could be an explanation, maybe in combination with the cutaneous route of immunization.

In previous investigations, the IgG subclass reactivity with whole virus particles or complex viral antigens was examined. Recent studies have shown that antiviral subclass reactivity may differ against different purified subcomponent antigens from the same virus. In a recent study [19], IgG2 reactive with the G glycoprotein but not with the F glycoprotein of RS virus was found in sera from adults. This may be explained by different types of glycosylation of the two antigens [19].

We examined the IgG subclass reactivity with purified mumps antigens [9]. Mumps virus, grown in embryonated hens' eggs, was separated into envelope antigens consisting mainly of glycoproteins (GP), and nucleocapsid protein (NP). IgG1 was found against both antigens in all serum samples. During mumps infection, IgG1 appeared later against the GP than against the NP antigen, but IgG1 to the two antigens reached similar levels in late convalescent samples and in healthy individuals. IgG3 reactive with the NP antigen was found in sera from 58 of 60 patients with mumps infection, but IgG3 to mumps GP was detectable in only 6 of 60 sera. The earlier appearance of antibodies against the internal nucleocapsids than against the envelope GP of mumps virus has been known for 30 years [4], and the same type of delayed antibody response against envelope GP is known also for other viruses. The difference in IgG3 reactivity has, however, not been noted previously. We can only speculate on the reasons for the discrepancies. The glycosylation of the GP antigens may be of importance for the type of IgG subclass response. Part of the mumps envelope is host cell derived, which could hamper the recognition of those antigens as nonself and cause a delay of the antibody response. The initial designation of the NP and GP antigens was soluble (S) antigen and virus-bound (V) antigen, respectively [4]. The S antigen was recovered from the amniotic fluid of mumps infected, embryonated eggs, while the V antigen was cell bound in the chorioallantoic membranes. If NP antigen is secreted also in human fluids, it may be more easily available for antigen-presenting cells than cell-bound GP. Antiviral neutralizing efficacy is often correlated to antibody levels against envelope GP. The late response against those antigens, and the lack of the biologically active IgG3 antibody, seemingly is protective for the virus rather than for the host.

Synthetic viral peptides represent another type of subcomponent antigens. Five EBV-coded EBNA antigens are expressed in nuclei of all EBV-transformed cells [1]. We examined the IgG subclass reactivity

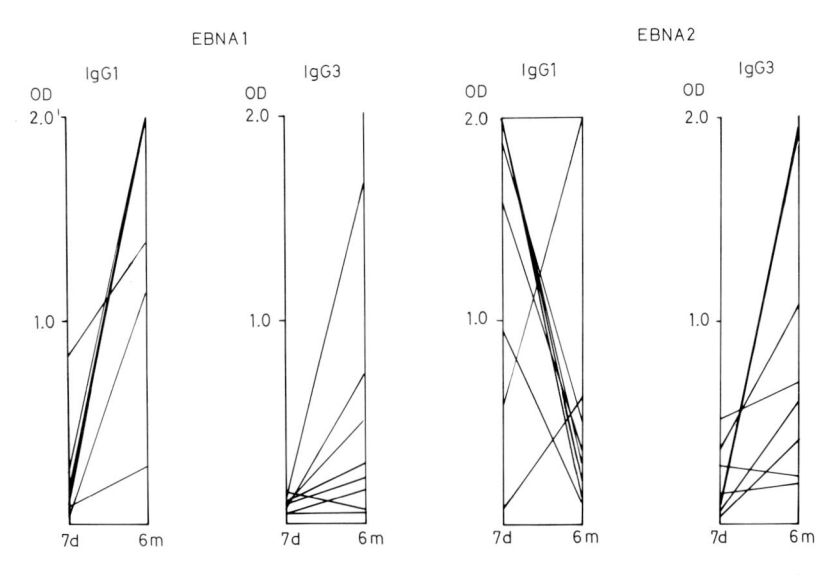

Fig. 1. Virus-specific IgG1 and IgG3 to synthetic EBNA1 and EBNA2 peptides in sera drawn at less than 7 days and 6 months after primary EBV infection.

against synthetic peptides consisting of around 20 amino acids from the EBNA1 and EBNA2 antigens. After the primary EBV infection, EBNA1 antibodies were found to appear later than EBNA2 antibodies. The EBNA1 IgG response was of subclasses IgG1 and 3. There was a rise of both subclasses during the first half year after EBV infection. During the same period EBNA2 IgG1 fell while EBNA2 IgG3 rose in 8 of 10 patients (fig. 1). We have not previously noted a disappearance of IgG1 and appearance of IgG3 late after a virus infection. We have no ready explanation for this phenomenon. Perhaps EBNA1 and EBNA2 are presented to B cells in different ways. However, the finding illustrates the complexity of the IgG subclass responses, and gives us a hint of the tremendous work that is left before we will reach complete knowledge on antiviral IgG subclass reactivity.

Today, analysis of antiviral IgG subclasses is valuable for diagnostic work in virology. For viruses without latency, specific IgG3 can be used as a marker for current or recent viral infections [3, 5, 8, 9]. It can also be used to differentiate between homologous and heterologous antiviral IgG titer increases [9, 13]. In many viral infections, memory antibody responses to heterologous but related viruses are induced. Thus, titer increases to parainfluenza 1–3 are often seen in a mumps infection, and vice versa. In sera from patients with parainfluenza infections, titer increases to the described mumps NP were restricted to IgG1 while NP IgG3 was found only in true mumps infections [9]. Likewise, titer increases to varicella zoster virus (VZV) induced by HSV infection were restricted to IgG1 [13]. A further important clinical use of antiviral IgG subclasses is for the diagnosis of herpes virus reactivations in immunosuppressed individuals [11, 20]. In around of 20% of bone marrow transplant (BMT) recipients, isolated increases of IgG3 or IgG4 against herpes viruses at one or more occasions were the only serological signs of herpes virus reactivations [11]. The increases were not measurable in assays for total antiviral IgG. High but stationary antiviral IgG1 titers may have concealed the fluctuations of the minor subclasses in examinations for total IgG. Also for separation of locally produced and passively transferred antibodies IgG subclass analysis is valuable. In 5 of 19 cases, herpes simplex encephalitis could be diagnosed earlier by comparison of HSV-reactive IgG subclasses in serum and cerebrospinal fluid (CSF) than by comparison of total IgG reactivity against HSV and other viral antigens [13]. Again, the reason was probably that the fluctuations of the minor subclasses were not noted in assays for total IgG. HSV IgG1, passively transferred to CSF, concealed the HSV IgG2–4 increases.

Analysis of Ig classes and subclasses is definitely valuable also as an indicator of the virus-host balance in an individual. With progression of human immunodeficiency virus (HIV) infections, a restriction of the anti-HIV subclass reactivity was seen [18]. HIV-specific IgG3 was rarely seen in AIDS patients, while it was found in asymptomatic infected persons and in patients with lymphadenopathy syndrome. A fall in CMV IgG3 was shown to be a sign of poor prognosis in CMV-infected BMT patients [20]. However, we do not know whether the disappearance of IgG3 per se has clinical consequences or if it is a result of cellular deteriorations that also cause the progress of the disease.

One aim of the studies of antiviral IgG subclasses is to evaluate their functional efficacy. Studies on the neutralizing capacity of IgG subclass fractions obtained by negative chromatography [14] are in progress. Those studies seem to corroborate the theoretical assumption that IgG3 has the best relative neutralizing efficacy while IgG1 fractions give the highest total neutralizing titers due to the abundance of specific IgG1. These studies may serve to bring about optimal IgG subclass concentrations in future antiviral immunoglobulin preparations.

References

1 Ernberg, I.; Kallin, B.; Dillner, J.: Epstein-Barr virus gene expression during primary B-lymphocyte infection in transformed and Burkitt lymphoma derived cell lines. Curr. Top. Microbiol. Immunol. *132:* 251 (1986).
2 Gilljam, G.; Sundqvist, V.-A.; Linde, A.; Pihlstedt, P.; Eklund, A.E.; Wahren, B.: Sensitive analytic ELISAs for subclass herpes virus IgG. J. Virol. Meth. *10:* 203 (1985).
3 Grauballe, P.C.; Hornsleth, A.; Hjelt, K.; Krasilnikoff, P.A.: Detection by ELISA of immunoglobulin G subclass specific antibody response in rotavirus infection in children. J. med. Virol. *18:* 277 (1986).
4 Henle, G.; Harris, S.; Henle, W.: The reactivity of various human sera with mumps complement fixation antigens. J. exp. Med. *88:* 133 (1948).
5 Hornsleth, A.; Bech-Tomsen, N.; Friis, B.: Detection of RS-virus IgG-subclass-specific antibodies: variation according to age in infants and diagnostic value in RS-virus-infected small infants. J. med. Virol. *16:* 329 (1985).
6 Jefferis, R.; Reimer, C.; Skvaril, F.; Lange, G. de; Ling, N.; Lowe, J.; Walker, M.; Phillips, D.; Aloisio, C.; Wells, T.; Vaerman, J.; Magnusson, C.; Kubagawa, H.; Cooper, M.; Vartdal, F.; Vandvik, B.; Haaijman, J.; Mäkelä, O.; Sarnesto, A.; Lando, Z.; Gergely, J.; Radl, J.; Molinaro, G.: Evaluation of monoclonal antibodies having specificity for human IgG subclasses: results of an IUIS/WHO collaborative study. Immunol. Lett. *10:* 223 (1985).
7 Linde, A.; Hammarström, L.; Persson, M.A.A.; Smith, C.I.E.; Sundqvist, V.-A.; Wahren, B.: Virus-specific antibody activity of different subclasses of immunoglobulins G and A in cytomegalovirus infections. Infect. Immunity *42:* 237 (1983).
8 Linde, A.: Subclass distribution of rubella virus-specific immunoglobulin G. J. clin. Microbiol. *21:* 117 (1985).
9 Linde, A.; Granström, M.; Örvell, C.: Serodiagnosis of mumps infections and immunity – a comparison of Ig class and IgG subclass ELISAs and microneutralization assay. J. clin. Microbiol. (submitted, 1987).
10 Linde, A.; Andersson, J.; Lundgren, G.; Wahren, B.: Subclass reactivity of Epstein-Barr virus capsid antigen in primary and reactivated EBV infections. J. med. Virol. *21:* 109 (1987).
11 Ljungman, P.; Linde, A.; Hinkula, J.; Sundqvist, V.-A.; Wahren, B.: IgG subclass responses to herpesvirus infections after bone marrow transplantation. Serodiagn. Immunother. (in press, 1987).
12 Ljungman, P.; Zetterqvist, L.; Sundqvist, V.-A.; Jeansson, S.; Heimdahl, A.; Wahren, B.: Anti-HSV antibodies and lymphocyte proliferation responses to diffe-

rent HSV antigens in patients with frequent HSV-1 reactivations. Scand. J. Immunol. (submitted, 1987).
13 Mathiesen, T.; Linde, A.; Olding-Stenkvist, E.; Wahren, B.: Specific IgG subclass reactivity strengthens the analysis of herpes simplex encephalitis. J. clin. Microbiol. (submitted, 1987).
14 Persson, M.A.A.: Preparation of human sera containing one single subclass using affinity chromatography. J. immunol. Methods (in press, 1987).
15 Skvaril, F.: IgG subclasses in viral infections. Monogr. Allergy, vol. 19, pp. 134–143 (Karger, Basel 1986).
16 Skvaril, F.; Joller-Jemelka, H.: IgG subclasses of anti-HBs antibodies in vaccinated and nonvaccinated individuals and in anti-HBs immunoglobulin preparations. Int. Archs Allergy appl. Immun. *73:* 330 (1984).
17 Sundqvist, V.-A.; Linde, A.; Wahren, B.: Virus-specific immunoglobulin G subclasses in herpes simplex and varicella-zoster virus infections. J. clin. Microbiol. *20:* 94 (1984).
18 Sundqvist, V.-A.; Linde, A.; Kurth, R.; Verner, A.; Helm, E.B.; Popovic, M.; Galli, R.C.; Wahren, B.: Restricted IgG subclass response to HTLV-III and CMV in patients with AIDS and lymphadenopathy syndrome. J. infect. Dis. *153:* 970 (1986).
19 Wagner, D.K.; Nelson, D.L.; Walsh, E.E.; Reimer, C.B.; Henderson, F.W.; Murphy, B.R.: Differential immunoglobulin G subclass antibody titers to respiratory syncytial virus F and G glycoproteins in adults. J. clin. Microbiol. *25:* 748 (1987).
20 Wahren, B.; Linde, A.; Sundqvist, V.-A.; Ljungman, P.; Lönnqvist, B.; Ringdén, O.: IgG subclass-specific CMV reactivity in bone marrow transplant recipients. Transplantation *38:* 479 (1984).

Annika Linde, MD, Department of Virology, National Bacteriological Laboratory, S-105 21 Stockholm (Sweden)

IgG Subclasses and Subclass Distribution in Allergic Disorders

R. Urbanek

Universitäts-Kinderklinik, Freiburg i.Br., FRG

The normal human immunoglobulin class G contains 4 subclasses with different biochemical characteristics. By using sensitive immunoquantitation techniques, it was demonstrated that normal IgG consisted of about 70% IgG1, 18% IgG2, 8% IgG3 and 3% IgG4. The route and duration of antigen exposure, type of antigen, and genetic background may all affect the subclass of IgG antibody produced. As the major class of immunoglobulin, a better insight into the role of IgG and IgG subclasses both in immunity and in disease is of considerable importance.

Because of the nature of the available polyclonal subclass-specific antisera, precise quantitation of IgG subclass antibodies has been difficult. The introduction of monoclonal subclass-specific antisera has also made it possible to develop equally sensitive and specific techniques. Recent studies enlarged our understanding of how different IgG subclass proteins interact in biological reactions, in the normal immune response and in a variety of clinical situations.

Already in 1968, Goodfriend and Perelmutter [1] had suggested that there is a homocytotropic antibody in man belonging to the IgG class able to sensitize skin mast cells and peripheral blood basophils to release histamine on challenge with allergen. Later on, contradictory findings on histamine release with anti-IgG4 were reported [2–4]. Although specific IgG4 antibodies to animal dander [5], honey-bee venom [6] and grass pollen [7] were found, it has been difficult to demonstrate allergen-induced histamine release from naturally sensitized basophils mediated by IgG4. In addition, specific IgG4 antibodies were detected in sera from bee-keepers who were frequently stung [8].

Comparing the total IgG subclass antibody concentrations with allergen-specific IgG subclass levels, different distributions can be found. Above all, IgG1 and IgG4 allergen-specific antibodies predominate in allergic individuals; no significant amounts of allergen-specific IgG2 and IgG3 antibodies has been reported. However, one has to consider that there is a definite age dependency in the synthesis of IgG subclass antibodies. Serum levels are lower in infants and young children than in adolescents and adults. IgG1 and IgG3 levels rise more rapidly with age than do IgG2 and IgG4. Also, whereas in the normal children there is a gradual rise in IgG4, there is a wide scattering of IgG4 with age in the atopics. Since children encounter different environmental antigens/allergens as they grow, and obtain immunological maturity at differing ages, they cannot be expected to follow a precise pattern in obtaining adult levels of serum IgG subclasses.

Therefore, the most interesting experiment in allergic individuals is to look upon IgG subclass response during a standardized immunization, a hyposensitization treatment. Since it has been suggested that specific immunization/allergen immunotherapy induces heat-stable serum IgG antibodies that blocked the ability of homologous reaginic antibodies to produce an immediate cutaneous reaction, many studies of the immunological mechanism of immunotherapy have been performed [9–11]. The aim of these investigations was to find out if specific IgG subclass antibodies were suitable indicators of a therapeutic effect in terms of protection from symptoms after an allergen exposure.

In the course of a successful therapeutic allergen administration, several immunological changes in sera of hyposensitized patients occur: (1) an increase in the concentration of allergen-specific IgG antibodies; (2) a suppression of the IgE antibody response to seasonal allergen exposure; (3) a decrease in specific IgE concentration after prolonged immunotherapy.

In connection with these immunological changes, a fall in sensitivity of the basophil leucocytes to the offending allergen, a rise of stimulation index of lymphocytes and an increase of allergen-specific T suppressor cell activity may be observed [11]. Investigating the subclass nature of the IgG antibody response during immunotherapy, we have studied the antibody response to a parenteral antigen bee venom [12]. 23 individuals (21 children and 2 adults) who had a history of severe systemic allergic reactions to bee stings were followed over a period of 5 years. All patients gave a positive intradermal prick skin test (>2 mm wheal) to 100 µg/ml or less of bee venom and a positive bee venom radio-allergo sorbent test for IgE. The treatment with bee venom was by a rush regime and the maintenance dose of 100 µg, an equivalent of approximately 2 bee stings, was reached after 7 days and continued by monthly injections of this amount of venom for the following 3–4 years. As an efficacy control of the performed hyposensitization treatment, all patients were sting-challenged annually after they had reached the maintenance dose. Venom immunotherapy was discontinued after 3–4 years and all individuals re-stung at 1 and 2 years after discontinuation of treatment.

Specific IgG subclass antibodies were measured by an enzyme-linked immuno sorbent assay as described elsewhere [12]. Following an initial rise in specific IgE antibodies, these fell below pre-treatment levels in all patients and remained low subsequently. Venom-specific IgG antibodies to whole bee venom rose and subsequently fell. Termination of therapy after 3 years had little effect on specific IgE or IgG antibody levels, and the live stings too did not effect these, although samples were taken shortly afterwards when a boost in antibody levels might be expected.

The subclass of IgG antibody to bee venom was restricted to IgG1 and IgG4. We were unable to detect any IgG2 or IgG3 anti-venom activity. During the early phase of treatment, the concentration of both IgG1 and IgG4 antibodies rose although the increase in IgG4 antibody was much higher (fig. 1). Continued administration of bee venom was paralleled by a marked fall in IgG1 antibody to pre-treatment levels while IgG4 antibody titres, in contrast, persisted. The proportion of IgG antibody in each subclass changed from predominantly IgG1 pre-treatment to predominantly IgG4 post-treatment. Similar findings have been reported by Aalberse et al. [8] and Wetterwald et al. [13] in beekeepers. All patients studied by us remained clinically protected, as demonstrated by sting challenge 1 and 2 years after termination of hyposensitization therapy. One can therefore assume that the lasting protection was mainly associated with decreased IgE and raised IgG4 antibodies to allergenic components of bee venom.

Comparable findings were reported by immunotherapy of allergy to inhalants [7, 14, 15]. Although a seasonal natural exposure to grass pollen has already induced a slight increase of specific IgG1 and IgG4 antibodies, only an appropriate immunotherapy revealed a substantial

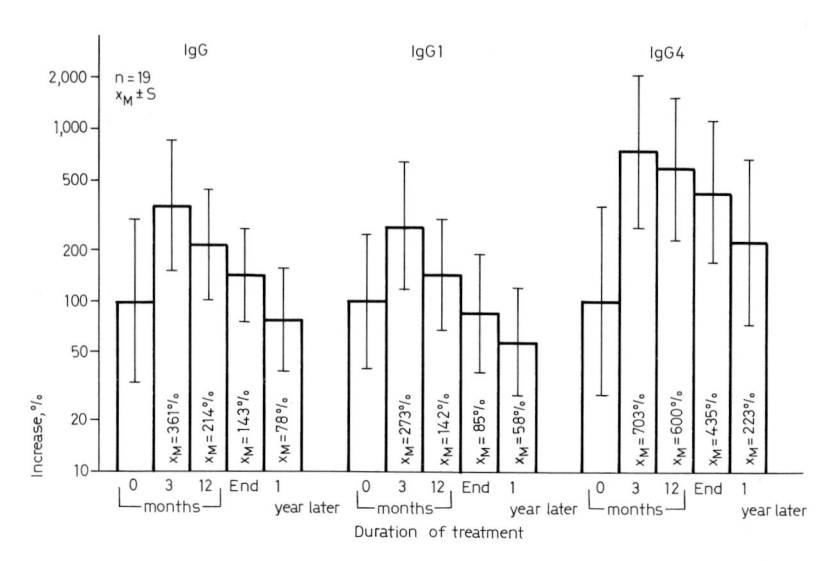

Fig. 1. Course of venom-specific IgG, IgG1 and IgG4 antibodies (AU/ml) in 19 successfully treated allergic patients on bee-venom immunotherapy. The most pronounced increase and the longest persistence is shown by the IgG4 antibody [12].

immune response restricted to the same subclasses. As in allergy to parenteral antigens and also in allergy to inhalants, specific IgG4 antibodies predominated and were a useful marker of effective immunotherapy. However, according to Djurup et al. [10], IgG1 may be of greater importance in the early treatment period.

Both inhalant and nutritive antigens are common allergens in our environment. Although an association between an immediate hypersensitivity and the presence of specific IgE antibodies was established, it is of interest to analyse the IgG subclass distribution to dietary proteins in allergic desease as well as in individuals with increased intestinal permeability and in healthy controls. We studied two types of adverse reactions to foods for which there are accepted criteria: (1) an immediate type of egg allergy, an IgE-mediated disorder, and (2) coeliac disease with its intolerance to gliadin [16, 17].

In agreement with other investigators, we have also found that, above all, persons with untreated coeliac disease had elevated IgG antibody levels to food antigens, such as gliadin, ovalbumin and casein.

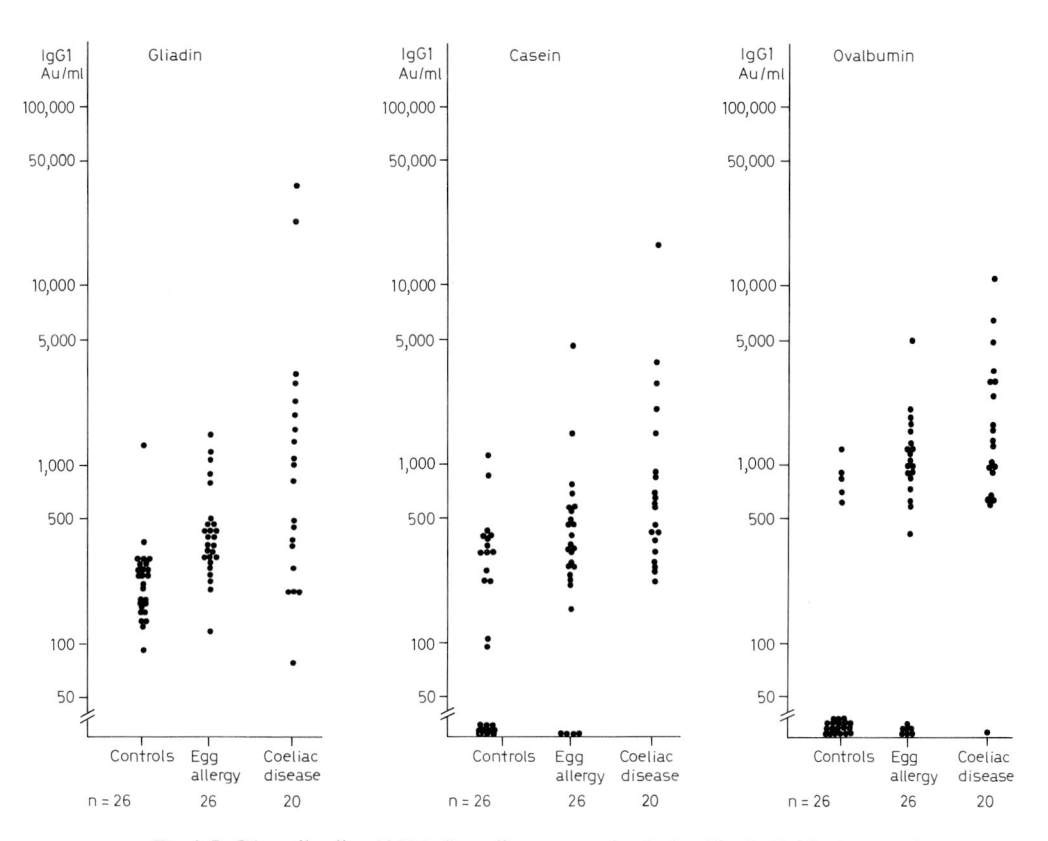

Fig. 2. IgG1 antibodies (AU/ml) to dietary proteins in healthy individuals, egg-allergic and coeliac disease patients. The highest antibody levels were achieved by coeliac disease patients without any diet.

For all three antigens studied, the dominant subclasses were IgG1 and IgG4; IgG2 and IgG3 antibodies were usually at low or undetectable levels. Only in untreated coeliac disease patients, concentrations of IgG1 antibodies to gliadin, ovalbumin and casein were significantly elevated (fig. 2). IgG4 antibodies were the same as controls for gliadin and ovalbumin and slightly increased for casein. In contrast, in egg-allergic persons, anti-ovalbumin IgG subclass antibodies were in the range of healthy adults. This finding suggests a predominant IgG1 subclass response to an antigenic stimulation, presumably caused by an increased penetration due to mucosal damage. Therefore, high lev-

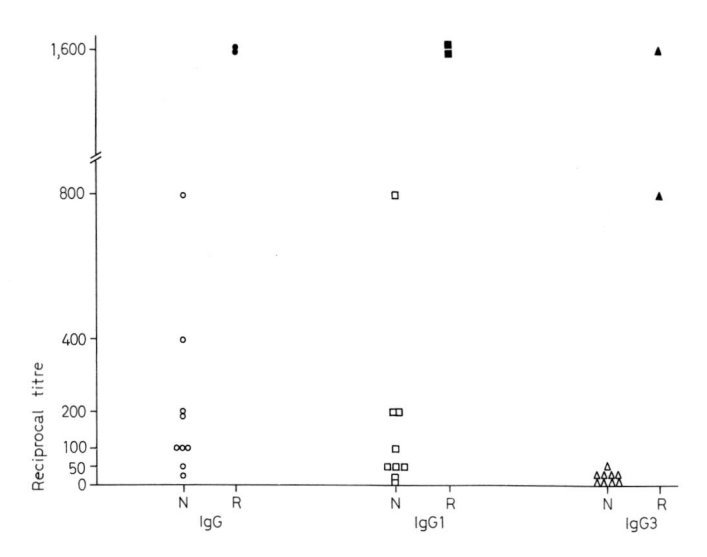

Fig. 3. Specific antibodies to *L*-asparaginase in 11 patients on chemotherapy for leukaemia. The highest levels (reciprocal titres) were achieved in 2 patients with anaphylaxis due to administration of *L*-asparaginase. The best segregation between reacting (R) and non-reacting (N) patients demonstrates the *L*-asparaginase-specific titre in IgG3 subclass.

els of IgG1 antibodies to gliadin and common dietary antigens, such as casein and ovalbumin, appear as valuable adjuncts in the diagnosis as well as in the follow-up of patients with coeliac disease. However, antibodies to dietary proteins may occur in several IgG subclasses in both in healthy persons and in individuals with food allergy [18].

Another field of application of IgG subclass measurements should be demonstrated by our recent investigation of anaphylactic reactions to *L*-asparaginase treatment in leukemic patients [19]. The employment of *L*-asparaginase in the chemotherapy of acute lymphoblastic leukemia may lead, in up to 30% of treated patients, to anaphylactic reactions. *L*-asparaginase is a bacterial protein with a molecular weight of 120,000 daltons. Formation of IgM, IgA and mainly IgG antibodies after repeated administration was described. Fabry et al. [20] reported in patients developing anaphylactic reactions a significant activation of the complement system. In most instances, elevated IgG antibodies to *L*-asparaginase activate the complement system and may induce anaphylactic reactions following L-asparaginase infusion. Although the dominant immune response to L-asparaginase treatment was in the IgG1 subclass, patients with anaphylactic reactions demonstrated an additional high level of specific IgG3 antibodies (fig. 3). Thus, IgG subclass-specific determination of antibodies to L-asparaginase enable us to estimate the risk of anaphylaxis prior to L-asparaginase administration. Although antibodies of the various IgG subclasses express different biological functions, we have to consider that the magnitude of the immune response to allergens is related to the type of antigen and the timing and route of administration rather than to the disease process itself. In addition, the future immunotherapy regimes will have to attempt to establish the value of IgG subclass antibody quantitation as a marker for the clinical outcome.

References

1 Goodfriend, L.; Perelmutter, L.: Properties of two chromatographically distinct reagins in the sera of ragweed atopic individuals. Int. Archs. Allergy Appl. Immun. *33:* 87 (1968).
2 Toorenenbergen, A.W. van; Aalberse, R.C.: IgG4 and release of histamine from human peripheral blood leukocytes. Int. Archs Allergy appl. Immun. *67:* 117–122 (1982).
3 Gwynn, C.M.; Morrison Smith, J.; Leon, G.L.; Stanworth, D.R.: Role of IgG4 subclass in childhood allergy. Lancet *i:* 910–911 (1978).
4 Fagan, D.L.; Slaughter, C.A.; Capra, J.D.; Sullivan, T.J.: Monoclonal antibodies to immunoglobulin G4 induce histamine release from human basophils in vitro. J. Allergy clin. Immunol. *70:* 399–404 (1982).
5 Berrens, L.; Koers, W.J.; Bruynzeel, P.L.B.: IgE and IgG4 antibodies in specific allergies. Lancet *ii:* 92 (1977).
6 Heiner, D.C.; De Weck, A.L.; Skvaril, F.; Muller, U.; Underdown, B.: IgG4 antibody responses to five bee venom antigens. J. Allergy clin. Immunol. *65:* 201 (1980).
7 Devey, M.E.; Wilson, D.V.; Wheeler, A.W.: The IgG sub-classes of antibodies to grass pollen allergens produced in hay fever patients during hyposensitization. Clin. Allergy *6:* 227 (1976).
8 Aalberse, R.C.; Gaag, R. van der; Leeuwen, J. van: Serological aspects of IgG4 antibodies. I. Prolonged immunization results in an IgG4-restricted response. J. Immun. *130:* 722–726 (1983).
9 Norman, P.S.: An overview of immunotherapy. J. Allergy clin. Immunol. *65:* 87 (1980).
10 Djurup, R.: The subclass nature and clinical significance of the IgG antibody responce in patients undergoing allergen-specific immunotherapy. Allergy *40:* 469–486 (1985).

11 Rocklin, R.E.: Clinical and immunologic aspects of allergen-specific immunotherapy in patients with seasonal allergic rhinitis and/or allergic asthma. J. Allergy clin. Immunol. 72: 323 (1983).
12 Urbanek, R.; Dold, S.: Schlüsselrolle der IgG4-Subklassen-Antikörper bei Schutzentstehung gegen allergische Reaktionen auf Insektenstiche. Mschr. Kinderheilk. 134: 536–540 (1986).
13 Wetterwald, A.; Skvaril, F.; Müller, U.; Blaser, K.: Isotypic and idiotypic characterization of anti-bee venom phospholipase A2 antibodies. Int. Archs Allergy appl. Immun. 77: 195–197 (1985).
14 Giessen, M. van der; Homan, W.L.; Kernebeck, G. van; Aalberse, R.C.; Dieges, P.H.: Subclass typing of IgG antibodies formed by grass-pollen-allergic patients during immunotherapy. Int. Archs Allergy appl. Immun. 50: 625 (1976).
15 Moss, R.B.; Hsu, Yao-Pi; Kwasnicki, J.M.; Sullivan, M.M.; Reid, M.J.: Isotypic and antigenic restriction of the blocking antibody response to ryegrass pollen: correlation of rye group I antigen-specific IgG1 with clinical response. J. Allergy clin. Immunol. 79: 387–398 (1987).
16 Kemeny, D.M.; Urbanek, R.; Samuel, D.; Richards, D.: Improved sensitivity and specificity of sandwich, competitive and capture enzyme-linked immunosorbent assays for allergen-specific antibodies. Int. Archs Allergy appl. Immun. 77: 198–200 (1985).
17 Ciclitira, P.J.; Ellis, H.J.; Richards, D.; Kemeny, D.M.: Gliadin IgG subclass antibodies in patients with coeliac disease. Int. Archs Allergy appl. Immun. 80: 258–261 (1986).
18 Husby, S.; Oxelius, V.-A.; Teisner, B.; Jensenius, J.C.; Svehag, S.-E.: Humoral immunity to dietary antigens in healthy adults. Occurence, isotype and IgG subclass distribution of serum antibodies to protein antigens. Int. Archs Allergy appl. Immun. 77: 416–422 (1985).
19 Urbanek, R.; Körholz, D.; Göbel, U.; Jobke, A.; Jürgens, H.; Wahn, V.: Can anaphylactic reactions to L-asparaginase be predicted by determination of specific IgG-antibodies of different subclasses? Eur. J. Pediat. 146: Abstr. 31, p. 104 (1987).
20 Fabry, U.; Körholz, D.; Jürgens, H.; Göbel, U.; Wahn, V.: Anaphylaxis to L-asparaginase during treatment for acute lymphoblastic leukemia in children – evidence of a complement-mediated mechanism. Pediat. Res. 19: 400–408 (1985).

PD Dr. R. Urbanek, Universitäts-Kinderklinik,
Mathildenstrasse 1, D-7800 Freiburg i. Br. (FRG)

Distribution of IgG Subclasses among Human Autoantibodies to Sm, RNP, dsDNA, SS-B and IgG Rheumatoid Factor[1]

William J. Yount, Philip Cohen, Robert A. Eisenberg

Department of Medicine and Department of Microbiology and Immunology, University of North Carolina, Chapel Hill, N.C., USA

Introduction

Certain autoantibodies are highly specific for the diagnosis of systemic lupus erythematosus (SLE). These include anti-Sm, directed at a small nuclear ribonuclear protein molecule [1, 2], and anti-double-stranded DNA [3]. Anti-Sm antibodies probably do not play a critical role in the pathogenesis of SLE, while anti-DNA antibodies are almost certainly important in the development of nephritis in many patients [4]. Nevertheless, the diagnostic specificity of both these antibodies strongly implies that their production is intimately linked with the basic immunoregulatory abnormalities that cause SLE. Antibodies to the nuclear antigen SS-B [5], which is also known as Ha [6] and La [7], are found in the sera of patients with SLE and with primary Sjögren's syndrome. SS-B is a soluble nuclear protein resistant to RNAase and DNAase but sensitive to trypsin. Its function in the cell is unknown, although it has been shown to form a complex with a variety of RNA that are the product of RNA polymerase III [8–10]. The SS-B polypeptides can associate with several viral RNA, a fact which may be related to the induction of anti-SS-B [11–13]. Rheumatoid factors (RF) are found in the serum of most patients with rheumatoid arthritis. RF of the IgG class have been suspected of having s special role in some of

---

[1] Supported by NIH grants AM26574, AM34156, AM33887, AM25733 and AR34976, a visiting scholar award from the Burroughs Wellcome Foundation (W.J.Y.) and a Kenan sabbatical grant (W.J.Y.). Drs. Cohen and Eisenberg were Senior Investigators of the Arthritis Foundation.

the pathological manifestations of this illness, and may be associated with vasculitis [14–17], but there is not universal agreement on this point [18, 19]. The presence of IgG RF in synovial fluids, especially in the form of intermediate complexes, together with decreased concentrations of intrasynovial complement, has lent support to the concept that this autoantibody has a special role in immune complex formation with consequent inflammation [20].

In the present communication, we have characterized the IgG subclass of 19 Sm-positive SLE sera, 9 RNP-positive sera, 26 ds-DNA-positive sera, 39 SS-B-positive sera and 23 sera and 40 synovial fluids positive for IgG rheumatoid factor. Portions of the work described herein have been described previously for anti-Sm [21], anti-RNP [21], anti-ds-DNA [21] for anti-SS-B (La) [22], and for IgG RF [23]. For each autoantibody response, a restricted polyclonal distribution of IgG subclasses was found, and compared to other humoral responses in the same patients. The results suggest that the formation of these autoantibodies is T-cell-dependent and may be driven by antigen or may reflect T cell influences of heavy chain constant region switching [24]. The immunoregulation of the response to several autoantigens may be quite similar. The demonstration of an important role for IgG4 as a RF is of special interest because of the relative inability of this subclass to fix complement or bind to Fc receptors, and because of its potential role as a mediator of increased vascular permeability.

Methods

Sera. Sera from patients with rheumatic disorders, other illnesses and normal volunteers were obtained from the clinics and wards of the North Carolina Memorial Hospital with informed consent according to protocols approved by the committee for the protection of the rights of human subjects. 42 anti-Sm-positive sera were identified by double diffusion using standard references [25]. All patients except one with diffuse interstitial pulmonary fibrosis had the clinical diagnosis of SLE. The 39 sera positive for anti-SS-B included 18 patients with SLE, 2 with probable SLE, 1 with discoid LE, 2 with subacute cutaneous LE, 1 with urticarial vasculitis and SLE, 7 with primary Sjögren's syndrome and 8 with miscellaneous disorders. Patients with SLE and classical or definite rheumatoid arthritis met criteria defined by the American Rheumatism Association.

Antigens for Enzyme-Linked Immunosorbent Assays (ELISA). Sm antigen was affinity purified from RNAase- and DNAase-digested rabbit thymus extract as previously described [26]. Pneumococcal polysaccharides were in the form of Pneumovax (Merck,

Table I. Isotype distribution of human anti-Sm antibody (µg/ml)

Patient	IgM	IgD	IgG4	IgG2	IgG3	IgG1	IgE	IgA
1	11	< 0.2	4	< 10	16	15,000	< 0.02	< 0.4
2	16	< 0.2	1	< 10	15	1,700	< 0.02	< 0.4
3	9	< 0.2	42	85	32	5,900	< 0.02	3
4	11	< 0.2	0.1	11	1	1,500	< 0.02	< 0.4
5	17	< 0.2	< 0.1	< 10	0.4	700	< 0.02	1
6	100	< 0.2	0.1	11	3	570	< 0.02	8
7	6	< 0.2	0.1	< 10	0.7	190	< 0.02	0.8
8	6	< 0.2	0.1	52	2	380	< 0.02	17
9	40	< 0.2	0.8	< 10	0.8	480	< 0.02	< 0.4
10	14	< 0.2	0.2	< 10	105	510	< 0.02	< 0.4
11	5	< 0.2	< 0.1	< 10	29	190	< 0.02	4
12	14	< 0.2	< 0.1	< 10	13	16	< 0.02	< 0.4
13	78	< 0.2	< 0.1	< 10	28	123	< 0.02	4
14	53	< 0.2	< 0.1	< 10	19	80	< 0.02	2
15	27	< 0.2	< 0.1	< 10	45	60	< 0.02	< 0.4
16	42	< 0.2	< 0.1	< 10	21	155	< 0.02	< 0.4
17	23	< 0.2	< 0.1	< 10	6	1,300	< 0.02	0.6
18	17	< 0.2	< 0.1	< 10	26	190	< 0.02	2
19	11	< 0.2	< 0.1	< 10	37	210	< 0.02	1
$\bar{X}$	26	< 0.2	2.6	16	20	1,540	< 0.02	3.3
SEM	6.0	–	2.2	4.4	5.7	808	–	1.2
% of total	1.6	< 0.01	0.16	1.0	1.2	96	< 0.001	0.2

Sharp & Dohme, West Point, Pa.) and were used at 10 µg/ml. Trinitrophenylated bovine serum albumin (TNP-BSA) was utilized in the ELISA at 10 µg/ml. Tetanus toxoid was obtained as a purified preparation from the Massachusetts Department of Public Health (Boston, Mass.) and was used at a concentration of 1 µg/ml. SS-B was purified from rabbit thymus extract by extraction with phosphate-buffered saline, RNAase and DNAase digestion and precipitation with 60% saturated ammonium sulfate [27]. For detection of RF, rabbit γ-globulin 10 µg/ml or alternatively purified human myeloma proteins, horse IgG or fragments of human IgG were used as antigen.

Isotype Reagents and Isotype-Specific Proteins. Myeloma proteins and polyclonal subclass antisera were prepared as previously described [28, 29]. Monoclonal anti-subclass reagents were the kind gift of Dr. Charles Reimer. The following clones were used (originally from Dr. R. Jefferis, Birmingham, England): 6012, anti-IgG1; 6014, anti-IgG2; 6051, anti-IgG3; and 6022, anti-IgG4.

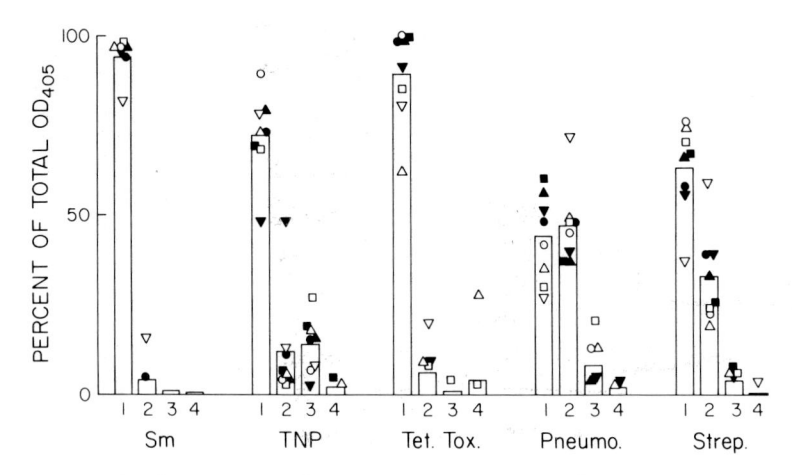

Fig. 1. IgG subclass distribution of anti-Sm and other antibodies determined with hybridoma reagents. ELISA assays for the indicated antigens were developed with standardized IgG subclass monoclonal antibodies. For each serum, the sum of the OD obtained in all four assays was divided into the results with each monoclonal to determine the percent contribution of each subclass to the total response. The bars indicate the mean percents for each subclass for all sera. Seven individual anti-Sm sera are shown and correspond to those listed in table I: ○ = patient 1; △ = patient 14; ▽ = patient 8; □ = patient 2; ● = patient 5; ▲ = patient 17; ▼ = patient 3; ☐ = normal human serum. Points < 3% were omitted from the graph for clarity. All sera were tested in all assays, except that the results of the normal serum in the anti-Sm assay did not give sufficient OD for analysis. Antigens utilized: Sm; TNP-BSA; tetanus toxoid (Tet. tox.); Pneumovax, pneumococcal polysaccharides (Pneumo.); group A streptococcal cell wall (Strep.).

ELISA. Antigens were added to polyvinyl chloride microtiter plates in 0.2 M borate-buffered saline, pH 8.4 with 5 protease inhibitors. After 5 h incubation at 4 °C, the plates were washed and were nonspecifically coated with BBS-PI plus 0.5% BSA and 0.4% Tween 80. After 1 h at 4 °C, the plates were aspirated and samples were added in the coating buffer. Each sample was tested at three dilutions for each isotype. The plates were incubated overnight at 4 °C. They were washed again, and affinity-purified anti-isotype biotinylated reagents were added for a further incubation at 4 °C for 3 h. The concentrations of the anti-isotype reagents were determined empirically to give comparable optical densities (OD). The plates were again washed, and avidin-alkaline phosphatase was added in coating buffer for a further 3-hour incubation. The plates were again washed, and the substrate paranitrophenylphosphate was added at a concentration of 1 mg/ml in 0.01 M diethanolamine, pH 9.8. The development of $O.D._{405}$ was followed at appropriate intervals with a Dynatech microELISA auto-reader (MR580; Dynatech Laboratories).

Anti-DNA Antibodies. Anti-ds-DNA antibodies were measured by a standard *Crithidia lucilia* assay using commercial slides (Kallestad Laboratories, Inc., Austin, Tex.).

Table II. IgG subclass distribution of anti-RNP antibodies

Patient	Dx	Percent of total OD				Total OD for 4 subclasses	
		IgG1	IgG2	IgG3	IgG4	$\Sigma(^{OD}RNP)$	$\Sigma(^{OD}Sm)$
1	PSS/DM	95	4	1	0	1.420	0.136
2	SLE	74	3	1	21	0.775	0.063
3	PSS	97	2	1	1	1.143	0.039
4	PSS/DM	93	2	4	0	0.461	0.044
5	MCTD	86	12	2	0	0.367	0.087
6	SLE	98	1	1	0	0.627	0.446
7	SLE	94	4	1	0	1.063	0.599
8	MCTD	96	1	2	1	0.353	0.131
9	Cervical dysplasia	92	1	2	4	0.752	0.305
$\bar{x}$		92±8	3±3	2±1	3±7	0.773 ±0.371	0.206 ±0.200

DM = Dermatomyositis; MCTD = mixed connective tissue disease; PSS = progressive systemic sclerosis.

Results

Isotype Analysis of Anti-Sm Antibodies. 19 anti-Sm-positive SLE sera gave strong enough results in the ELISA for isotype analysis. The overall isotype distributions are compiled in table I. In every case, the most prominent isotype was IgG1. All sera also had IgG3 and IgM anti-Sm antibodies detectable. Some sera had IgA, IgG2, or IgG4 antibodies present, usually in very low amounts. No IgD or IgE anti-Sm antibodies were seen. The IgG1 isotype was represented far out of proportion to its expected concentration in total serum IgG and comprised 96% of total Sm antibody and 98% of total IgG anti-Sm. Despite the prominence of IgG1, the light chain distributions were similar to those expected for total IgG, with a κ/λ ratio of approximately 2:1. In contrast (fig. 1), pneumococcal polysaccharide antibodies in these

Table III. Ig isotypes in human systemic lupus erythematosus double-stranded DNA antibodies as determined by indirect immunofluorescence using *Crithidia luciliae* (1/titer)

Patient	Polyvalent	IgM	IgD	IgG4	IgG2	IgG3	IgG1	IgE	IgA	kappa	lambda	C3 fixation
McK	20,000	320	–	20	4	20	80	–	–	80	160	128
Ba	5,120	640	–	–	–	40	160	–	–	80	160	8
Th	1,280	320	–	–	–	80	640	–	–	320	640	–
Va	1,280	10	–	–	–	40	320	–	–	80	160	ND
Gr	640	160	–	–	–	80	160	–	–	320	640	512
He	640	10	–	4	–	40	10	–	–	20	20	–
Mu	640	80	–	20	–	80	40	–	–	80	80	32
Gi	640	80	–	–	–	4	10	–	–	80	–	–
Ed	512	640	–	–	–	40	320	–	–	80	160	–
Ra	320	4	–	–	–	10	4	–	–	20	4	–
Hal	320	4	–	–	–	10	80	–	–	80	80	–
Br	320	4	–	–	–	4	–	4	–	–	80	–
Fi	320	80	–	–	–	–	80	–	–	–	–	–
Har	320	640	–	–	–	–	40	–	–	80	320	–
Wi	320	40	–	–	–	80	640	–	–	320	320	ND
Pe	160	20	–	–	–	20	20	–	–	40	20	–
Br	160	–	–	–	–	20	–	4	–	40	40	–
Mo	160	40	–	–	–	–	–	–	–	–	–	–
Les	160	4	–	–	–	1	40	–	–	80	80	ND
McP	80	–	–	–	–	4	4	4	–	4	4	ND
Oa	80	40	–	–	–	–	–	–	–	–	–	4
Pe	80	–	–	–	–	4	80	–	–	–	–	–
Ph	40	10	–	–	–	–	–	–	–	–	–	–
Al	40	80	–	–	–	1	10	4	–	40	10	2
Lea	40	4	–	–	–	10	4	4	–	4	4	–
McD	20	–	–	–	–	–	–	–	–	–	80	–

ND = Not determined.

same sera were mainly IgG2 and IgG1, while anti-TNP and antigroup A streptococcal cell wall were of several isotypes. Tetanus toxoid antibodies in these sera were mainly IgG1. In 12 sera from other individuals hyperimmunized for antiragweed or house dust mite IgG4 antibodies were readily identified in one antiragweed and one antimite serum.

Table IV. Anti-SS-B isotypes and IgG subclasses in serum

Patient number	Anti-SS-B antibody, µg/ml				
	IgG	IgM	IgA	IgG1	IgG3
1	120	–[1]	–[2]	100	6
2	25	–	–	34	–[3]
3	72	–	–	140	3
4	47	–	–	25	3
5	18	–	–	30	–
6	25	–	–	22	2
7	11	–	–	–[4]	–
8	8	–	–	7	5
9	29	–	–	44	4
10	15	–	–	50	–
11	–[5]	–	–	–	–
12	–	–	–	–	–
13	–	–	–	–	–
14	31	–	9	52	–
15	–	–	–	3	–
16	14	–	–	48	–
17	–	–	–	–	–
18	–	–	–	–	–
19	20	–	–	28	–
20	5	3	–	–	–
21	44	–	–	56	4
22	29	–	–	23	–
23	–	–	–	–	2
24	51	–	–	140	2
25	36	–	9	26	2
26	40	–	8	56	3
27	5	–	–	–	3
28	–	–	–	7	5
29	36	7	8	140	6
30	–	–	–	3	–
31	16	–	–	100	5
32	35	2	10	62	2
33	11	–	–	4	6
34	6	–	–	–	–
35	–	–	–	–	–
36	–	–	–	19	2
37	6	–	–	22	–
38	–	–	–	–	–
39	4	–	–	38	–
Normals, n = 7–10	–	–	–	–	–

[1] < 2 µg/ml; [2] < 5 µg/ml; [3] < 1 µg/ml; [4] < 3 µg/ml; [5] < 4 µg/ml.

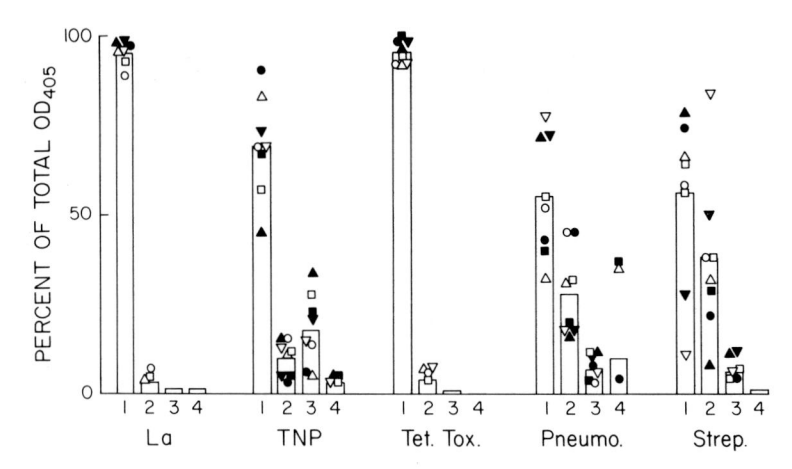

Fig. 2. IgG subclass distribution of anti-SS-B (La) and other antibodies is shown in a manner similar to that described for figure 1. Ten individual anti-SS-B (La) sera are shown and correspond to those listed in table II: ○ = patient 21; △ = patient 2; ▽ = patient 4; □ = patient 25; ● = patient 5; ▲ = patient 3; ▼ = patient 24; ■ = normal. Antigens utilized correspond to those indicated in figure 1. The preponderance of the IgG1 subclass in anti-SS-B is apparent.

IgG Subclass of Anti-RNP Antibodies. In like fashion, anti-RNP antibodies were characterized in 9 sera known to be negative for anti-Sm (table II). Again, greater than 90% of the reactivity was found in the IgG1 isotype.

Isotype of Anti-ds-DNA Antibodies. The anti-ds-DNA response was generally restricted to IgM, IgG1 and IgG3 (table III). Occasional sera had low titers of IgG4, IgG2 or even IgE anti-ds-DNA antibodies.

Isotype of Anti-SS-B. In all cases, IgG was the predominant isotype (table IV). Only 4 patients had detectable IgA or IgM anti-SS-B. No IgE anti-SS-B was detected. Anti-SS-B was predominantly or exclusively IgG1 subclass in all but 3 sera. Smaller amounts of IgG3 anti-SS-B were also found. No IgG2 or IgG4 response was detected in any serum. The distribution of IgG subclasses for anti-SS-B versus antibodies to TNP, tetanus toxoid, pneumococcal vaccine and group A streptococcal cell walls in these same patient's sera is illustrated in

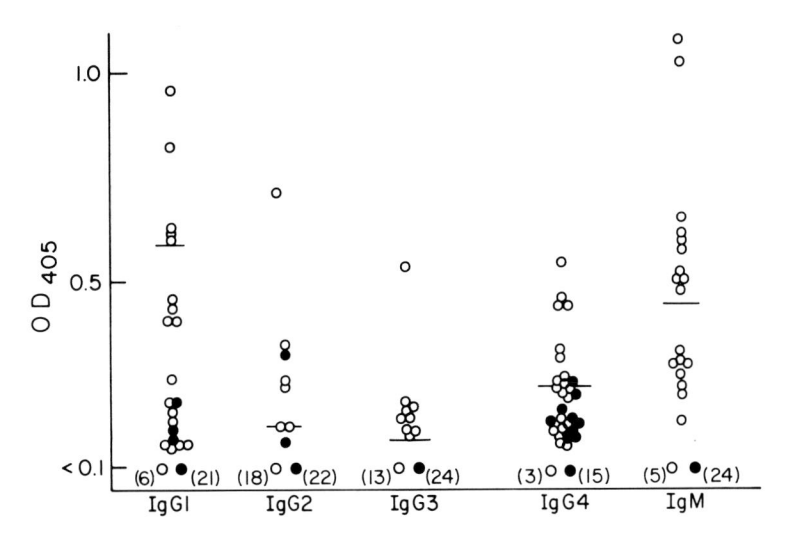

Fig. 3. IgG RF subclass distribution. IgG RF was quantitated in sera from 23 patients with RA (○) and in 24 controls (●). Horizontal lines indicate the means for the RA sera. Note that the IgG assay was not standardized against the IgG assays.

figure 2. Antibodies to SS-B, and to a lesser extent tetanus toxoid, were relatively restricted to IgG1, unlike antibodies to TNP, pneumococcal vaccine, and group A streptococcal cell walls. Again, a mixture of light chains was seen in most anti-SS-B with an overall κ/λ ratio of 1.4.

Subclass Distribution of IgG Rheumatoid Factor. As is indicated in figure 3, IgG1 and IgG4 were the most abundant subclasses, followed by IgG2 and IgG3. It is noteworthy that IgG RF was also detected in some normal sera. Similar results were obtained with two other anti-IgG4 monoclonal antibodies (6024 and 6025). In contrast, these same sera showed very different proportions of antibodies to TNP and tetanus toxoid (fig. 4). The same preponderance of IgG1 and IgG4 was noted when horse IgG was used as antigen in the IgG RF assay and when human myeloma proteins were used as targets (data not shown). The IgG RF was shown to bind to cross-linked Fc with little binding to Fab. Synovial fluid samples also exhibited IgM and IgG RF with a similar skewing to IgG4.

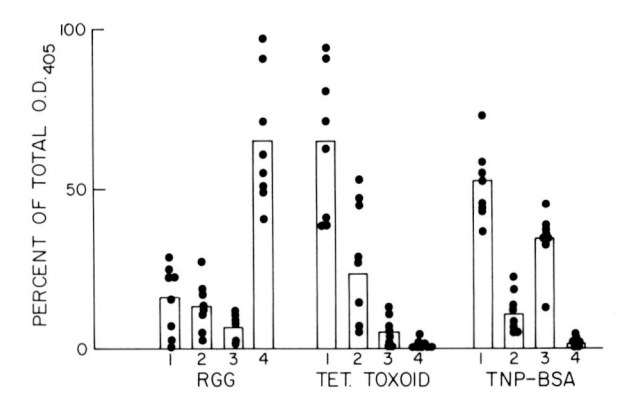

Fig. 4. IgG subclass distribution of other antibodies in eight RA sera with high levels of IgG4 RF. Antigens are similar to those depicted in figure 1. No preponderance of IgG4 to these antigens was noted.

Discussion

We have determined that anti-Sm autoantibodies in sera of patients with SLE were relatively restricted to the IgG1 isotype. In spite of this subclass restriction, these antibodies were polyclonal, as judged by the presence of both κ- and λ-light chains and also by diffuse patterns on isoelectric focusing (data not shown). The related specificity anti-RNP was also nearly entirely IgG1. Anti-ds-DNA antibodies were mainly of the IgM, IgG1, and IgG3 isotypes and, like the anti-Sm antibodies, contained both κ- and λ-light chains. The subclass distribution of human autoantibodies has been examined by several investigators previously. Sontheimer and Gilliam [30] found that anti-DNA antibodies are mainly of the IgG1 and IgG3 subclass, in accord with our results. Zouali et al. [31] also confirmed the distribution of anti-DNA antibodies. However, they reported that anti-RNP antibodies were of the IgG2 subclass, in contrast to our finding of an IgG1 restriction similar to that of anti-Sm. Antinuclear antibodies detected by immunofluorescence have been characterized as unrestricted [31, 32], or as mainly IgG1 [33] or IgG1 and IgG3 [34]. Antithyroglobulin has been found to be unrestricted [35], while acetylcholine receptor antibodies in certain myasthenic patients were restricted to the IgG3 subclass [36]. The antibodies to SS-B herein reported were mainly of the IgG1 subclass. A unique enrichment of IgG4 in addition to IgG1 was found for IgG RF. Finally, in our earlier work with the anti-Sm response in mice, we found a relative restriction to the IgG2a subclass [37].

The isotype restriction and polyclonality of the anti-Sm response suggests certain conclusions regrading their production in vivo. First, since the anti-Sm, anti-RNP, anti-SS-B and anti-DNA responses are all relatively restricted to the same T cell-dependent isotype (IgG1), it is probable that T cells play an important role in the production of these antibodies in vivo and their immunoregulation may be similar. Second, the polyclonality of the anti-Sm response, like that of the anti-SS-B response, suggests that it is not the result of a small number of mutations creating 'forbidden clones' [38]. Rather, it is more probable that the response is antigen-driven. This is consistent with interpretations based on the antigen specificity of these responses [39, 40]. The current work is also consistent with previous studies which showed that anti-Sm was mainly IgG and could fix complement [41].

The present results may also explain the old observation of restricted electrophoretic mobility of anti-Sm antibodies [25]. This is probably due to their subclass restriction, rather than to oligoclonality. In addition, the relatively normal distribution of κ- and λ-light chains in the anti-Sm, as well as the anti-RNP, anti-SS-B and anti-ds-DNA responses indicates that neither chain is uniquely essential for these specificities. Further investigations will emphasize the definition of anti-Sm idiotypes with anti-idiotypic reagents and the determination of the relationship of these idiotypes to specificity of anti-Sm antibodies for different Sm polypeptides.

The pathogenetic significance of the IgG1 antibodies against SS-B seen in Sjögren's syndrome and SLE is unclear. It seems likely, however, that this restriction also reflects basic immunoregulatory defects which underlie these diseases. A number of theories, primarily based on work done with mice, could account for the subclass restriction. Mayumi et al. [42] have suggested that T cells can influence the terminal differentiation of precommitted B cell precursors. The restriction may be due to T cells which preferentially help or suppress the B cells which express a particular isotype. T cells may also play an important role in forcing IgG subclass switching toward certain isotypes [43]. It is furthermore possible that heavy chain hypervariable regions associate with heavy chain constant regions nonrandomly. Although we cannot at present choose among these alternative explanations, the striking class and subclass restrictions of anti-Sm, anti-RNP, anti-ds-DNA, anti-SS-B and RF provide important clues to in vivo regulatory events.

The data presented for IgG RF indicate that IgG4 is an important subclass, responsible for a significant fraction of the IgG RF in rheumatoid serum and synovial fluid. The IgG4 RF was not accompanied in these patients by an aberrant distribution of IgG antibodies to exogenous antigens. Previous work by Shakib and Stanworth [44] also supports a special role for IgG4 anti-immunoglobulin. In this study, as in the present study, IgG1 and IgG4 RF activity was more frequently in RA sera that IgG2 or IgG3. The finding both in rheumatoid synovial fluid and in serum of elevated levels of IgG4 RF is evidence against the preferential clearance of complexes containing RF of other IgG subclasses. IgG4 is often the subclass of the clonally restricted antibodies to coagulation factors found in hemophiliacs [45]. IgG4 antibodies arise upon prolonged antigenic stimulation associated with allergy immunotherapy [46, 47]. IgG4 antibodies may have lower avidity than antibodies of other IgG subclasses [48]. Antibasement membrane antibodies in bullous pemphigoid have been found to be restricted to the IgG4 subclass [49], and there is evidence for the participation of the IgG4 subclass in other autoantibodies deposited in tissues [50–52]. Some investigators have observed binding of IgG4 to mast cells, implying a role for this subclass in immediate hypersensitivity [53, 54], and monoclonal antibodies to IgG4 provoke histamine release by mast cells [55]. Thus, the IgG4 RF may be of importance in causing the release in the joint or elsewhere of mediators of immediate hypersensitivity, and thus augment vasodilatation and immune complex deposition. The presence of significant amounts of IgG4 RF in these sera gives an attractive explanation for the reduced complement-fixing activity in isolated IgG RF preparations, because IgG4 is a noncomplement-fixing subclass. It also fails to bind to monocyte Fc receptors another biologic property of potential pathogenetic significance regarding Fc-mediated clearance by the macrophage-phagocytic system. The interesting enrichment of IgG RF with IgG4 thus may reflect both immunoregulatory as well as pathogenetic implications.

Summary

The IgG subclass distribution of human autoantibodies to Sm, double-stranded DNA (ds-DNA), ribonucleoprotein (RNP), SS-B (La), and IgG rheumatoid factor (RF) have been determined using sensitive ELISA or by indirect immunofluorescence on *Crithidia lucilia* in sera from patients with systemic lupus erythematosus (SLE), Sjögren's syndrome, and rheumatoid arthritis. For anti-Sm and anti-RNP, IgG1 was the predominant isotype. For anti-ds-DNA and anti-SS-B, IgG1 and a lesser contribution of IgG3 was found. In contrast, IgG1 and IgG4 were the predominant isotypes of human IgG RF. The preponderance of isotypes noted for these autoantibodies did not extend to the IgG subclass distribution for antibodies to trinitrophenol-bovine serum albumin (TNP), tetanus toxoid (Tet. tox.), pneumococcal polysaccharides (Pneumo.), and group A streptococcal cell walls (Strep.). The restriction of human humoral responses as well as autoantibodies has both pathogenetic and immunoregulatory implications, and suggests that for these autoantibodies, T-cell-dependent responses, probably driven by antigen, are of importance.

References

1 Notman, D.D.; Kurata, N.; Tan, E.M.: Profiles of antinuclear antibodies in systemic rheumatic diseases. Ann. intern. Med. *83:* 464–469 (1975).
2 Lerner, M.R.; Steitz, J.A.: Antibodies to small nuclear RNAs complexed with proteins are produced by patients with systemic lupus erythematosus. Proc. natn. Acad. Sci. USA *76:* 5495–5499 (1979).
3 Swaak, A.J.; Groenwold, G.J.; Aarden, L.A.; Feltkamp, T.E.W.: Detection of anti-ds-DNA as diagnostic tool. Ann. rheum. Dis. *40:* 45–49 (1981).
4 Koffler, D.; Schur, P.H.; Kunkel, H.G.: Immunological studies concerning the nephritis of systemic lupus erythematosus. J. exp. Med. *126:* 607–631 (1967).
5 Alspaugh, M.A.; Tan, E.M.: Antibodies to cellular antigens in Sjögren's syndrome. J. clin. Invest. *55:* 1067–1073 (1975).
6 Akizuki, M.; Powers, R.; Holman, H.R.: A soluble acidic protein of the cell nucleus which reacts with serum from patients with systemic lupus erythematosus and Sjögren's syndrome. J. clin. Invest. *59:* 264–272 (1977).
7 Mattioli, M.; Reichlin, M.: Heterogeneity of RNA protein antigens reactive with sera of patients with systemic lupus erythematosus. Description of a cytoplasmic nonribosomal antigen. Arthritis Rheum. *17:* 421–429 (1974).
8 Hendrick, J.P.; Wolin, S.L.; Rinke, J.; Lerner, M.; Steitz, J.A: Ro small cytoplasmic ribonucleoproteins are a subclass of La ribonucleosomes: further characterization of the Ro and La small ribonucleoproteins from uninfected mammalian cells. Mol. cell. Biol. *1:* 1138–1149 (1981).
9 Rinke, J.; Steitz, J.A.: Precursor molecules of both human 5S ribosomal RNA and transfer RNAs are bound by a cellular protein reactive with anti-La lupus antibodies. Cell *29:* 149–159 (1982).
10 Hashimoto, C.; Steitz, J.A.: Sequential association of nucleolar 7-2 RNA with two different autoantigens. J. biol. Chem. *258:* 1379–1382 (1983).

11 Francoeur, A.M.; Mathews, M.B.: Interaction between VA RNA and the lupus antigen La: formation of a ribonucleoprotein particle in vitro. Proc. natn. Acad. Sci. USA 79: 6772–6776 (1982).
12 Wilusz, J.; Kurilla, M.G.; Keene, J.D.: A host protein (La) binds to a unique species of minus-sense leader RNA during replication of vesicular stomatitis virus. Proc. natn. Acad. Sci. USA 80: 5827–5831 (1983).
13 Mathews, M.B.; Bernstein, R.M.: Myositis autoantibody inhibits histidyl-tRNA synthetase: a model for autoimmunity. Nature, London 304: 177–179 (1983).
14 Theofilopoulos, A.N.; Burtonboy, G.; LoSpalluto, J.J.; Ziff, M.: IgG rheumatoid factor and low molecular weight IgM: an association with vasculitis. Arthritis Rheum. 17: 272–284 (1974).
15 Allen, C.; Elson, C.J.; Scott, D.G.I.; Bacon, P.A.; Bucknall, R.C.: IgG antiglobulins in rheumatoid arthritis and other arthritides: relationship with clinical features and other parameters. Ann. rheum. Dis. 40: 127–131 (1981).
16 Westedt, M.L.; Herbrink, P.; Molenaar, J.L.; deVries, E.; Verlaan, P.; Stinjen, T.; Cats, A.; Lindeman, J.: Rheumatoid factors in rheumatoid arthritis and vasculitis. Rheumatol. int. 5: 209–214 (1985).
17 Pope, R.M.; Fletcher, M.A.; Mamby, A.; Shapiro, C.M: Rheumatoid arthritis associated with hyperviscosity syndrome and intermediate complex formation. Archs intern. Med. 135: 281–285 (1975).
18 Wernick, R.; Merryman, R.; Jaffe, I.; Ziff, M.: IgG and IgM rheumatoid factors in rheumatoid arthritis. Quantitative response to penicillamine therapy and relationship to disease activity. Arthritis Rheum. 26: 593–598 (1983).
19 Jakle, C.; Feigal, D.W.; Robbins, D.L.; Shapiro, R.; Wiesner, K.: Serum IgG and IgM rheumatoid factors and complement activation in extraarticular rheumatoid disease. J. Rheumatol. 12: 227–232 (1985).
20 Winchester, R.J.; Agnello, V.; Kunkel, H.G.: Gamma globulin complexes in synovial fluids of patiens with rheumatoid arthritis. Partial characterization and relationship to lowered complement levels. Clin. exp. Immunol. 6: 689–706 (1970).
21 Eisenberg, R.A.; Dyer, K.; Craven, S.Y.; Fuller, C.R.; Yount, W.J.: Subclass restriction of the systemic lupus erythematosus marker antibody anti-Sm. J. clin. Invest. 75: 1270–1277 (1985).
22 Pearce, D.C.; Yount, W.J.; Eisenberg, R.A.: Subclass restriction of anti-SS-B (La) autoantibodies. Clin. Immunol. Immunopathol. 38: 111–119 (1986).
23 Cohen, P.L.; Cheek, R.L.; Hadler, J.A.; Yount, W.J.; Eisenberg, R.A.: Subclass distribution of IgG rheumatoid factor. Arthritis Rheum. 29: S73 (1986).
24 Theze, J.; Lowy, I.; Seman, M.; Brezin, C.; Neauport-Santes, C.; Fridman, W.H.: Control of isotype expression by helper T-cell clones and suppressor cells. Ann. Immunol, Paris 134D: 55 (1983).
25 Tan, E.M.; Kunkel, H.G.: Characteristics of a soluble nuclear antigen precipitating with sera of patients with systemic lupus erythematosus. J. Immun. 96: 464–471 (1966).
26 Eisenberg, R.A.; Fox, A.; Greenblatt, J.; Anderle, S.K.; Cromartie, W.J.; Schwab, J.H.: Measurement of bacterial cell wall in tissues by solid phase radioimmune assay. Correlation of the distribution and persistence of streptococcal cell wall fragments with experimental arthritis in rats. Infect. Immunity 38: 127–135 (1982).

27 Eisenberg, R.A.; Klapper, D.G.; Cohen, P.L.: The polypeptide structure of the Sm and RNP antigens. Molec. Immunol. *20:* 187–195 (1983).
28 Yount, W.J.; Hong, R.; Seligmann, M.; Good, R.; Kunkel, H.G.: Imbalances of gamma globulin subgroups and gene defects in patients with primary hypogammaglobulinemia. J. clin. Invest. *49:* 1957–1966 (1970).
29 Puritz, E.M.; Yount, W.J.; Newall, M.; Utsinger, P.D.: Immunoglobulin classes and IgG subclasses of human antinuclear antibodies. Clin. Immunol. Immunopathol. *2:* 98–113 (1973).
30 Sontheimer, R.D.; Gilliam, J.N.: DNA antibody class, subclass, and complement fixation in systemic lupus erythematosus with and without nephritis. Clin. Immunol. Immunopathol. *10:* 459 467 (1978).
31 Zouali, M.R.; Jefferis, R.; Eyquem, A.: IgG subclass distribution of autoantibodies to DNA and to nuclear ribonucleoproteins in autoimmune diseases. Immunology *51:* 595–600 (1984).
32 Tojo, T; Friou, G.J.; Spiegelberg, H.L.: Immunoglobulin G subclass of human antinuclear antibodies. Clin. exp. Immunol. *6:* 145–151 (1970).
33 Kacaki, J.N.; Callerame, M.L.; Blomgren, S.E.; Vaughan, J.H.: Immunoglobulin G subclasses of antinuclear antibodies and renal deposits. Comparison of systemic lupus erythematosus, drug-induced lupus and rheumatoid arthritis. Arthritis Rheum. *14:* 276–282 (1971).
34 Schur, P.H.; Monroe, M.; Rothfield, N.: The IgG subclass of antinuclear and antinucleic acid antibodies. Arthritis Rheum. *15:* 174–182 (1972).
35 Hay, F.C.; Torrigiani, G.: The distribution of antithyroglobulin antibodies in the immunoglobulin G subclasses. Clin. exp. Immunol. *16:* 517–521 (1974).
36 Lefvert, A.K.; Bergstrom, K.: Immunoglobulins in myaesthenia gravis: effect of human lymph IgG3 and F(ab')$_2$ fragments on a cholinergic receptor preparation from *Torpedo marmorata*. Eur J. clin. Invest. *7:* 115–119 (1977).
37 Eisenberg, R.A.; Winfield, J.B.; Cohen, P.L.: Subclass restriction of anti-Sm antibodies in MRL mice. J. Immun. *129:* 2146–2149 (1982).
38 Burnet, M.: Auto-immunity and auto-immune disease (Davis, Philadelphia 1972).
39 Fisher, D.E.; Conner, G.E.; Reeves, W.H.; Blobel, G.; Kunkel, H.G.: Synthesis and assembly of human small nuclear ribonucleoproteins generated by cell-free translation. Proc. natn. Acad. Sci. USA *80:* 6356–6360 (1983).
40 Boyer, C.; Cohen, P.L.; Eisenberg, R.A.: Quantitation of the Sm nuclear antigen. Arthritis Rheum. *25:* Abstr., p. S22 (1982).
41 Sabharwal, U.K.; Fong, S.; Hoch, S.; Cook, R.D.; Vaughan, J.H.; Curd, J.G.: Complement activation by antibodies to Sm in systemic lupus erythematosus. Clin. exp. Immunol. *51:* 317–324 (1983).
42 Mayumi, M.; Kuritani, T.; Kubagawa, H.; Cooper, M.D.: IgG subclass expression by human B lymphocytes and plasma cells: B lymphocytes precommitted to IgG subclass can be preferentially induced by polyclonal mitogens with T cell help. J. Immun. *130:* 671–677 (1983).
43 Mongini, P.K.; Paul, W.E.; Metcalf, E.S.: T cell regulation of immunoglobulin class expression in the antibody response to trinitrophenyl-ficoll. Evidence for T cell enhancement of the immunoglobulin class switch. J. exp. Med. *155:* 884–902 (1982).
44 Shakib, F.; Stanworth, D.R.: Antigammaglobulin (rheumatoid factor) activity of human IgG subclasses. Ann. rheum. Dis. *37:* 12–17 (1978).

45 Briet, E.; Reisner, H.M.; Roberts, H.L.: Inhibitors in Christmas VII inhibitors, pp. 123–129 (Liss, New York 1984).
46 Devey, M.E.; Wilson, D.V.; Wheeler, A.W.: The IgG subclasses of antibodies to grass pollen allergens produced in hay fever patients during hyposensitization. Clin. Allergy 6: 227–236 (1976).
47 Aalberse, R.C.; Van der Gaag, R.; Van Leeuwen, J.: Serologic aspects of IgG4 antibodies. I. Prolonged immunization results in an IgG4-restricted antibody response. J. Immun. 130: 722–726 (1983).
48 Devey, M.E.; Bleasdale, K.M.; French, M.A.H.; Harrison, G.: The IgG4 subclass is associated with a low affinity antibody response to tetanus toxoid in man. Immunology 55: 565–567 (191985).
49 Bird, P.; Friedman, P.S.; Ling, N.; Bird, A.G.; Thompson, R.A.: Subclass distribution of IgG antibodies in bullous pemphigoid. J. invest. Derm. 86: 21–25 (1986).
50 Lewis, E.; Busch, G.; Schur, P.H.: Gamma G globulin subgroup composition of the glomerular deposits in human renal disease. J. clin. Invest. 49: 1103–1113 (1970).
51 Roberts, J.L.; Wyatt, R.J.; Schwartz, M.M.; Lewis, E.J.: Differential characteristics of immune-bound antibodies in diffuse proliferative and membranous forms of lupus glomerulonephritis. Clin. Immunol. Immunopathol. 29: 223–241 (1983).
52 Bannister, K.M.; Howarth, G.S.; Clarkson, A.R.; Woodroffe, A.J.: Glomerular IgG subclass distribution in human glomerulonephritis. Clin. Nephrol. 19: 161–165 (1983).
53 Vijay, H.M.; Perelmutter, L.: Inhibition of reagin-mediated PCA reactions in monkeys and histamine release from human leukocytes by human IgG4 subclass. Int. Archs. Allergy appl. Immun. 53: 78–87 (1977).
54 Van Toorenbergen, A.W.; Aalberse, R.C.: IgG4 and release of histamine from human peripheral blood leucocytes. Int. Archs. Allergy appl. Immun. 67: 117–122 (1982).
55 Fagan, D.L.; Slaughter, C.A.; Capra, J.D.; Sullivan, T.J.: Monoclonal antibodies to immunoglobulin G4 induce histamine release from human basophils in vitro. J. Allergy clin. Immunol. 70: 399–404 (1982).

William J. Yount, MD, University of North Carolina,
School of Medicine, Division of Rheumatology and Immunology,
932 FLOB Building 231H, Chapel Hill, NC 27514 (USA)

Restrictive Murine Monoclonal IgG Subclass Antisera Revealing Antigenic Variants of Human IgG Subclasses

Vivi-Anne Oxelius

Department of Pediatrics, University of Lund, Lund, Sweden

Monoclonal antibodies to human γ-chain determinants are now available [5]. In an earlier report with an extensive study of 59 monoclonal antibodies of putative specificity for human IgG subclasses, tested by different methods, the results were discouraging with IgG1 and particularly IgG2 demonstrating assay restriction [3]. It has also been shown that murine monoclonal antibodies recognize only a limited number of the unique epitopes of the IgG subclasses [4].

Murine monoclonal IgG subclass antisera were compared with rabbit polyclonal IgG subclass antisera by immunoelectrophoresis, by double immunodiffusion and by absorption experiments [7]. 0.6% agarose with 6% PEG 3000 and temperature +4 °C was used throughout all experiments. The polyclonal specific IgG subclass antisera were produced in rabbits according to the method described before [6], and the murine monoclonal antisera: anti-IgG1 (BAM 09), anti-IgG2 (BAM 10), anti-IgG3 (BAM 08) and anti-IgG4 (BAM 11 and BAM 16) were bought from Unipath Ltd, Bedford, England.

By immunoelectrophoresis, it was shown that none of the IgG subclasses could precipitate along the whole electrophoretic distance with the monoclonal antisera compared to the polyclonal antisera (fig. 1). By immunodiffusion it was shown that the rabbit polyclonal antisera spurred over the respectively monoclonal antisera when investigated against a normal serum pool and individual sera (fig. 2). The polyclonal antisera were thus detecting molecules of the IgG subclasses not precipitated by the monoclonal antisera. Absorption experiments confirmed these findings [7].

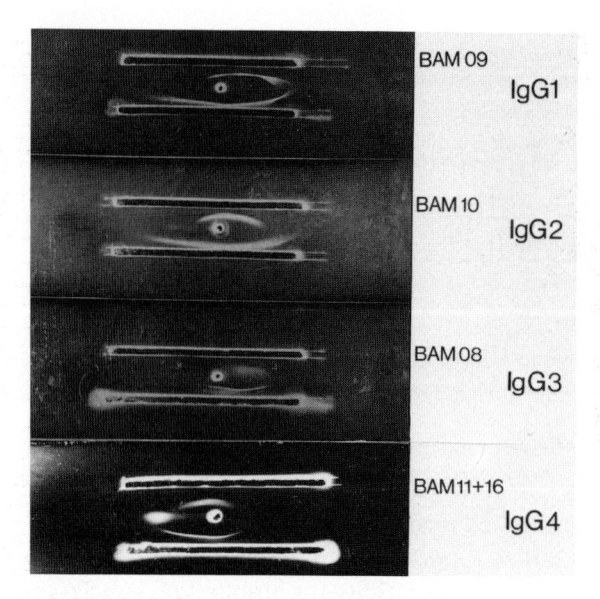

Fig. 1. Immunoelectrophoresis of a normal serum pool against the various murine monoclonal antisera (above) and polyclonal rabbit antisera (below). Photographed directly after 24 h of diffusion at +4 °C. Anode to the left.

The experiments demonstrated a restriction of the murine monoclonal anti-IgG subclass antisera. In all papers about monoclonal anti-IgG subclass antisera their restrictivity is discussed [1–5]. There are many examples of monoclonal antisera detecting only narrow sequences or not detecting sequences of the IgG subclass molecule: e.g. antibodies with specificity for the Glm(f) allotype recognizing an IgG Fab epitope [1] and although there are six IgG1 unique residues within the Cγ1 domain, no specific monoclonal antibody has exhibited reactivity to this region [4].

The murine monoclonal IgG subclass antisera which were tested here are known to be some of the best available. Anyhow, they were too restrictive and did not detect all antigenic variants within the IgG subclass. Therefore, they cannot be used as universally reacting agents. Neither can the standards with known contents of IgG subclasses be used nor reference values found with polyclonal antisera when wor-

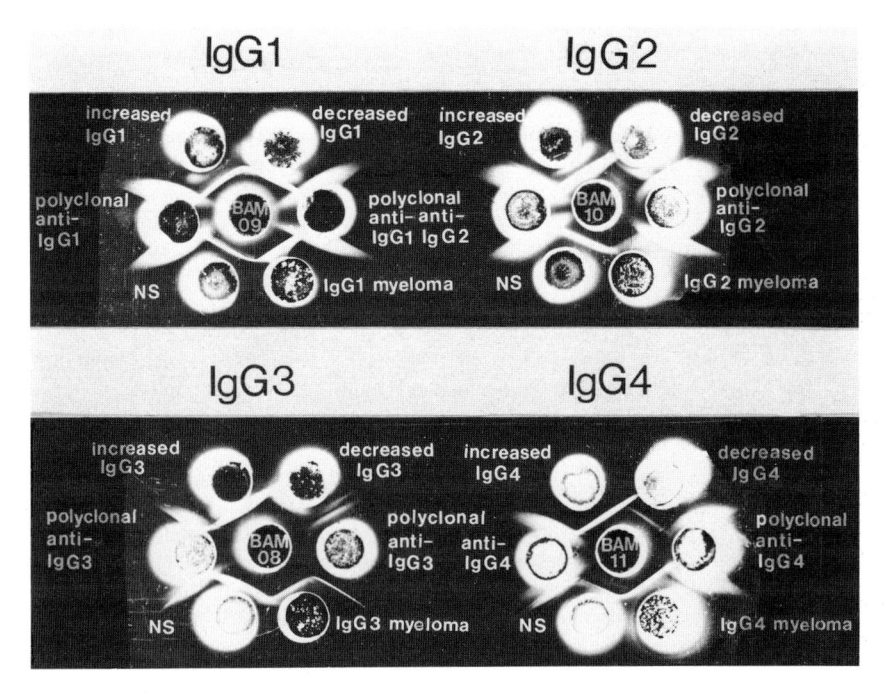

Fig. 2. Immunodiffusion of the various murine monoclonal and rabbit polyclonal anti-IgG subclass antisera against a normal serum pool (NS), purified myeloma proteins and sera with decreased and increased levels of IgG subclasses. Photographed directly after 24 h of diffusion at +4 °C.

king with restrictively reacting monoclonal antisera. The reactivity of monoclonal antisera should always be standardized against polyclonal antisera before used.

The comparison of polyclonal and monoclonal IgG subclass antisera also revealed further antigenic variants within all the IgG subclasses: at least two antigenic variants in IgG1, two in IgG2, two in IgG3 and beside IgG4a and IgG4b a third in IgG4. These antigenic variants could not be referred to Gm allotypic variation. Antigenic variants of IgG4 has been shown among IgG4 myeloma proteins, but these have not as yet been shown to be present in sera of normal individuals [8]. The physical and functional properties of the antigenic variants found within the IgG subclasses need further investigation.

References

1 Bird, P.; Lowe, J.; Jefferis, R.; Ling, N.R.: Monoclonal antibodies to an immunoglobulin allotype marker Glm(f). Vox Sang. *47:* 366–372 (1985).
2 Jefferis, R.; Ling, N.R.: More pitfalls in the use of antibodies. Immunol. Today *5:* 127 (1984).
3 Jefferis, R.; Reimer, C.B.; Skvaril, F.; deLange, G.; Ling, N.R.; Lowe, J.: Evaluation of monoclonal antibodies having specificity for human IgG subclasses: results of an IUIS/WHO collaborative study. Immunol. Lett. *10:* 223–252 (1985).
4 Jefferis, R.: Human IgG subclass specific epitopes recognized by murine monoclonal antibodies. Monogr. Allergy, vol. 20, pp. 26–33 (Karger, Basel 1986).
5 Lowe, J.; Bird, P.; Hardie, D.; Jefferis, R.; Ling, N.R.: Monoclonal antibodies (McAbs) to determinants on human gamma chains: properties of antibodies showing subclass restriction or subclass specificity. Immunology *47:* 329–336 (1982).
6 Oxelius, V.-A.: Crossed immunoelectrophoresis and electroimmuno assay of human IgG subclasses. Acta path. microbiol. scand., C, Immunol. *86:* 109–116 (1978).
7 Oxelius, V.-A.: Antigenic variants of human IgG subclasses. Restriction of murine monoclonal IgG subclass antisera. Scand. J. Immunol. *25:* 169–174 (1987).
8 Wahler, M.R.; Bird, P.; Uacaeto, D.O.; Vartdal, F.; Goodall, D.M.; Jefferis, R.: Immunogenic and antigenic epitopes of immunoglobulins. XIV. Antigenic variants of IgG4 proteins revealed with monoclonal antibodies. Immunology *57:* 25–28 (1986).

Vivi-Anne Oxelius, MD, PhD, Department of Pediatrics,
University Hospital, S-221 85 Lund (Sweden)

IgG Subclass Assays with Polyclonal Antisera and Monoclonal Antibodies[1]

Antonio Ferrante, Lorraine J. Beard[2]

University Department of Paediatrics and Department of Immunology, The Adelaide Children's Hospital, Adelaide, South Australia

Introduction

Despite unanimous recognition of the importance of identifying IgG subclass levels in patients with recurrent infections, persistent infections and certain disorders, the method of assay and the use of either polyclonal antisera or monoclonal antibodies (McAb) in the assays has remained highly controversial. The existing uncertainties are further complicated by the possible need for measuring IgG subclass 'specific' antibodies in patients suspected of having IgG subclass deficiency.

The Assays – Polyclonal Antisera – Monoclonal Antibodies

It is unequivocally agreed that appropriate polyclonal antisera for measuring human IgG subclasses is available in only a few specialized laboratories. Production of such antisera is extremely complex, requiring highly involved and meticulous preparation procedures. Extensive adsorption protocols are required which guarantee not only specificity but maintenance of high titres and an absence of immune complexes. Antisera can be raised in rabbits and monkeys using myeloma proteins of IgG subclasses [1, 2]. A convenient approach in

---

[1] This work was supported by a grant from the Children's Medical Research Foundation of South Australia.

[2] We are particularly grateful to Julie Hagedorn and Brenton Rowan-Kelly for technical help.

raising the antisera is to make the animals tolerant to three of the IgG subclasses prior to immunization with myeloma proteins of the fourth.

Recently the hybridoma technology has enabled the preparation of reagents (McAb) which can be made more readily and widely available, and which can be suitably standardized and prepared in high titres [3]. Evaluation of McAb which have specificity for human IgG subclasses has been undertaken by an IUIS/WHO collaborative study group [4]. More recently, 16 McAb have been identified for IgG subclass measurements (information shortly to be made available by IUIS/WHO study group).

It is clear that both polyclonal antisera and McAb are suitable for the same types of assays, although the assay conditions for either type of reagent may differ. The assays include radial immunodiffusion (RID), radioimmunoassay (RIA) and enzyme-linked immunosorbent assay (ELISA) methods. Indeed commercial kits for measuring IgG subclasses using either polyclonal antisera or McAb have recently become available. While the original methods used electroimmune assays for measuring IgG subclass concentrations, RID has been the recent method of choice. In the RID both polyclonal antisera and McAb have been used [2-5]. Our own experience with polyclonal antisera and RID methods has shown this assay to have some limitations. The first approach was to prepare RID plates using the Netherland Red Cross Transfusion Service reagents. Using these plates the measurement of IgG2 and IgG4 was obtained only with difficulty. The former presented precipitin rings which were hazy and partly indistinguishable, and the latter with rings which bordered the edge of the wells. A similar observation was made when commercial RID plates from two sources were used. Also at present conditions have been defined for using McAb in RID assays [3-5].

Most recently a number of ELISA or competitive ELISA for measuring IgG subclasses have been described [6-9]. Some difficulties have been encountered in ELISA methods in which microtitre plate surfaces were coated directly with subclass-specific McAb. Thus, other means have been used to immobilize McAb. For example, plates can be coated with anti-mouse IgG (Fc-specific) antibodies which are used to capture subclass-specific McAb (fig. 1a) [7]. Following the addition of serum samples or standards, the bound immunoglobulin subclass is detected with horseradish peroxidase (HRP)-anti-human Ig conjugate. The assay offers good sensitivity down to 1 ng/ml and the standard

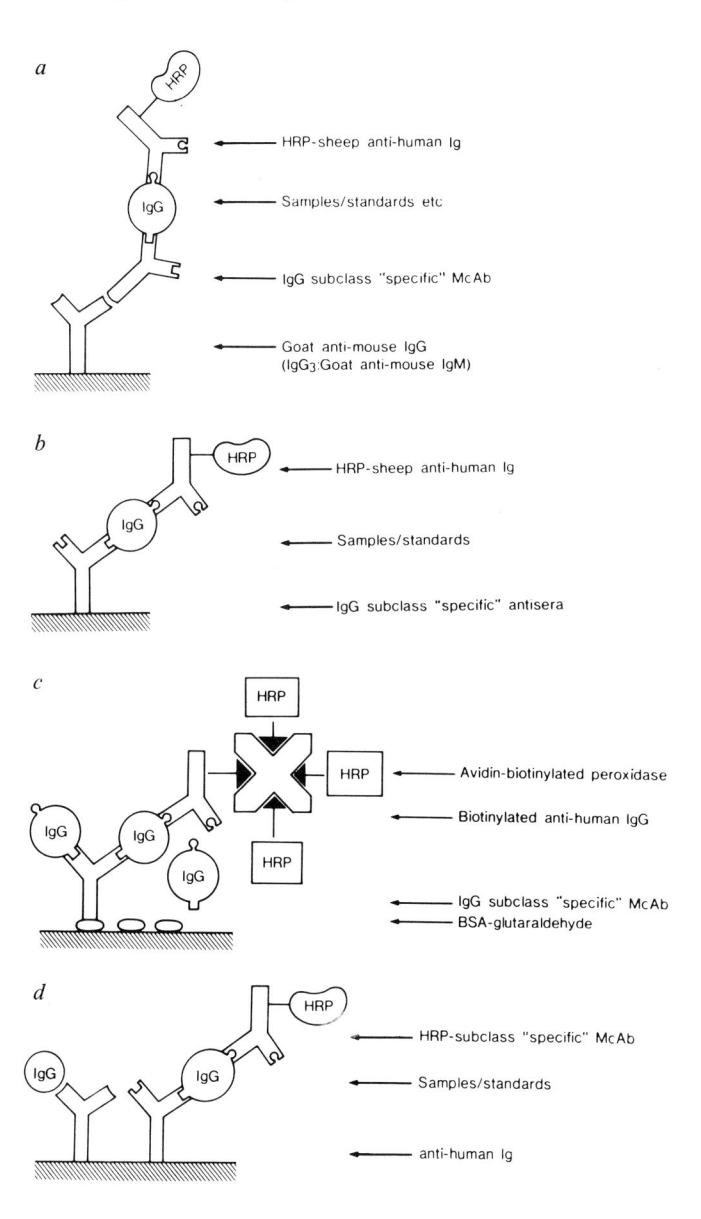

Fig. 1. ELISA methods for measuring IgG subclasses (see text for description).

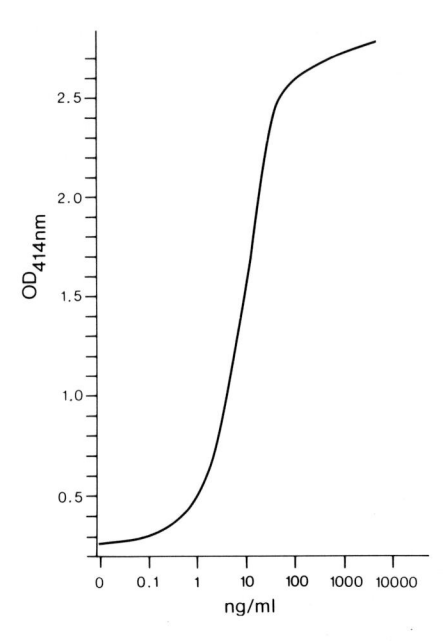

Fig. 2. A typical standard curve obtained with an ELISA assay for measuring IgG subclasses using subclass-specific McAb (in this case using an antibody directed against human IgG4; SK44).

curve is linear over a two-log immunoglobulin concentration (fig. 2) [7]. In this assay variability may be encountered between plates from different manufacturers and from batch to batch. This can be overcome by appropriate blocking of sites on plastic surfaces with serum. Greater uniformity of results is obtained if the outer-most wells of microtitre plates are excluded. Inaccuracy in dilutions can add to variability and this may be overcome by diluting samples in triplicates or using automated diluting systems.

Polyclonal subclass specific antisera can also be used in ELISA assays [Ferrante, unpublished]. In this case the subclass-specific antisera can be used as the coating reagent, as illustrated in figure 1b. In addition to these systems, an ELISA method using gluteraldehyde-treated bovine serum albumin (BSA) as the coating agent for capturing the IgG subclass specific McAb has proven useful (fig. 1c) [6]. An

ELISA kit for measuring IgG subclasses is also available commercially. This system involves coating plates with an anti-human immunoglobulin which then permits the binding of all IgG subclasses (fig. 1d). The bound IgG is then identified and quantitated by using HRP subclass specific McAb conjugates. When this kit was examined in our laboratory, we found great variability between kits and the IgG2 standard curves were poor by our criteria. To some degree the problems were overcome by modifying the serum blocking step.

Competitive ELISA methods using McAb have been described [8, 9]. These may involve coating plates with the purified monoclonal IgG subclass and subsequent addition of a mixture of samples (or standards) plus the IgG subclass specific McAb (incubated together prior to addition) [8]. The ability of serum samples to inhibit binding of the McAb to the IgG on the plastic surface can be used to compute IgG subclass concentrations. Alternatively, a competitive ELISA has been described in which the subclass-specific McAb are bound to the microtitre plates followed by the addition of serum samples [9]. The concentration of subclasses is related to the degree of inhibition of binding of alkaline phosphatase-human (myeloma) IgG subclass conjugates.

Other sensitive IgG subclass measuring assays have been established, such as RIA [10, 11] or particle concentration fluorescence immunoassays [12].

The Dilemma in IgG Subclasses Measurements and Defining Subclass Deficiencies

A list of relevant questions that need to be addressed are presented in table I. Many laboratories including those in which IgG subclass measurements have been recently attempted, or in which such measurements are being considered, face the dilemma of choice of assay method. In general, two alternatives are probably being considered: RID and ELISA. Since IgG1 is present in relatively high concentrations, perhaps the RID can be utilized for this isotype, and ELISA for IgG2, IgG3 and IgG4. However, this will make comparisons (such as expression as relative percentages) of IgG1 and the other three isotypes difficult. Alternatively, the RID could be used as a first screen, and final quantitation made with ELISA. Unfortunately, this can be an expensive exercise because of the duplication. Nevertheless, it could

Table I. The dilemma in laboratory diagnosis of IgG subclass deficiency

1	Which IgG subclass method is to be used? RID? ELISA, RIA, etc.
2	The choice – monoclonal antibodies or polyclonal antisera?
3	What is the approach to paediatric serum samples?
4	Do patients' IgG subclass levels need to be compared to a normal range established with the same technique, in the same laboratory, in the same race, and with the same reagents?
5	Does one measure total IgG subclass immunoglobulin or IgG subclass 'specific' antibodies?
6	Antibodies to which antigens should be measured?
7	Definition of IgG subclass deficiency?

be considered as an approach involving the less specialized laboratory running RID and subsequent referral of the more 'interesting' samples for further analysis to the more specialized laboratory for ELISA quantitation.

It is inevitable that the assay systems will employ McAb in all laboratories. However, some laboratories are meeting such changes with grave reservations and often criticize subclass McAb as being 'too specific'. Thus, it is important that good standardization of IgG subclass-specific McAb is undertaken. At this stage in the ELISA the following McAb can be used: IgG1, HP6012; IgG2, HP6009, HP6014; IgG3, HP6010, SJ33; IgG4, HP6011, SK44.

The problem of assay method selection may be further compounded in those laboratories which have a paediatric service. In infants the immunoglobulin concentrations may be low and can require a more sensitive assay. Thus we can see certain advantages in using the ELISA methods.

The additional advantage of the ELISA is the ability to measure the low concentrations of IgG subclasses which may be encountered in secretions such as saliva (table II), and those produced by lymphocytes in culture [7].

A comparison using RID (with polyclonal antisera) and ELISA (with McAb) showed that while the relative percentages were close, the absolute values were different (table III). This leads one to conclude that comparisons of patients' serum samples need to be made with a

Table II. IgG subclass levels in adult saliva samples as measured by ELISA

Individual		IgG1	IgG2	IgG3	IgG4
1	mg/l	20.22	14.70	3.59	6.39
	R%	(44.8)	(32.5)	(8.0)	(14.1)
2	mg/l	1.93	0.99	0.13	0.15
	R%	(60.3)	(31.0)	(3.9)	(4.8)
3	mg/l	1.85	2.39	0.21	0.80
	R%	(35.2)	(45.6)	(4.0)	(15.2)
4	mg/l	3.70	3.01	0.20	1.91
	R%	(42.0)	(34.1)	(2.3)	(21.7)
5	mg/l	3.79	4.28	0.24	0.40
	R%	(43.5)	(49.1)	(2.8)	(4.6)
Means ± SD		6.30 ± 7.0	5.07 ± 4.93	0.87 ± 1.36	1.93 ± 2.3
		(45.2 ± 8.3)	(38.5 ± 4.93)	(4.2 ± 2.0)	(12.1 ± 6.6)

R% = Relative percentage.
IgG1, IgG2, IgG3 and IgG4 were identified with McAb study code HP6012, HP6014, SJ33 and SK44, respectively.

Table III. A comparison of IgG subclass measurements using RID with polyclonal antisera and ELISA

Subclass	RID polyclonal antisera	ELISA monoclonal antibodies
IgG1	6.12 ± 1.57 61.29%	7.41 ± 2.41 64.64%
IgG2	2.78 ± 1.75 26.34%	2.55 ± 0.94 22.32%
IgG3	0.62 ± 0.29 6.30%	0.77 ± 0.35 6.70%
IgG4	0.61 ± 0.40 6.07%	0.75 ± 0.49 6.35%

Results are mean ± SD in g/l of 39 healthy adults.
RID was conducted with commercially available plates (Serotec, Oxon, England).
Monoclonal antibodies used: HP6012 (IgG1), HP6014 (IgG2), SJ33 (IgG3) and SK44 (IgG4).

Table IV. Serum IgG subclass levels in normal adults

Reference	Method	Antibodies	Number of sera	IgG1	IgG2	IgG3	IgG4
Yount et al. [13]	RID	polyclonal		9.4 ± 1.9	3.2 ± 1.3	1.0 ± 0.45	0.62 ± 0.48
Morell et al. [14]	RIA	polyclonal	108	6.63 ± 1.70 (3.5 – 11.5)	3.22 ± 1.08 (1.3 – 6.8)	0.58 ± 0.30 (0.10 – 2.11)	0.46 (0.03 – 2.90)
Shakib et al. [15]	RID	polyclonal	111	8.01 (3.7 – 12.3)	2.17 (0.46 – 4.3)	0.94 (0.15 – 2.45)	0.08 (0.015 – 0.185)
Oxelius [16]	EIA	polyclonal	20	7.55 ± 2.45 (4.22 – 12.92)	3.80 ± 1.5 (1.7 – 7.47)	0.73 ± 0.26 (0.41 – 1.29)	0.55 ± 0.63 (<0.01 – 2.91)
Kaschka et al. [17]	RID	polyclonal	23	6.13 ± 2.89 (2.43 – 13.29)	3.00 ± 1.49 (1.21 – 5.71)	0.74 ± 0.71 (0.16 – 2.67)	0.44 ± 0.39 (0.03 – 1.38)
French and Harrison [5]	RID	McAb	172	5.91 ± 2.64 (2.86 – 13.46)	3.04 ± 2.52 (1.00 – 7.25)	0.61 ± 0.56 (0.09 – 3.16)	0.24 ± 0.90 (<0.03 – 5.39)
Aucouturier et al. [8]	ELISA	McAb	122–129	6.35 ± 1.50 (3.0 – 10.5)	2.61 ± 1.36 (0.4 – 6.3)	0.414 ± 0.17 (0.12 – 1.14)	0.385 ± 0.392 (<0.01 – 2.10)
Ferrante et al. [7]	ELISA	McAb	41	7.41 ± 2.41 (3.82 – 14.27)	2.55 ± 0.94 (1.24 – 4.96)	0.77 ± 0.35 (0.30 – 1.57)	0.75 ± 0.49 (0.18 – 2.01)
Shackelford et al. [11]	RIA	McAb (IgG1) polyclonal (IgG2)	41	6.56 (3.44 – 12.07)	2.55 (0.88 – 7.40)	ND	ND
Mayus et l. [12]	PCFIA (IgG1, IgG2, IgG3) RIA (IgG4)	McAb	186 32	6.03 (2.87 – 12.65)	2.49 (0.92 – 6.72)	0.52 (0.17 – 1.62)	0.34 (0.028 – 4.06)

Means ± SD and ranges or range presented as 2 SDS.
PCFIA = Particle concentrate fluorescence immunoassay; EIA = electroimmune assay.

normal range established with the same technique. Furthermore, consideration needs to be given to findings that IgG subclass measurements may depend on race [11], laboratory handling and reagents. Therefore, some form of standardization is required if comparisons from different laboratories are to be made.

Table IV presents adult normal ranges obtained by various laboratories using a range of assay methods and either polyclonal antisera or McAb. The mean IgG1, IgG2, IgG3 and IgG4 in these studies varied from 5.91–9.4, 2.17–3.80, 0.41–1.0 and 0.08–0.75 g/l. It also illustrates that RID is not going to be useful for measuring IgG4 levels.

Even more complications will arise in attempts to establish a paediatric normal range and measurement of paediatric serum samples. A comparison of the paediatric range obtained by two different methods is presented (fig. 3). One represents the normal range published by Oxelius [16] using an electroimmunoassay with polyclonal antisera. The other represents a normal range obtained in our laboratory using the ELISA with McAb. The graph demonstrates that the IgG1 results are very similar between the two laboratories. However, the IgG2 and IgG3 were higher and IgG4 lower in Oxelius' range. This clearly illustrates the need to standardize methodologies from laboratory to laboratory.

IgG Subclass 'Specific' Antibodies

The isotype characteristic of IgG subclass antibodies to different antigens may vary [18]. Generally, antibodies to protein antigens are of the IgG1 and IgG3 isotype while those to polysaccharide antigens are mainly IgG2. An urgent consideration needs to be made regarding whether, for the identification of an immunodeficiency, it is necessary to measure both total serum IgG subclass levels and IgG subclass antibodies. The results of Granoff et al. [19] would suggest that individuals may show normal IgG subclasses but fail to produce an antibody response to *Haemophilus influenzae* type B polysaccharide vaccine. It is therefore important to measure antibody responses and possibly the isotype distribution of the antibodies. If IgG subclass antibodies are to be measured, which approach should be taken? It is likely that antibodies to a range of antigens should be measured. Some of these antigens may be part of an immunization programme and others may be anti-

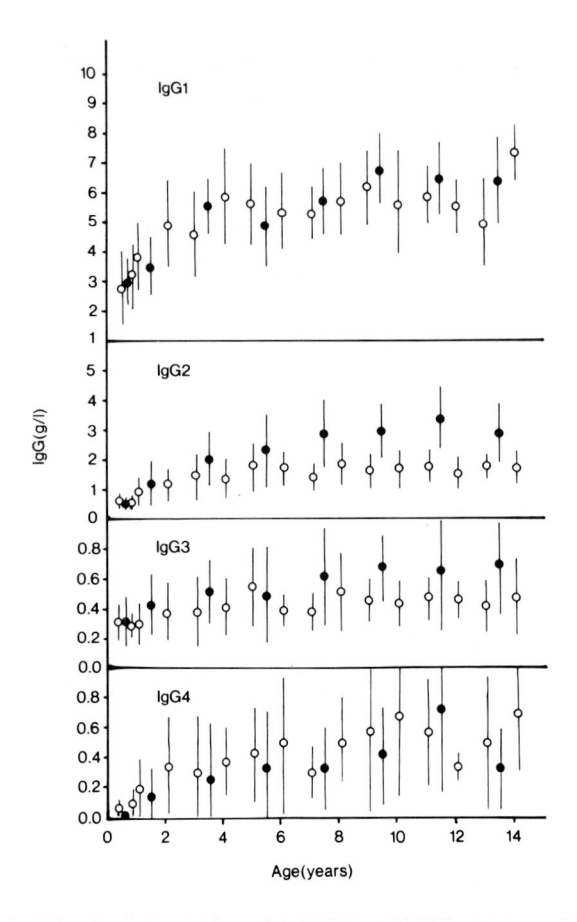

Fig. 3. A comparison of paediatric normal range obtained in Swedish (●) and South Australian (○) children. Samples in the Swedish population were assayed with polyclonal antisera in EIA while those from South Australia were assayed with McAb (as listed in table I) using ELISA. The results are expressed as mean ± SD.

gens to which we become continuously exposed, of microbial or food origin. Ideally, it would be appropriate to consider making a standard antigen mixture which may be used to measure antibodies to a variety of antigens. The ELISA has been used for measuring IgG subclass antibodies to a range of antigens and appears to be a useful method [20, 21]. IgG subclass-specific McAb were used to identify the isotype and this appears to be the future approach to such determinations. One of the problems is going to be associated with defining the normal range.

Concluding Remark

It is likely that the ELISA technique is going to be the method of choice in a number of laboratories for the measurement of IgG subclasses and subclass antibodies. The use of McAb instead of polyclonal antisera is seen as an advantage. It is therefore suggested that this is the most logical avenue for future directions to achieve standardization in measurement of IgG subclasses and identification of subclass deficiencies.

References

1. Oxelius, V.-A.: Crossed immunoelectrophoresis and electroimmunoassay of human IgG subclasses. Acta pathol. microbiol. scand., C, Immunol. *86:* 109–113 (1978).
2. Schur, P.H.; Rosen, F.; Norman, M.E.: Immunoglobulin subclasses in normal children. Pediat. Res. *13:* 181–183 (1979).
3. Lowe, J.; Bird, P.; Hardie, D.; Jefferis, R.; Ling, N.R.: Monoclonal antibodies (McAbs) to determinants on human gamma chains.: properties of antibodies showing subclass restriction or subclass specificity. Immunology *47:* 329–336 (1982).
4. Jefferis, R.; Reimer, C.B.; Skvaril, F.; et al.: Evaluation of monoclonal antibodies having specificity for human IgG sub-classes: results of an IUIS/WHO collaborative study. Immunol. Lett. *10:* 223–252 (1985).
5. French, M.A.H.; Harrison, G.: Serum IgG subclass concentrations in healthy adults: a study using monoclonal antisera. Clin. exp. Immunol. *56:* 473–475 (1984).
6. Papadea, C.; Check, I.J.; Reimer, C.B.: Monoclonal antibody-based solid-phase immunoenzymometric assays for quantifiying human immunoglobulin G and its subclass in serum. Clin. Chem. *31:* 1940–1945 (1985).
7. Ferrante, A.; Rowan-Kelly, B.; Beard, L.J.; Maxwell, G.M.: An enzyme-linked immunosorbent assay for the quantitation of human IgG subclasses using monoclonal antibodies. J. immunol. Methods *93:* 207–212 (1986).
8. Aucouturier, P.; Mounir, S.; Preud'homme, J.-L.: Distribution of IgG subclass levels in normal adult sera as determined by a competitive enzyme immunoassay using monoclonal antibodies. Diagnostic Immunol. *3:* 191–196 (1985).
9. Skvaril, F.: Immunoglobulin G subclasses. Methods of enzymatic analysis, vol. 10, 60–71 (VCH Verlagsgesellschaft, Weinheim 1986).
10. Heiner, D.C.: Significance of immunoglobulin G subclasses. Am. J. Med. *76:* 1–6 (1984).
11. Shackelford, P.G.; Granoff, D.M.; Nahm, M.H.; Scott, M.G.; Suarez, B.; Pandey, J.P.; Nelson, S.J.: Relation of age, race and allotype to immunoglobulin subclass concentrations. Pediat. Res. *19:* 846–849 (1986).
12. Mayus, J.; Macke, K.; Shackelford, P.; Kim, J.; Nahm, M.: Human IgG subclass assays using a novel assay method. J. immunol. Methods *88:* 65–73 (1986).

13 Yount, W.J.; Hong, R.; Seligmann, M.; Good, R.; Kunkel, H.G.: Imbalances of gamma globulin subgroups and gene defects in patients with primary hypogammaglobulinemia. J. clin. Invest. *49:* 1957–1966 (1970).

14 Morell, A.; Skvaril, F.; Steinberg, A.G.; Van Loghem, E.; Terry, W.D.: Correlation between the concentration of the four subclasses of IgG and Gm allotypes in normal human sera. J. Immun. *108:* 195–201 (1972).

15 Shakib, F.; Stanworth, D.R.; Drew, R.; Catty, D.: A quantitative study of the distribution of IgG subclasses in a group of normal human sera. J. immunol. Methods *8:* 17–28 (1975).

16 Oxelius, V.-A.: IgG subclass levels in infancy and childhood. Acta paediat. scand. *68:* 23–27 (1979).

17 Kaschka, W.P.; Hilgers, R.; Skvaril, F.: Humoral immune response in Epstein-Barr virus infections. I. Elevated serum concentration of the IgG1 subclass in infectious mononucleosis and nasopharyngeal carcinoma. Clin. exp. Immunol. *49:* 149–156 (1982).

18 Skvaril, F.: Clinical relevance of IgG subclasses; in Morrell, Nydegger, Clinical Use of intravenous immunoglobulins, pp. 37–45 (Academic Press, London 1986).

19 Granoff, D.M.; Shackelford, P.G.; Suarez, B.K., et al.: Hemophilus influenza type B disease in children vaccinated with type B polysaccharide vaccine. New Engl. J. Med. *315:* 1584–1990 (1986).

20 Persson, M.A.A.; Hammarström, L.; Smith, C.I.E.: Enzyme-linked immunosorbent assay for subclass distribution of human IgG and IgA antigen-specific antibodies. J. immunol. Methods *78:* 109–121 (1985).

21 Husby, S.; Jensenius, J.C.; Svehag, S.-E.: ELISA quantitation of IgG subclass antibodies to dietary antigens. J. immunol. Methods *82:* 321–331 (1985).

Dr. A. Ferrante, University Department of Paediatrics and Department of Immunology, The Adelaide Children's Hospital, Adelaide 5006 (South Australia)

The Biological Significance of Specific Antibody IgG Subclass Profiles

R. Jefferis, M.R. Walker

University of Birmingham Medical School, Birmingham, England

The structural diversity of potentially pathogenic organisms is reflected in the recognition diversity of antibody molecules and the evolution of multiple isotypes that, in concert, provide humoral immune protection throughout the intact vertebrate. Recognition and binding of antibody to an organism at external surfaces may provide protection by preventing colonisation, penetration and infection, e.g. secretory IgA. However, when non-specific and specific immune barriers are penetrated, recognition and binding of antibody is only the first essential interaction necessary for the killing and elimination of the infectious agent. The antigen/antibody complexes formed may potentiate effector functions dependent on the activation of the C1 and/or C3 components of complement or killing and clearance mechanisms mediated through Fc receptors expressed on a wide range of cell types (table I).

The predominant immunoglobulins in the blood and interstitial fluids of higher vertebrates is IgG and in man each of the four subclasses has been demonstrated to express a unique profile of effector functions [Burton et al., 1986]. However, our current understanding of the functional activity of the IgG subclasses in vivo is an extrapolation from studies using myeloma proteins of unknown antigen specificity, and often doubtful purity, that have been aggregated by physical and chemical means in attempts to simulate immune complexes [Spiegelberg, 1974]. We are entering a new era when human (and mouse) monoclonal antibodies will become increasingly available for in vivo applications. Also, the techniques of molecular biology and peptide chemistry have the potential to provide a wide range of new vaccines. It is essential therefore to gain a complete understanding of the opti-

Table I. Effector/interaction sites on human IgG subclasses

Fc receptors		Subclass specificity			
Monocytes/macrophages (FcRI, high affinity)		IgG1,	IgG3>	IgG4	
Monocytes					
Neutrophils					
Eosinophils	(FcRII, low affinity)	IgG1,	IgG3>	IgG2,	IgG4
Platelets					
B cells					
Neutrophils					
Eosinophils					
Macrophages	(FcR$_{10}$ low affinity)	IgG1,	IgG3		
NK, K					
T cells		IgG1:	IgG2:	IgG3:	IgG4
Syncytiotrophoblast	(intermediate affinity)	IgG1,	IgG2,	IgG3,	IgG4
Kupffer cells		IgG1,	IgG2,	IgG3,	IgG4
Complement C1		IgG3>	IgG1	≫IgG2	
Rheumatoid factor		IgG1,	IgG2,	IgG4	
Staphylococcal protein A		IgG1,	IgG2,	IgG4,	IgG3 allo-type

mal pathway(s) for resolution of each infectious agent to allow selection of the right antibody or immunisation protocol.

The IgG molecule is multifunctional with the Fab region determining antigen-binding specificity and the Fc region determining effector functions. Whilst subclass-specific residues are present in the CH1 domain, Fab fragments derived from each of the IgG subclasses may be equivalent in their biological activity. Their value as therapeutic reagents may be limited to the neutralisation of toxins since they equilibrate rapidly between blood and other body fluids, but do not activate secondary effector functions. Fab fragments may also be optimal reagents for in vivo imaging since they do not interact with Fc receptors and therefore localise to target cells more specifically. It is possible that (Fab')2 fragments that can form large complexes may activate the complement cascade through the alternative pathway.

Uncomplexed monomer IgG is not inert in vivo since catabolism is a specific Fc-mediated mechanism. The half-life for IgG1, 2 and 4 is 21–23 days, whilst for IgG3 it is only 7 days. This consideration will obviously have an important bearing on the duration of prophylactic or therapeutic activity and the required interval between antibody administration. Monomer IgG is also the active species in the transmission of immunity from mother to foetus and is mediated through Fc receptors on cells of the syncytiotrophoblast. IgG subclass levels in the cord blood of normal term infants is equal to or greater than that in maternal blood and the receptor involved is presumed to recognise an Fc structure common to each subclass. In contrast, the high-affinity receptor expressed on monocytes and macrophages binds IgG1 and IgG3 subclasses preferentially with a K_{ass} of $5 \times 10^8 M^{-1}$ [Burton, 1985]. It has been calculated that at physiological concentrations of IgG all high-affinity receptors will be occupied. Since aggregated IgG does not bind with increased avidity, it is not apparent that immune complexes will displace monomer IgG to activate these cell types via FcRI. Whilst IgG4 binds with a K_{ass} one order of magnitude lower than IgG1 or IgG3, it should allow activation of monocytes and macrophages through FcRI. In contrast, monomer IgG2 has been shown to have negligible binding affinity for FcRI. Assuming no increase in binding by complexed multivalent IgG2, it would appear not to activate FcRI-mediated effector functions.

It can be appreciated that it would be entirely inappropriate and indeed harmful for protective mechanisms to be continously activated by uncomplexed monomer IgG. Thus, these mechanisms are dependent on low-affinity interactions that result in high-avidity binding of multivalent antigen/antibody complexes. The biological consequences of immune complex formation may depend on the size, IgG subclass composition and steric orientation of IgG molecules; parameters that will influence multi-site attachment.

Probably the most defined system available for study of the in vivo activity of IgG antibody is the anti-rhesus-D system. Anti-D therapy is successfully applied worldwide, however, despite extensive study the effector mechanism(s) essential for red cell clearance is not unequivocally determined. In both naturally immunised mothers and volunteer donors, the anti-D response is confined to IgG1 and IgG3 with the relative proportion differing from individual to individual. Anti-D sensitised human R^0R^0 red cells do not activate or fix complement and there is not evidence for the participation of this effector mechanism in immune clearance. Mechanisms remaining for consideration are (1) antibody-dependent cellular cytotoxicity (ADCC) mediated by κ cells; (2) extracellular killing by monocytes or polymorphonuclear cells activated through Fc receptors, and (3) intracellular killing following Fc-receptor-mediated phagocytosis.

Several studies have suggested that the most reliable indicator for possible haemolytic disease of the newborn is the efficacy of maternal anti-D antibody in sensitising R^0R^0 red cells for ADCC. Maternal or donor sera having the same anti-D titre may vary widely in this activity, however, ADCC activity has been observed to correlate with predominance of anti-D antibody of the IgG3 subclass [Urbaniak and Greiss, 1980].

Several laboratories have established cell lines or (hetero)hybridomas producing human monoclonal anti-D antibody and there is considerable interest in commercialising an effective reagent. We have had access to monoclonal anti-D antibody produced by Epstein-Barr virus transformation of peripheral blood lymphocytes [Doyle et al., 1985] or mouse/human heterohybridomas [Thompson et al., 1986]. Using a panel of mouse monoclonal anti-human IgG antibodies [Nik Jaafar et al., 1983], we were able to demonstrate that each antibody studied expressed the appropriate class, subclass and allotypic determinants and therefore apparently represented native molecules. However, it was reported to us [Thompson and Kumpel, personal communication] that early studies showed that these antibodies did not sensitise red cells for either ADCC or phagocytosis.

We have further investigated several of these anti-D antibodies for interaction with Fc receptors on the monocytic cell line U937 shown to express both FcRI and FcRII [Anderson and Looney, 1986]. Human R^0R^0 were sensitised with monoclonal anti-D antibody by incubation with cell culture supernate. The sensitised red cells were further incubated with U937 cells at a ratio of 100:1 and the percentage of U937 cells forming rosettes counted. Rosette formation was observed for IgG3 sensitised cells but not for IgG1 sensitised cells. An inhibition system was established in which sensitised red cells were incubated with U937 cells in the presence of unbound anti-D antibody. Under these conditions, both IgG1 and IgG3 antibodies inhibited rosette formation between U937 cells and IgG3-sensitised R^0R^0 cells.

Our interpretation of these data is that in this system we are investigating interactions between IgG and the FcRI receptor since monomer IgG is able to inhibit rosette formation. FcRII and FcR_{lo} are low-affinity receptors that do not bind monomer IgG. We have previously predicted that the FcRI interaction site is located at the N-proximal end of the Cγ2 domain and that accessibility may be critically dependent on the relative orientation of the Fab arm to the Fc region and the length of the hinge region. It is likely therefore that interaction between R^{0}R^0 cells sensitised with IgG1 anti-D and FcRI on U937 cells would require too close an approach resulting in charge repulsion, similar to the effect that prevents IgG1 anti-D antibody from agglutinating red cells. However, IgG3 has an extended hinge region, of the order 50–70 Å, which allows access to the FcRI binding site without requiring such a close approach of the two cell surfaces. It appears that FcRII is not involved in these interactions because the level of sensitisation of the R^{0}R^0 cells is too low, due to the low density of the D antigen, to yield a high-avidity interaction.

This study represents the beginning of an attempt to rationalise functional activity with defined structural features. However, recent experiences suggest that even with monoclonal human antibodies the functional heterogeneity appears to exceed the known structural variants.

References

Anderson, C.L.; Looney, R.J.: Human leucocyte IgG Fc Receptors. Immunol. Today 7: 264–266 (1986).

Burton, D.R.; Gregory, L.; Jefferis, R.: Aspects of the molecular structure of IgG subclasses. Monogr. Allergy, vol. 19, pp. 7–35 (Karger, Basel 1986).

Doyle, A.; Jones, T.J.; Bidwell, J.L.; Bradley, B.A.: In vitro development of human monoclonal antibody secreting plasmacytomas. Hum. Immunol. 13: 199–209 (1985).

Nik Jaafar, M.I.; Lowe, J.A.; Ling, N.R.; Jefferis, R.: Immunogenic and antigenic epitopes of immunoglobulins. V. Reactivity of a panel of monoclonal antibodies with sub-fragments of human Fc and abnormal proteins having deletions. Molec. Immunol. 20: 679–686 (1983).

Spiegelberg, H.L.: Biological activity of immunoglobulins of different classes and subclasses. Adv. Immunol. 19: 259–294 (1974).

Thompson, K.M.; Hough, D.W.; Maddison, P.J.; Melamed, M.D.; Hughes-Jones, N.: The efficient production of stable, human monoclonal antibody-secretion hybridomas from EBV-transformed lymphocytes using the mouse myeloma X63-Ag8.653 as a fusion partner. J. immunol. Methods 94: 7–12 (1986).

Urbaniak, S.J.; Greiss, M.A.: ADCC (k cell) lysis of human erythrocytes sensitised with Rhesus autoantibodies. III. Comparison of IgG anti-D agglutinating and lytic (ADCC) activity and the role of IgC subclasses. Br. J. Haemat. 46: 447–453 (1980).

Dr. R. Jefferis, Department of Immunology, The Medical School,
Vincent Drive, Birmingham, B15 2TJ (England)

IgG Subclass Representation within Homogeneous Immunoglobulins in Immunodeficiency Diseases

J. Radl[a], C.M. Jol-van der Zijde[b], M.J.D. van Tol[b], J.M. Vossen[b]

[a] TNO Institute for Experimental Gerontology, Rijswijk;
[b] Department of Pediatrics, University of Leiden, Leiden, The Netherlands

It has been shown in both clinical and experimental studies [1, 2] that in immunodeficiencies (ID), characterized by impaired T cell functions and preserved B cell functions, transient monoclonal gammopathies (MG) frequently occur. These conditions are listed in the 3rd category according to our recent classification of MG [3] (table I). The homogeneous immunoglobulins (H-Ig) in this group are often multiple and belong to the IgM and IgG classes. For their detection, the use of a reliable, highly sensitive technique is necessary, because the monoclonal immunoglobulin components in the patients' sera are often present at a very low concentration. To demonstrate this point, four examples from our study on IgG subclass representation within H-Ig in some ID diseases are shown.

The techniques used for the detection of H-Ig were: (1) agar electrophoresis (agar EP) according to Wieme [4], with the lower detection sensitivity limit for H-Ig on a heterogeneous background at about 100 µg/ml, and (2) immunoblotting, Western blotting, on the Wieme agar EP (IMBL) [5], with the detection sensitivity for H-Ig in the same material of <1 µg/ml. In the latter technique, the following reagents were used: Mouse monoclonal antibodies anti-human (MAHu) IgG common determinants (IgG-c), 164–7.1 Rijswijk [6], asc. dil. 1/50,000; MAHu IgG1, BAM 15, HP 6012, Unipath, GB, dil. 1/5,000; MAHu IgG2, HP 6014 [7], dil. 1/2,000; MAHu IgG3, 86–2.4, HP 6080, Rijswijk [6], dil. 1/10,000; MAHu IgG4, 315–1.1.1, Rijswijk [6], dil. 1/25,000; MAHu IgM, 89–1.1.11, Rijswijk [6], dil. 1/10,000. As a secondary reagent, the rabbit anti-mouse Ig serum, labelled with alkaline phosphatase (DAKO) was used in the dilution 1/2,000.

Table I. Monoclonal gammopathies

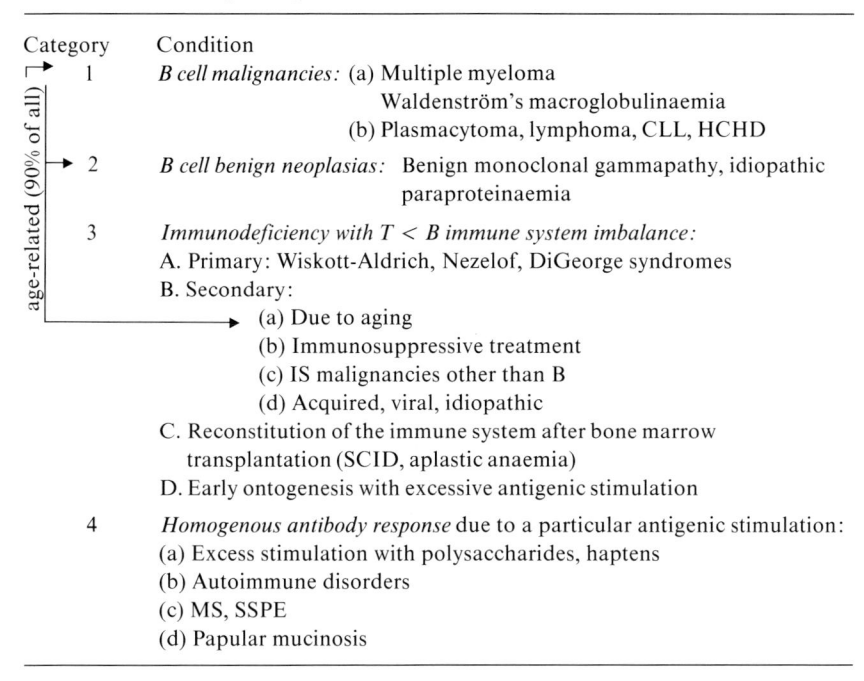

Category	Condition
1	*B cell malignancies:* (a) Multiple myeloma, Waldenström's macroglobulinaemia (b) Plasmacytoma, lymphoma, CLL, HCHD
2	*B cell benign neoplasias:* Benign monoclonal gammapathy, idiopathic paraproteinaemia

3	*Immunodeficiency with T < B immune system imbalance:*
	A. Primary: Wiskott-Aldrich, Nezelof, DiGeorge syndromes
	B. Secondary:
	  (a) Due to aging
	  (b) Immunosuppressive treatment
	  (c) IS malignancies other than B
	  (d) Acquired, viral, idiopathic
	C. Reconstitution of the immune system after bone marrow transplantation (SCID, aplastic anaemia)
	D. Early ontogenesis with excessive antigenic stimulation

4	*Homogenous antibody response* due to a particular antigenic stimulation: (a) Excess stimulation with polysaccharides, haptens (b) Autoimmune disorders (c) MS, SSPE (d) Papular mucinosis

Categories 1 and 3 are age-related (90% of all).

CLL = chronic lymphocytic leukaemia; HCHD = heavy chain disease; IS = immune system; SCID = severe combined immunodeficiency; MS = multiple sclerosis; SSPE = subacute sclerosing panencephalitis.

Figure 1 shows an analysis of the serum from patient H.M. (Nezelof syndrome) at 8 months of age. On agar EP, 3–4 clear-cut H-Ig bands are seen; by IMBL the H-Ig were detected as: 2 × IgG1, 1 × IgG3 and 3 × IgM.

In the second analysis (fig. 2), serum from the patient P.B. with Wiskott-Aldrich syndrome was tested when the boy was 9 years of age. While the agar EP showed a clear-cut H-Ig band in the γ-region and 3 very weak bands with a more anodic mobility, the IMBL technique demonstrated ten H-Ig components: 3 × IgG1, 3 × IgG2, 1 × IgG3, 1 × IgG4, and 2 × IgM.

An even more illustrative example offers an analysis of the serum from patient R.G. (7 years of age), 6 months after bone marrow transplantation performed for acute lymphocytic leukaemia (ALL) (fig. 3).

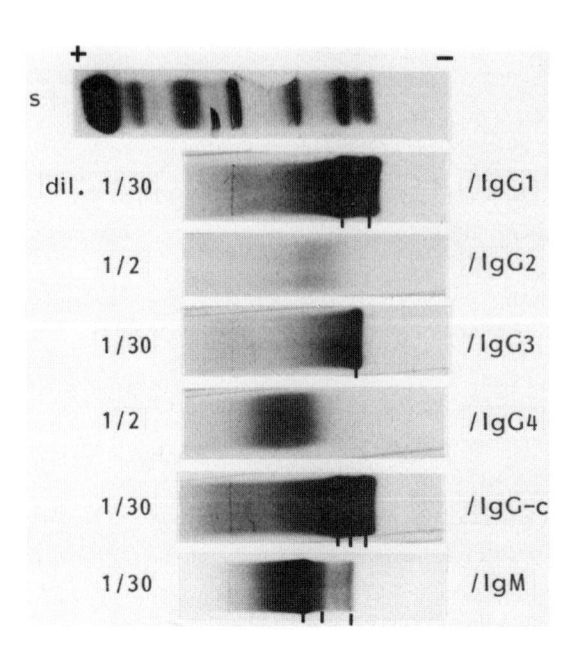

Fig. 1. Agar EP and IMBL of serum (s) from a patient (H.M.) with Nezelof syndrome. The dilutions in which the serum was tested are indicated on the left side. The individual reagents applied in the IMBL are shown on the right side. Homogeneous Ig components are indicated by the black marks.

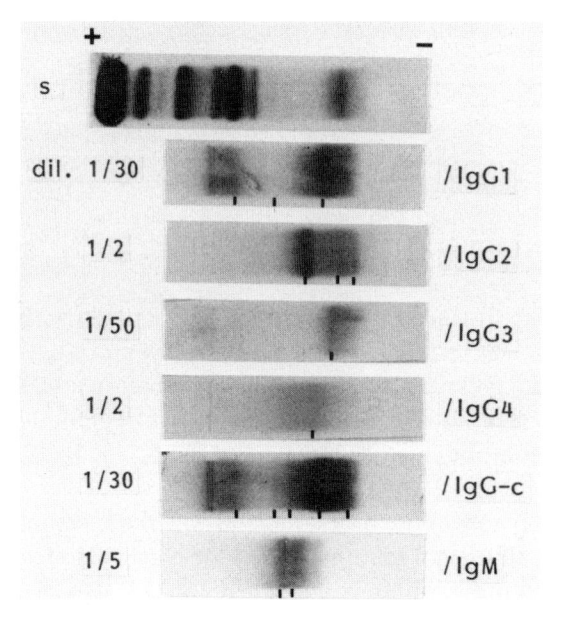

Fig. 2. Agar EP and IMBL of serum from a patient (P.B.) with Wiskott-Aldrich syndrome. (Further legend as in fig. 1.)

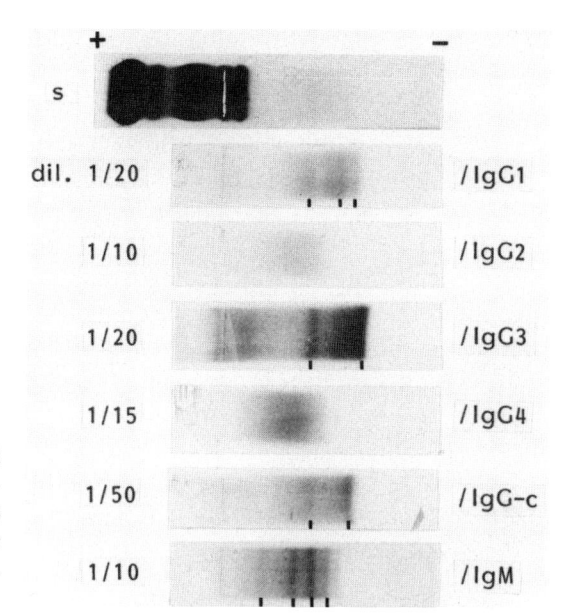

Fig. 3. Agar EP and IMBL of serum from a patient (R.G.) with ALL, 6 months after bone marrow transplantation. (Further legend as in fig. 1.)

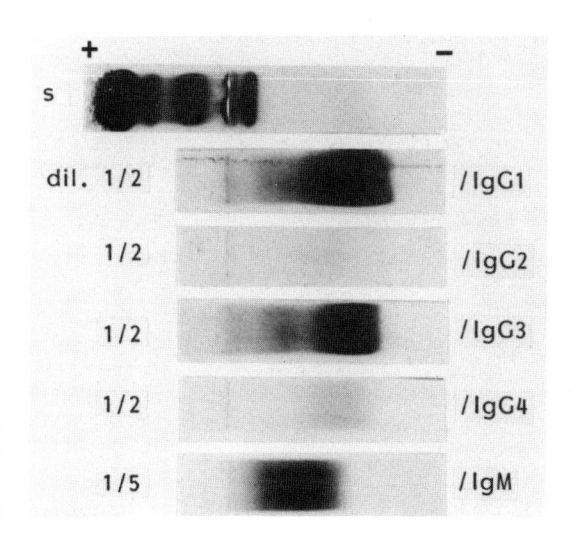

Fig. 4. Agar EP and IMBL of serum from a patient (P.N.) with a late onset agammaglobulinaemia. (Further legend as in fig. 1.)

In the agar EP plate, the γ-globulin region shows only a very low heterogeneous staining. By IMBL, however, 9 distinct H-Ig components can be discerned: 3 × IgG1, 2 × IgG3 and 4 × IgM.

The last example (fig. 4) shows a serum pattern in a late onset agammaglobulinaemia (patient P.N., 11 years of age), where the B cell failure caused a severe depression in Ig of all isotypes which, however, retained a heterogeneous pattern.

In conclusion, our data indicate that: (1) various ID diseases show small multiple H-Ig in high frequencies; it seems that individual subclasses within these H-Ig may have different frequency distribution in different disorders; (2) consequently, when testing sera from ID patients for IgG subclasses by quantitative technique only, the results in some situations may be misleading; the level of a given subclass may be found to fall within normal range, but this subclass may clonally be highly restricted and therefore deficient.

References

1 Vossen, J.M.: Monoclonal gammapathies in immunodeficiencies; in Radl, Hijmans, van Camp, Monoclonal gammapathies, clinical significance and basic mechanisms, pp. 41–48 (Eurage, Rijswijk 1985).
2 Benner, R.; Akker, T.W. van den; Radl, J.: Monoclonal gammapathies in immunodeficient animals – a review; in Radl, Hijmans, van Camp, Monoclonal gammapathies, clinical significance and basic mechanisms, pp. 97–102 (Eurage, Rijswijk 1985).
3 Radl, J.: Monoclonal gammapathies – an attempt at a new classification. Neth. J. Med. *28:* 134–137 (1985).
4 Wieme, R.J.: Studies on agar gel electrophoresis, techniques-applications (Arscia, Brussels 1959).
5 Gerritsen, E.J.A.; Vossen, J.M.; Van Tol, M.J.D.; Jol-Van der Zijde, C.M.; Van der Weijden-Ragas, C.P.M.; Radl, J.: Monoclonal immunoglobulins in childhood; in Radl, Hijmans, van Camp, Monoclonal gammapathies, clinical significance and basic mechanisms, pp. 175–178 (Eurage, Rijswijk 1985).
6 Haaijman, J.J.; Coolen, J.; Deen, C.; Kröse, C.J.M.; Zijlstra, J.J.; Radl, J.: Monoclonal antibodies directed against human immunoglobulins. Reviews on immunoassay technology (Macmillan, London, in press).
7 Jefferis, R.; Reimer, C.B.; Skvaril, F.; and 22 other authors: Evaluation of monoclonal antibodies having specificity for human IgG subclasses: results of an IUIS/WHO collaborative study. Immunol. Lett. *10:* 223–252 (1985).

J. Radl, MD, TNO Institute for Experimental Gerontology,
PO Box 5815, NL-2280 HV Rijswijk (The Netherlands)

Clinical Aspects of IgG Subclasses

Hypergammaglobulinemia Associated with Human Immunodeficiency Virus Infection

Charles B. Reimer, Charlotte M. Black, Robert C. Holman, Thomas W. Wells, Romelia M. Ramirez, Jose Antonio Sa-Ferreira, Janet K.A. Nicholson, J. Steven McDougal [1]

Division of Host Factors, Center for Infectious Diseases, Centers for Disease Control, Public Health Service, US Department of Health and Human Services, Atlanta, Ga., USA

Numerous studies have demonstrated the hypergammaglobulinemia following human immunodeficiency virus (HIV) infection [1, 4, 7, 14, 27, 30]. Primarily IgG and IgA concentrations are elevated. Only two published studies evaluate the subclasses of IgG [2, 5]. The strongest association with (or prediction of) progression to AIDS was lower numbers of T-helper cells as shown in a companion study [15] by a multivariate analysis of laboratory tests that included the titers of HIV antibody of various immunoglobulin (Ig) isotypes specific for Western blot defined HIV antigens, total lymphocyte count, T-helper cell count, T-suppressor/cytotoxic cell count, and the T4/T8 cell ratios for the same patient groups used in this study.

The purpose of this retrospective study is to quantitatively evaluate the serum concentration of all Ig isotypes in a representative sample of anti-HIV-seropositive patients to explore the possibility that a relatively inexpensive Ig-isotype assay could help predict the likelihood of progressive HIV disease.

Materials and Methods

Study Subjects. Blood specimens obtained from 82 anti-HIV-seropositive homosexual or bisexual men were collected from late 1982 through 1984 from participants in

---

[1] We thank Bryan Plikaytis, PhD for help with the statistics, Gerald A. Ebert, PhD for his help in producing the computer graphics, and Mrs. Joann Forney for typing the manuscript.

Table I. Assay characteristics

Assay specificity	Solid-phase, capture Monoclonal antibody	Source[a]	References	Conjugate specificity[b]	Overall CV(%)[c]
IgG	HP6064 (8a4)	UH	11	K,L	9.4
IgG1	HP6069 (2B6)	UB	11	K,L(HP6064/6044)	9.6
IgG2	HP6014	CDC	11,20	(HP6064)	5.8
IgG3	HP6047/6050	CDC/CDC	11,20	K,L(HP6064)	7.2
IgG4	HP6025	CDC	11,20	K,L	4.2
IgA	HP6107	CDC	–	K,L	4.3
IgA1	HP6126	CDC	–	K,L	8.0
IgA2	HP6109/14-3-26	CDC/UA	–/6	K,L(HP6111)	8.8
IgM	HP6083	CDC	19	K,L	4.8
IgD	delta-TA4-1	ATCC-HB70	13	K,L	3.8
IgE	HP6061	CDC	18	K,L	7.4

[a] UH = University of Helsinki, Finland; UB = University of Birmingham, England; CDC = Centers for Disease Control, Atlanta, Ga, USA; UA = University of Alabama, Birmingham, Ala., USA; ATCC = American Type Culture Collection, Rockville, Md, USA.
[b] K,L = anti-kappa (HP6053), anti-lambda (HP6054), CDC(20); (HP6064) = anti-IgG$_{Fc}$, UB(11); (HP6044) = anti-IgG$_{Fab}$, CDC(20); (HP6111) = anti-IgA, CDC.
[c] CV% = $100 \; (N \; (x_1-x_2)^2)^{1/2} / (x_1+x_2)$, when N is the number of pairs of value x_1 and x_2.

ongoing clinical studies of HIV infection conducted by the Centers for Disease Control (CDC) in Atlanta and San Francisco [8, 10]. From subsequent follow-up studies, we identified 25 of these men whose condition had progressed to acquired immunodeficiency syndrome (AIDS) (progressors) from whom we had previously collected specimens when they were asymptomatic (n = 7) or had had persistent generalized lymphadenopathy (PGL) (n = 18). The average interval from specimen collection to onset of AIDS was 14 months (median 10 months; range 2–38 months). For comparison, we selected anti-HIV-sero-positive specimens that had been collected over the same calendar time from 37 asymptomatic men and 20 men with PGL whose clinical status had not changed (nonprogressors) during an average interval between specimen collection and a follow-up examination 29 months later (median 24 months, range 17–46 months). Additionally, specimens were examined from 25 men who fulfilled the CDC case definition for AIDS [3] and from 31 healthy, married HIV-seronegative men who were CDC employees with normal biochemical profiles.

Assay Methodology. We assayed appropriate dilutions of each patient's serum with recent modifications [Black et al., J. immunol. Methods, in press] of our previously published [9, 17], two-site immunoenzymometric assays specific for each of the human Ig isotypes. Briefly, we captured the patient's Ig with a human Ig-isotype-specific, mouse monoclonal antibody that had been bound to the plastic surface of Immulon II plates[1] (Dynatech, Alexandria, Va.), then quantified its presence with a mixture of peroxidase-conjugated monoclonal antibodies to κ, λ, and/or other appropriate human Ig epitopes (table I). A single 60-μl sample of each patient's serum was used to perform all dilutions for all 11 isotype assays using a calibrated positive liquid displacement diluter where the (previously measured) cumulative inaccuracy for any serial dilution was less than 2%. Specificity of the definitive assay, predicted on our knowledge of the individual specificity of each of the monoclonal antibodies used [11, 20], was reconfirmed here by assay of purified immunoglobulins of each isotype.

The WHO International Standard for Human IgG, IgA, and IgM (67/97) [24] was used to establish the numerical basis for our IgG, IgG1, IgG2, IgG3, and IgG4 assays, using the mass units tentatively assigned to these analytes by Klein et al. [12], and for IgA and IgM, using the mass units per international unit (IU) estimated for these two analytes by Reimer et al. [21]. Our IgA1 and IgA2 results are calibrated comparatively based on their (unspecified) concentrations in the US National Reference Preparation for Human Serum Proteins (USNRP) [21].

For our IgD assays, the British research standard for human IgD (67/37) was used as the calibrator, assuming 141 μg of IgD per vial before reconstitution [25]. An 'in-house' pool of seven individuals with elevated IgE, appropriately calibrated (in IU) against the WHO International Reference Standard for Human IgE (75/502) was the calibrator used for our IgE assays [26].

Statistics. The sigmoidal shape of the working curve when plotted on an optical density versus log concentration scale was analyzed by a four-parameter logistic model algebraically equivalent to the one presented by Rodbard and Hutt [23]. This allowed accurate computer interpolation of unknowns to be extended into curvilinear portions of the regression to provide an approximate 150-fold dynamic range for most working curves. A public domain BASIC computer program detailing our ELISA curve-fitting procedure suitable for an IMB-XT or IBM-AT is described by Black et al. [J. immunol. Methods, in press]. The overall coefficient of variation (CV), based on the imprecision of duplicate assays of all the specimens [22], is summarized for all 11 assays in table I. The assay concentration sensitivity, based on the limiting dilution of the specimen where the CV degenerated to 50%, was less than 10 ng/ml for all analytes.

Immunoglobulin concentrations were distributed more symmetrically around a central measure when logarithmically transformed. Therefore, the geometric mean rather than the arithmetic mean was used to express our results graphically, and the analysis was performed on the log-transformed data. Limits for the range of values were obtained by taking the antilog of the arithmetic sum of the mean logarithm ± two standard deviations of the logarithms of all values. Study groups were compared using Student's t-test, assuming unequal variances [29]. Comparisons between groups were specified before the analysis; therefore, the probabilities were not adjusted for multiple comparisons.

---

[1] Use of trade names is for identification only and does not constitute endorsement by the Public Health Service or the US Department of Health and Human Services.

Linear regression analysis by the unweighted least squares method [29] was used to examine the relationships among immunoglobulin concentrations, T cell concentrations, and the T4/T8 cell ratio. The *all-possible-regressions* selection procedure, with the R^2 statistic as the selection criterion, was used to examine related variables distinguishing progressors from nonprogressors [16].

Results

The distributions of T-helper cells, T-suppressor/cytotoxic cells, and the individual T4/T8 cell ratios for these anti-HIV-seropositive patient study groups [15] are shown in figure 1 for comparison with the Ig-isotype serum concentrations reported here.

Although large overlaps in the distributions are apparent, comparisons between the study groups show that the geometric mean number of T-helper cells (per μl of blood) in all anti-HIV-seropositive patients was significantly lower than normal. There was also a significant difference between any two of these five study groups (fig. 1). The geometric mean number of T-suppressor cells also was significantly different for all comparisons except for those of PGL-nonprogressors and progressors and of normals and AIDS patients. The geometric means of the individual T4/T8 cell ratios were significantly different for all comparisons except for those of asymptomatic-nonprogressors and PGL-nonprogressors. The geometric mean T4 cell concentrations from pooled nonprogressors (asymptomatic plus PGL) was significantly higher ($p \leq 0.0001$) than that found in progressors. The same was true for the T4/T8 cell ratio ($p = 0.0003$). The geometric mean T8 cell concentration from pooled nonprogressors bordered on being significantly higher ($p = 0.06$) than in progressors.

The distributions of Ig-isotype concentrations in our five study groups overlap relatively more than the distributions of the cellular

Fig. 1. Distributions of the number of T-helper cells (T4) and T-suppressor/cytotoxic cells (T8) per μl of blood and their ratios (T4/T8) in five study groups (see text). The geometric mean and geometric mean x/− (geometric standard deviation)² are shown for each group. The abscissa is drawn through the geometric mean of the anti-HIV-seronegative control population. The probability (using Student's t-test) that any study group mean is significantly different from that of the group indicated by an asterisk (*) is listed on the same line as the *. n.s. = Not statistically significant at the 5% level. (Individuals comprising the normal control study group used for obtaining the cellular data are not the same as those in the Ig-isotype-normal control study group; cellular data were not collected from the latter group.)

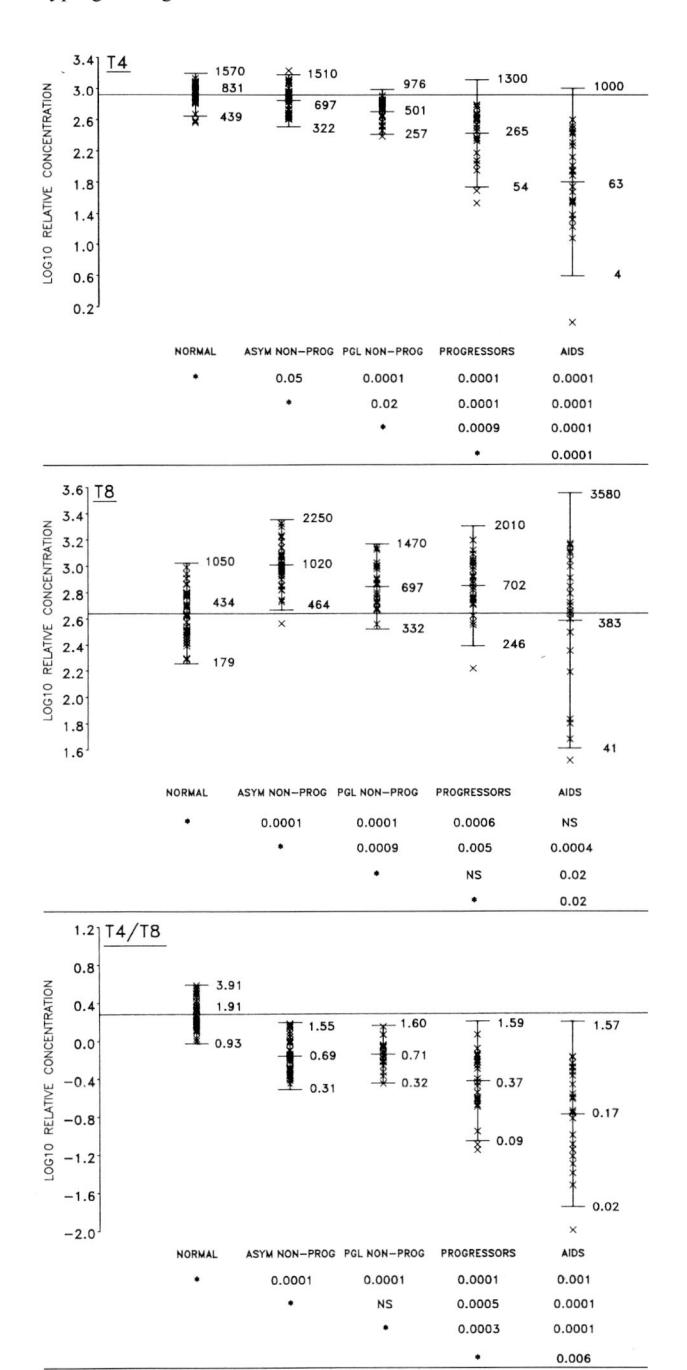

Hypergammaglobulinemia Associated with HIV Infection

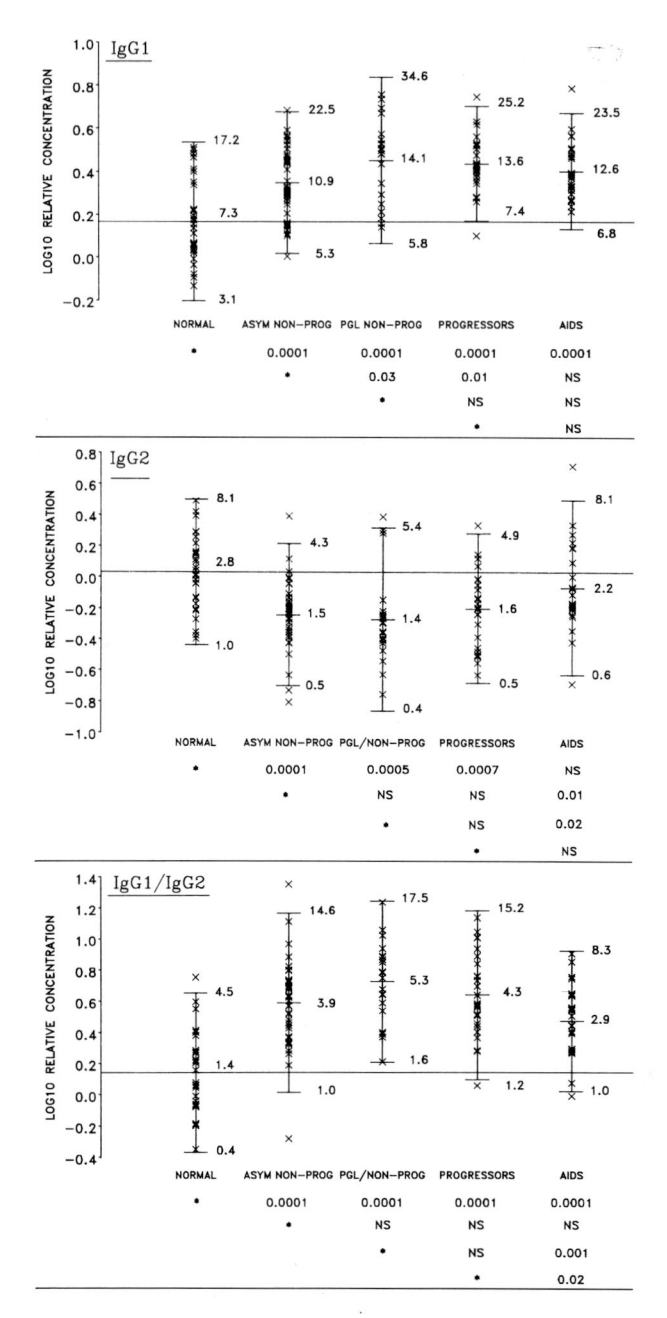

Fig. 2. Distribution of the serum concentrations of IgG1 and IgG2 (in mg/ml), and their ratio (IgG1/IgG2) in five study groups (see text). Scale shows $\log_{10}$ concentration relative to that of WHO (67/97). Also see legend to figure 1.

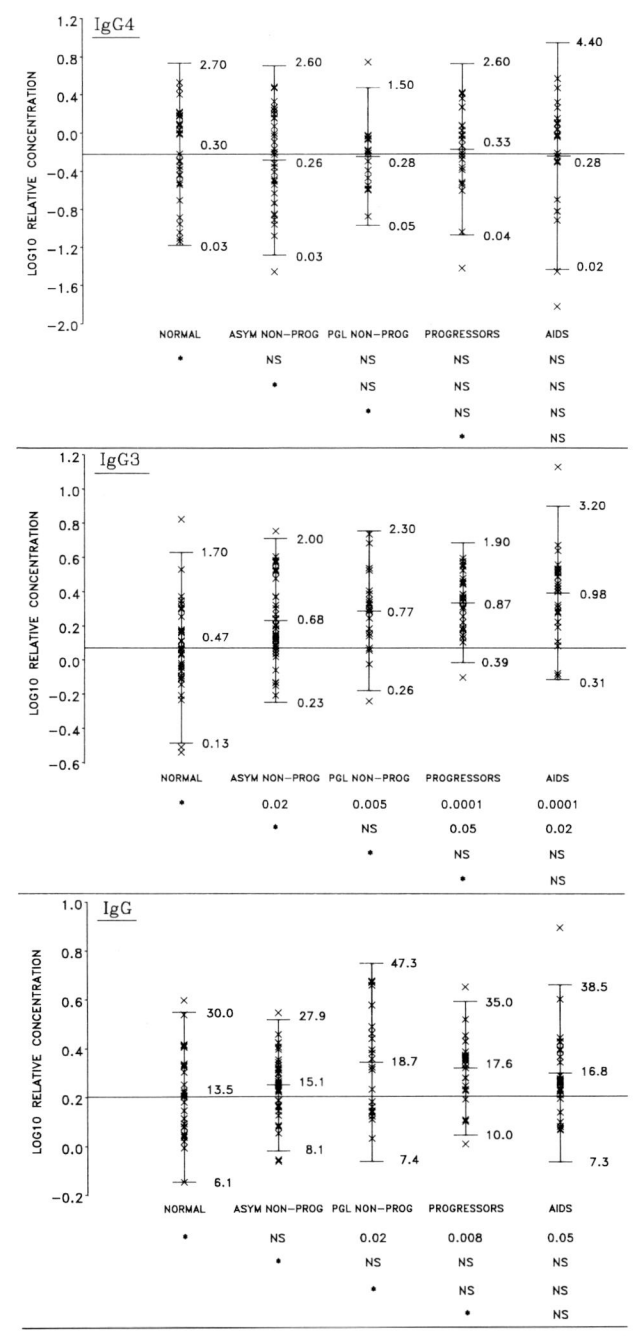

Fig. 3. Distribution of the serum concentration of IgG3, IgG4, and IgG (in mg/ml) in five study groups (see text). Scale shows $\log_{10}$ concentration relative to that of WHO (67/97). Also see legend to figure 1.

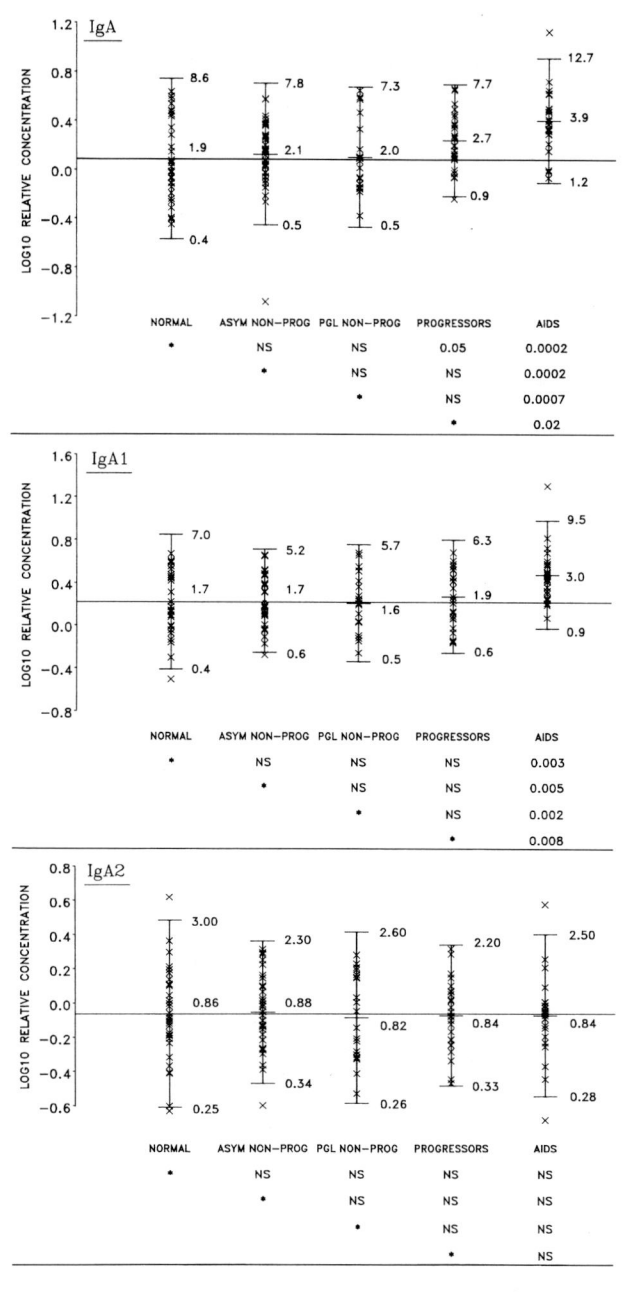

Fig. 4. Distributions of the serum concentrations of IgA (in mg/ml) in five study groups (see text). Scale shows $\log_{10}$ concentration relative to that of WHO (67/97). Distributions of the serum concentrations of IgA1 and IgA2 relative to their (undefined) concentrations in USNRP. Also see legend to figure 1.

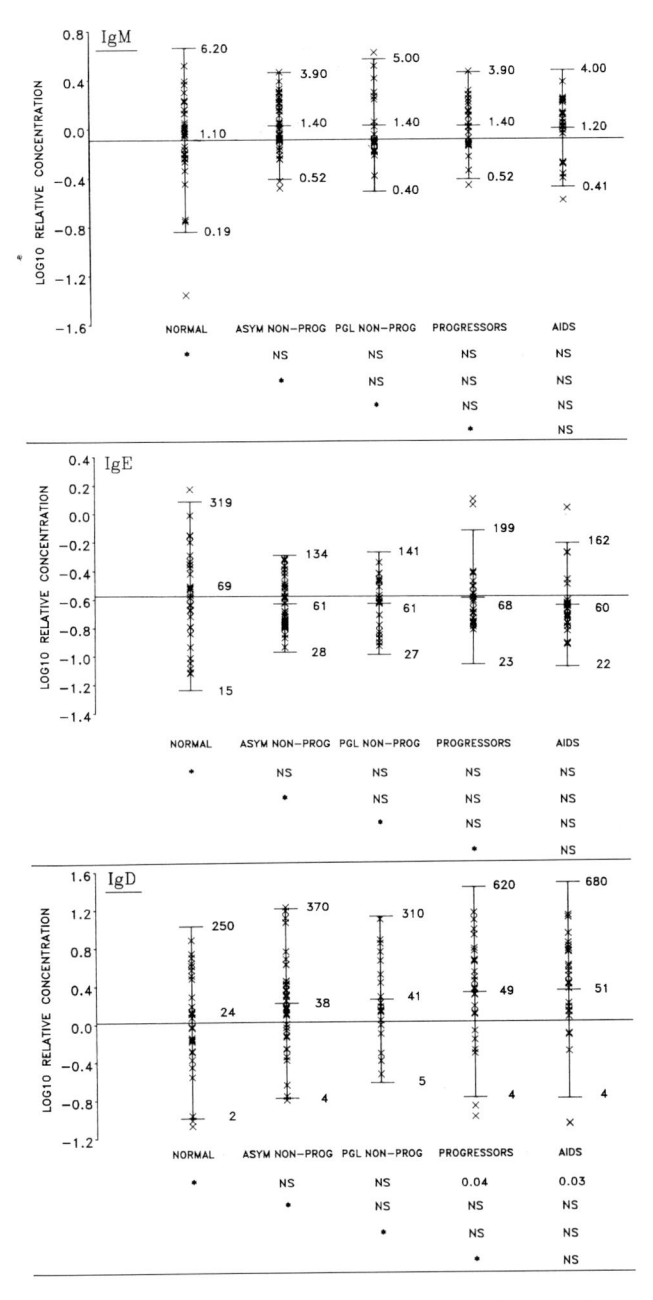

Fig. 5. Distributions of the serum concentrations of IgM (in mg/ml), IgE (in IU/ml), and IgD (in µg/ml) in five study groups (see text). Scales show $\log_{10}$ concentration relative to WHO (67/97) for IgM, WHO (75/502) for IgE, and the British standard (67/97) for IgD.

parameters. Depending on the Ig isotype, figure 2 shows both hyper- and hypogammaglobulinemia associated with progression towards AIDS. The geometric mean IgG1 serum concentration is significantly higher in asymptomatic nonprogressors, PGL-nonprogressors, progressors, and AIDS patient groups than that in HIV-seronegative normals. In contrast, the geometric mean IgG2 serum concentration is depressed in all the anti-HIV-seropositive patients (but not significantly with the AIDS group). Other contrasts showing significant differences were: the geometric means of IgG1 in progressors and PGL-nonprogressors were significantly higher than in asymptomatic nonprogressors, and the geometric mean IgG2 concentration in AIDS patients was significantly higher than in either the asymptomatic nonprogressors or PGL-nonprogressors.

Figure 3 shows the concentration distributions for the remaining IgG subclasses, IgG3 and IgG4, and for total IgG. As with IgG1, the geometric mean IgG3 concentration is significantly elevated in all anti-HIV-seropositive patients. Significant differences were not found for IgG4 concentrations in our five study groups.

The total concentration of IgG is the sum of concentrations of the four IgG subclasses. Logically, specific assay of the dominant IgG subclasses, IgG1 and IgG2, and their ratio (fig. 2) should be more discriminatory than measurement of total IgG, which is evidenced by comparison of the results for the latter (fig. 3) with those of the former (fig. 2). Nevertheless, measurement of the serum concentrations of any of the IgG subclasses, their ratios, or their sums did not statistically discriminate progressors from nonprogressors.

Figure 4 shows the concentration distributions for IgA and its two subclasses. The geometric mean IgA concentration of AIDS patients was more markedly elevated over normal controls than any of the other study groups. This was almost entirely due to increases in the IgA1 subclass concentration. The geometric mean IgA concentration was significantly higher ($p = 0.05$) in progressors than in pooled nonprogressors (asymptomatic plus PGL). This was the only Ig isotype where this contrast was statistically significant, but it was not significant for the IgA individual subclasses.

Figure 5 shows the distributions of IgM, IgE, and IgD concentrations. None of the geometric means of IgM or IgE were significantly different among our study groups. (However, the geometric mean IgM concentration of 13 anti-HIV-seropositive hemophiliac patients [a smaller study group not otherwise discussed here] was significantly elevated [p = 0.04] over our anti-HIV-seronegative control group, as was IgG1 [p ≤ 0.0001]. IgA in these hemophiliac patients, who, in contrast to our other study groups acquired their HIV infection via a nonmucosal route, was indistinguishable from that of our anti-HIV-seronegative controls.)

Significant linear relationships were found between T-helper cells and IgA (r = –0.35, p = 0.003), IgG2 (r = –0.22, p = 0.02), and IgG3 (r = –0.21, p = 0.03). The *all-possible-regressions* procedure selected the T-helper cells as the 'best' predictive variable ($R^2 = 0.377$).

Discussion

No current laboratory test can reliably predict when or even whether any given anti-HIV-seropositive patient will develop progressive disease culminating in clinical AIDS. Estimates of the fraction of current anti-HIV-seropositive patients who eventually will develop AIDS are uncertain and have been revised upward as more follow-up time has elapsed. Inspection of the overlap in the distributions of cellular data from our relatively small anti-HIV-seropositive study groups (fig. 1) shows that some progressors had more T4 cells, fewer T8 cells, and a higher T4/T8 ratio than did many nonprogressors, although the opposite was more often the case. Graphic analysis of the Ig-isotype assays showed relatively more overlap than with the cellular data; multivariate analysis showed the Ig-isotype assays to have much less predictive power for progression to AIDS than the T-helper cell assays.

Why hypergammaglobulinemia is associated with HIV infection is not easily understood. If the process is under T cell control, superficially one would expect to find more rather than fewer T4-helper cells and fewer rather than more T8-suppressor/cytotoxic cells. However, to characterize T4 cells only as helpers and T8 cells only as suppressors is oversimplification. For example, some subsets of T4 cells can exhibit a suppressor/cytotoxic function [31]. Several authors have suggested a primary activation of a polyclonal response in B cells by HIV or activation of another virus, such as Epstein-Barr virus in B cells [28, 32]. Whatever final understanding of the underlying control mechanisms is attained, the facts of humoral immunodeficiency for antigens not seen before HIV infection and selectivity toward certain Ig isotypes (e.g. IgG1/IgG2) must be accounted for by any acceptable control model.

Summary

The serum concentrations of 11 Ig isotypes (IgG, IgG1, IgG2, IgG3, IgG4, IgA, IgA1, IgA2, IgM, IgD, and IgE) were measured in four relatively small groups of homosexual (or bisexual) males. All these patients were seropositive for HIV. Two of the groups (nonprogressors) were clinically stable for approximately 2 years and were characterized either as asymptomatic or with PGL. The third group (progressors) developed AIDS 2-38 months after blood specimens were taken. The fourth group had AIDS. A fifth group of anti-HIV-seronegative heterosexual males completed the study. The geometric mean IgA serum concentration was more markedly elevated over normal control sera than any of the other study groups and was the only Ig isotype that was significantly higher in the progressor than in the nonprogressor group. The geometric IgG1 serum concentration was significantly higher in asymptomatic nonprogressors, PGL-nonprogressors, progressors, and AIDS patient groups than that in HIV-seronegative normals. In contrast, the geometric mean IgG2 serum concentration is depressed in all the anti-HIV-seropositive patients (but not significantly with the AIDS group). Multivariate analysis showed the Ig-isotype assays to have much less predictive power for progression to AIDS than the T-helper cell assays.

References

1 Ammann, A.; Abrams, D.; Conant, M.; Chudwin, D.; Cowan, M.; Volberding, P.; Lewis, B.; Casavant, C.: Acquired immuno dysfunction in homosexual men: immunologic profiles. Clin. Immunol. Immunopath. 27: 315 (1982).
2 Aucouturier, P.; Couderc, L.; Gouet, D.; Danon, F.; Gombert, J.; Matheron, S.; Saimot, A.; Clauvel, J.; Preud'homme, J.: Serum immunoglobulin G subclass dysbalances in the lymphadenopathy syndrome and acquired immune deficiency syndrome. Clin. exp. Immunol. 63: 234-240 (1986).
3 Centers for Disease Control: Revision of the case definition of acquired immunodeficiency syndrome for national reporting-United States. Morbidity and Mortality Weeklly Report 34: 373-375 (1985).
4 Chess, Q.; Daniels, J.; North, E.; Macris, N.: Serum immunoglobulin elevations in the acquired immunodeficiency syndrome (AIDS): IgG, IgA, IgM, and IgD. Diagn. Immunol. 2: 148-153 (1984).
5 Church, J.; Lewis, J.; Spotkov, J.: IgG subclass deficiencies in children with suspected AIDS. Lancet i: 279 (1984).
6 Conley, M.; Kearney, J.; Lawton, A. III; Cooper, M.: Differentiation of human B cells expressing the IgA subclasses as demonstrated by monoclonal hybridoma antibodies. J. Immun. 125: 2311-2316 (1980).

7 El-Sadr, W.; Stahl, R.; Sidhu, G.; Zolla-Pazner, S.: The acquired immune deficiency syndrome: laboratory findings, clinical features, and leading hypotheses. Diagn. Immunol. *2:* 73–85 (1984).
8 Fishbein, D.; Kaplan, J.; Spira, T.; Miller, B.; Schonberger, L.; Pinsky, P.; Getchell, J.; Kalyanaraman, V.; Braude, J.: Unexplained lymphadenopathy in homosexual men: a longitudinal study. J. Am. med. Ass. *254:* 930–935 (1985).
9 Hussain, R.; Poindexter, R. ; Wistar, R.; Reimer, C.: Use of monoclonal antibodies to quantify subclasses of human IgG. I. Development of twosite immunoenzymometric assays for total IgG subclass determinations. J. immunol. Methods *93:* 89–96 (1986).
10 Jaffe, H.; Feorino, P.; Darrow, W.; OMalley, P.; Getchell, J.; Warfield, D.; Jones, B.; Echenberg, D.; Francis, D.; Curran, J.: Persistent infection with HTLV-III/LAV in apparently healthy homosexual men. Ann. intern. Med. *102:* 627–628 (1985).
11 Jefferis, R.; Reimer, C.; Skavril, F.; deLange, G.; Ling, N.; Lowe, J.; Walker, M.; Phillips, D.; Aloisio, C.; Wells, T.; Vaerman, J.; Magnusson, C.; Kubagawa, H.; Cooper, M.; Vardtal, F.; Vandvi, B.; Haaijman, J.; Makela, O.; Sarnesto, A.; Lando, Z.; Gergely, J.; Rajnavolgyi, E. ; Laszlo, G.; Radl, J.; Molinaro, G.: Evaluation of monoclonal antibodies having specificity for human IgG subclasses: results of an IUIS/WHO collaborative study. Immunol. Lett. *10:* 223–252 (1985).
12 Klein, F.; Skvaril, F. ; Vermeeren, R.; Vlug, A.; Duimel, W.: The quantification of human IgG subclasses in reference preparations. Clinica chim. Acta *150:* (1985).
13 Kubagawa, H.; Gathings, W.; Levitt, D.; Kearney, J.; Cooper, M.: Immunoglobulin isotype expressions of normal pre-B cells as determined by immunofluorescence. J. clin. Immunol. *2:* 264–268 (1982).
14 Lane, H.; Masur, H.; Edgar, L.; Whalen, G.; Rook, A.; Fauci, A.: Abnormalities of B-cell activation and immunoregulation in patients with the acquired immunodeficiency syndrome. New Engl. J. Med. *309:* 453–458 (1983).
15 McDougal, J.; Kennedy, M.; Nicholson, J.; Spira, T.; Jaffe, H.; Kaplan, J.; Fishbein, D.; O'Malley, P.; Aloisio, C.; Black, C.; Hubbard, M.; Reimer, C.: Antibody response to human immunodeficiency virus in homosexual men. Relation of antibody specificity, titer, and isotype to clinical status, severity of immunodeficiency, and disease progression. J. clin. Invest. *80:* 316–324 (1987).
16 Neter, J.; Wasserman, W.; Kutner, M.: Applied linear statistical models (Irwin, Homewood 1985).
17 Papadea, C.; Check, I.; Reimer, C.: Monoclonal antibody-based solid phase enzyme immunoassays for quantitating human serum immunoglobulin G and its subclasses. Clin. Chem. *31:* 1940–1945 (1985).
18 Reimer, C.: Five hybridomas secreting monoclonal antibodies against human IgE. Monoclonal Antibody News *4:* 31 (1986).
19 Reimer, C.: Seven monoclonal antibodies against human IgM. Monoclonal Antibody News *5:* 1–2 (1987).
20 Reimer, C.; Phillips, D.; Aloisio, C.; Moore, D.; Galland, G.; Wells, T.; Black, C.; McDougal, J.: Evaluation of thirty-one mouse monoclonal antibodies to human IgG epitopes. Hybridoma *3:* 263–275 (1984).

21 Reimer, C.; Smith, S.; Wells, T.; Nakamura, R.; Keitges, P.; Ritchie, R.; Williams, G.; Hanson, D.; Dorsey, D.: Collaborative calibration of the US National and the College of American Pathologists' reference preparations for specific serum proteins. Am. J. clin. Path. 77: 12–19 (1982).
22 Rodbard, D.: Statistical quality control and routine data processing for radioimmunoassays and immunoradiometric assays. Clin. Chem. 20: 1255–1270 (1974).
23 Rodbard, D.; Hutt, D.: Statistical analysis of radioimmunoradiometric (labelled antibody) assays. A generalized weighted, iterative, least-squares method for logistic curve fitting; in Symp. on RIA and Related Procedures in Medicine. Int. Atomic Energy Agency, Vienna, p. 165 (Unipub, New York 1974).
24 Rowe, D.; Grab, B.; Anderson, S.: An international reference preparation for human serum immunoglobulins G, A, and M: content of immunoglobulin by weight. Bull. Wld Hlth Org. 46: 67–79 (1972).
25 Rowe, D.; Anderson, S.; Tackett, L.: A research standard for human serum immunoglobulin D. Bull. Wld Hlth Org. 43: 607–609 (1970).
26 Rowe, D.; Grab, B.; Anderson, S.: An international reference preparation for human serum immunoglobulin E. Bull Wld Hlth Org. 49: 320–321 (1973).
27 Rubinstein, A.; Sicklick, M.; Gupta, A.; Bernstein, L.; Klein, N.; Rubinstein, E.; Spigland, I.; Fruchter, L.; Litman, N.; Lee, H.; Hollander, M.: Acquired immunodeficiency with reversed T_4/T_8 ratios in infants born to promiscuous and drug-addicted mothers. J. Am. med. Ass. 249: 2350–2356 (1983).
28 Schnittman, S.; Lane, H.; Higgins, S.; Folks, T.; Fauci, A.: Direct polyclonal activation of human B lymphocytes by the acquired immune deficiency syndrome virus. Science 233: 1084–1086 (1986).
29 Snedecor, G.; Cochran, W.: Statistical methods (Iowa State University Press, Ames. 1980).
30 Stahl, R.; Friedman-Kien, A.; Dubin, R.; Marmor, M.; Zolla-Pazner, S.: Immunologic abnormalities in homosexual men: relationship to Kaposi's sarcoma. Am. J. Med. 73: 171–178 (1982).
31 Thomas, Y.; Rogozinski, L.; Irigoyen, O.; Friedman, S.; Kung, P.; Goldstein, G.; Chess, L.: Functional analysis of human T cell subsets defined by monoclonal antibodies. IV. Induction of suppressor cells within the OKT4+ population. J. exp. Med. 154: 459–467 (1981).
32 Zolla-Pazner, S.: B cells in the pathogenesis of AIDS. Immunol. Today 5: 289–291 (1984).

Charles B. Reimer, PhD, Division of Host Factors 1–1354 D03, Center for Infectious Diseases, Centers for Disease Control, Atlanta, GA 30333 (USA)

IgG Antibody Response to Polysaccharides in Children with Recurrent Infections

Raif S. Geha

The Children's Hospital, Boston, Mass., USA

Introduction

Many children with recurrent sinopulmonary infections present to the physician with serum IgG levels that are within the normal range. Over the last 3 years, we have been interested in examining the IgG subclass distribution and the specific antibody response of these children to immunization with polysaccharide antigens. The results we have obtained indicate that many of these children have an IgG subclass deficiency and/or an impaired capacity to respond to polysaccharide antigens. The latter may be an excellent indicator of a subtle antibody deficiency in these children. These investigations are clinically important because they will determine the modality of therapy which progresses, depending on the clinical response, from simple prophylaxis with antibiotics to intravenous γ-globulin replacement.

IgG2 Subclass Deficiency

We initially reported on 20 children with IgG2 subclass deficiency [1]. Since then, many more children were seen in our clinic, which is a referral clinic. All these children had a history of recurrent infections which consisted of recurrent otitis media of four or more per year, recurrent sinusitis diagnosed on the basis of radiographic examination of the sinus prompted by the presence of cough, foul-smelling breath, and purulent nasal discharge. In addition, some of these children had already suffered from pneumonia. The clinical characteristics of these children are found in table I.

Table I. Patient characteristics

Characteristic	Deficient subclass		
	IgG2	IgG3	IgG2 + IgG3
Number of patients	12	5	3
Sex, M/F	8/4	3/2	2/1
Age, years			
Mean ± SD	4.6 ± 3.4	9 ± 2.5	5 ± 9.4
Range	2 – 13	7 – 12	2 – 10
Age at onset of symptoms (years)			
– mean ± SD	1.5 ± 0.7	1.6 ± 0.8	2.8 ± 2.0
Patients with recurrent infections, %			
Otitis media	100	100	100
Sinusitis	100	100	100
Pneumonia	42	80	67
Recurrent asthma	42	80	33

Table II. Post-immunization response to Hib-CP: geometric mean (ng/ml)

	IgG2 deficiency (n = 15)	IgG3 deficiency (n = 5)	Controls (n = 15)
Anti-PRP IgG	1,714	58,550	18,570
Anti-PRP IgG1	199	–	258
Anti-PRP IgG2	1,219	–	15,842

Of the initial children studied, 12 were IgG2-deficient, 5 were IgG3-deficient and 3 had combined deficiency in IgG2 and IgG3. Because low serum levels of antibody to *Haemophilus influenzae* type b (Hib) capsular polysaccharide (CP) present before intentional immunization may reflect inadequate exposure to antigen rather than poor antibody responsiveness, these children were intentionally immunized with Hib-CP. The results of the immunization are shown in table II. These results show that children with an IgG2 subclass deficiency responded very poorly to immunization to the Hib-CP vaccine. In contrast, the children with IgG3 deficiency responded normally to that vaccine. Furthermore, table II shows that the majority of the antibody response to polyribosylribitolphosphate (PRP) in the normal siblings studied resided in the IgG2 subclass. This was not surprising, since IgG antibody responses to most bacterial polysaccharide antigens reside predominantly within the IgG2 subclass [2–4]. Furthermore, we studied the response of these children to meningococcus immunization. There was a lower response in the children with IgG2 subclass deficiency. This was statistically significant from the response of normal siblings. In addition, there was also a statistically significant decrease in the pneumococcal antibody response of these children to immunization with pneumococcus bacterial polysaccharide. The antibody response to polysaccharide antigen was not a reflection of a general failure of the immune system to respond to all antigens because antibody responses to bacterial protein antigens such as tetanus toxoid and diphtheria toxoid were completely normal.

Patients with Recurrent Infections, Normal IgG2 and Poor Antibody Response to Hib Antigen

More recently, we studied 15 children with recurrent infections and normal serum IgG, IgM, IgA, and IgG subclass levels that also fell within the normal range. These children suffered from the same type of infections as the children with IgG2 subclass deficiency. Following immunization, the geometric mean serum IgG antibody concentration to Hib of these children was 8-fold lower than that of age-matched controls. The significance level was $p = 0.002$. The patients also had a low geometric mean concentration of serum IgM and IgA directed to Hib although these differences did not reach significance. To confirm these findings, an additional 11 patients were identified and immunized. The geometric serum IgG anti-Hib for this group of patients was also significantly lower than normals ($p = 0.004$).

In these children, the serum IgG antibody response to pneumococcus types 3 and 23 was also examined. Although the geometric mean of these patients was lower than that of normal control, the results did not reach statistical significance. There was no significant difference when the geometric mean of IgG antibody concentration to diphtheria toxoid was compared between the patients and the controls.

The degree of impairment of the anti-Hib polysaccharide response in the second group of patients was equivalent to that seen in children with IgG2 subclass deficiencies. We propose that the impaired antibody response to Hib may be a marker for a poor antibody response to a variety of bacterial and viral antigens which results in an increased susceptibility to infections. The selectivity range of this response is not known. It appears that the response to a protein antigen such as diphtheria and tetanus was definitely normal, whereas the responses to some of the pneumococcal strains may be lower than normal. To further examine the selectivity of the impaired antibody response, it will be necessary to study the response of a large number of children with recurrent infections to a wide variety of antigens. It should be noted that within the group of 15 children we studied, some of the responses to Hib overlapped with those of normal children. In those cases, selective antibody deficiency, if present, may have involved antigens other than Hib polysaccharide. Alternatively, in such cases the recurrent infections may not have been due to an immunologic defect.

Treatment of Children with Poor Response to Polysaccharide Antigens

The identification of children with selective antibody deficiency is important for diagnostic and therapeutic reasons. In our experience, about 70% of children with either IgG2 antibody deficiency and/or poor response to polysaccharide antigens and recurrent infections respond well with the institution of prophylactic antibiotic therapy during the winter time. Another 25–35% of these children will require intravenous replacement therapy. We have recently conducted a study comparing the incidence of infections before and after immunoglobulin therapy in 11 children who had failed to improve on antibiotic prophylaxis [5]. The number of episodes of sinusitis, otitis, and pneumonia were recorded in the 12 months preceding the institution of intravenous γ-globulin as well as in the 12 months following the institution of γ-globulin levels. In all cases, institution of γ-globulin has resulted in an increase in the total IgG level and IgG2 level as well as in the level of the anti-PRP titer. The 11 children entered in this study showed a significant improvement by the following criteria: the number of episodes of otitis media was reduced from 7.9 ± 3.4 to 2.55 ± 1.60 per year (p < 0.001). The incidence of pneumonia decreased from 1.74 ± 1.4 to 0.25 ± 0.29 per year (p < 0.001). The incidence of ear infections decreased from 8.80 to 2.33 per year (p < 0.001). No patient developed infections which had not been previously experienced prior to intravenous γ-globulin, and all patients had reduction in the total number of infections. Those patients in this group who had severe asthma requiring multiple intensive care admissions and institution of corticosteroid therapy also showed a marked improvement in the course of their disease.

Summary

IgG2 subclass deficiency associated with poor antibody response to polysaccharide antigen is a now well-described entity. A newer entity which appears to be at least as common is the recurrent infection with a selective deficiency in the antibody response. At the present time, the antibody response to *Haemophilus influenzae* type b (Hib) is a good marker for the selective antibody deficiency in these children, as the vast majority of such children made a very poor antibody response to Hib. The data suggest that treatment of these children with prophylactic antibiotics and/or with IV γ-globulin, depending on the clinical situation, is beneficial. This reinforces the view that the observed abnormality in the antibody response may be causally related to the recurrent infections. Prospective studies of the 10% of 'normal' children who fail to respond to soluble polysaccharide antigen would reveal if there is within this group a higher incidence of recurrent infections. The result of such studies will be important in our understanding of normal as well as abnormal selective antigen-specific antibody deficiencies in children.

References

1 Umetsu, D.T.; Ambrosino, D.M.; Quinti, I.; Siber G.R.; Geha R.S.: Recurrent sinopulmonary infection and impaired antibody response to bacterial capsular polysaccharide antigen in children with selective IgG-subclass deficiency. New Engl. J. Med. *313:* 1247–1251 (1985).
2 Yount, W.J.; Dorner, M.M.; Kunkel, H.G.; Kabat, E.A.: Studies on human antibodies. IV. Selective variations in subgroup composition and genetic markers. J. exp. Med. *127:* 633–646 (1968).
3 Riesen, W.F.; Skvaril, F.; Braun, D.G.: Natural infection of man with group A streptococci; levels, restriction in class, subclass, and type, and clonal appearance of polysaccharide-group-specific antibodies. Scand, J. Immunol. *5:* 383–390 (1975).

4 Siber, G.R.; Schur, P.H.; Aisenberg, A.C.; Weitzman, S.A.; Schiffman, G.: Correlation between serum IgG2 concentrations and the antibody response to bacterial polysaccharide antigens. New Engl. J. Med. *303:* 178–182 (1980).
5 Silk, H.J.; Geha, R.S.: Intravenous gammaglobulin (IVGG) prophylaxis in children with IgG2 deficiency. J. Allergy clin. Immunol. *79:* 188 (1987).

Raif S. Geha, MD, Immunology Program, The Children's Hospital,
300 Longwood Avenue, Boston, MA 02115 (USA)

The Cellular Basis of Selective Defects in IgG Subclass Responses

I.C.M. Mac Lennan, A. Chandramukhi, P.J.L. Lane, S. Oldfield

Department of Immunology, University of Birmingham Medical School, Birmingham, England

Selective Defects in Subclass Responses to Certain Antigens

Patients have been identified with selective defects in their ability to respond to certain antigens but not others. In addition, these defective antibody responses may affect some subclasses more than others. Oxelius et al. [1] have described patients with combined IgG2 and IgA deficiency. These patients are far more susceptible to recurrent infection than patients with IgA deficiency alone. We have identified a group of patients who share many of the features of this deficiency [2]. The patients are IgA-deficient and are unable to produce IgG2 and in one case also IgG1 antibodies against pneumococcal capsular polysaccharides. However, they have both IgG2 and IgG1 in their serum and can produce normal IgG subclass responses to tetanus toxoid. Ambrosino et al. [3] have recently described a patient with defective IgG production against capsular polysaccharides but normal immunoglobulin levels. We have noted in patients with chronic lymphocytic leukaemia an association between splenic involvement and selective depression in levels of IgG1 and IgG2 but not IgM antibody against pneumococcal capsular polysaccharides (fig. 1).

Clinical observation indicates that selective deficiency of IgG antibody production against bacterial capsular saccharides is associated with increased susceptibility to infection with encapsulated bacteria. Briles et al. [4] have provided experimental evidence in mice that IgG antibodies are substantially more protective than IgM or IgA in this context. Patients with dysgammaglobulinaemia rather than hypogammaglobulinaemia are most unlikely to have deletions of heavy chain

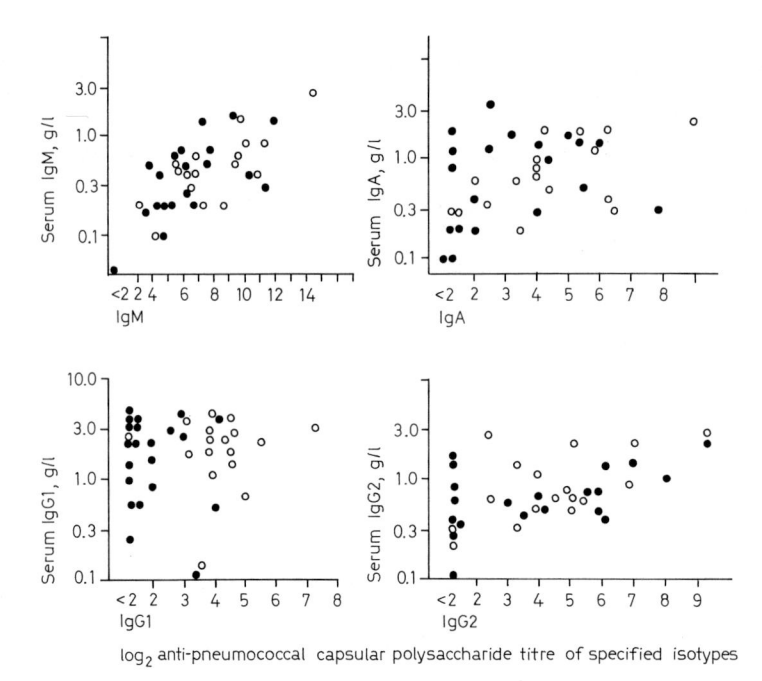

Fig. 1. Selective defect in levels of IgG1 and IgG2 antibody to pneumococcal capsular polysaccharides in patients with chronic lymphocytic leukaemia and splenomegaly. ● = Patients with palpable splenomegaly; ○ = patients without palpable splenomegaly. The levels shown are those in patients who have not been immunised with polyvalent vaccine against pneumococcal capsular polysaccharides. The total serum immunoglobulin class and subclass levels were measured as described in [30]. The class and subclass anti-pneumococcal capsular polysaccharide antibody levels were determined by solid-phase radio-immunoassay using Microwell plates coated with a mixture of capsular polysaccharides as described in ref. [26].

Table I. Characteristics of different classes of antigen

Antigen type	Chemical nature of core structure of most antigens of type	Site of activation	B cells activated	Typical immunoglobulin class and subclass profile (rat)	Response in infancy
TD in period immediately following exposure to antigen	polypeptide	secondary lymphoid organs outside follicles	newly produced virgin B cells and recirculating B cells	IgM IgA IgG2a = IgG1 > IgG2b > IgG2c	yes
TD after onset antibody production	polypeptide	secondary lymphoid organs in follicles	recirculating B cells	IgA IgG2a = IgG1 > IgG2b > IgG2c	yes
TI-1	lipopolysaccharide	adjacent to macrophages	? but includes a high proportion of newly produced virgin B cells	IgM IgA IgG2b > IgG2c > IgG1 = Ig2a	yes
TI-2	polysaccharide	marginal zones	marginal zone B cells	IgM IgA IgG2c > IgG2b > IgG1 > IgG2a	no

subclass genes, for this would imply a duplication of genes for which there is no evidence. However, studies of the cellular basis of antibody responses to different classes of antigen do point to ways in which defects of the sort listed above may occur.

The Main Classes of Antigen

Three main types of antigen have been identified. Congenitally athymic rats and mice have provided a means for identifying antigens which can induce antibody production in the absence of T cell help [5]. These T-cell-independent (TI) antigens in turn have been subclassified using two criteria: (a) the time during ontogeny when an antibody response can first be elicited, and (b) the ability of a TI antigen to evoke specific antibody production in CBA/N mice [6, 7]. (CBA/N mice have an X-linked immunodeficiency associated with poor or absent responses to certain TI antigens.) Responses in CBA/N mice and perinatal or even fetal responses in normal rodents are a feature of TI-1 antigens. Conversely, TI-2 antigens provoke little or no antibody production in CBA/N mice and are associated with poor antibody responses in early post-natal life in normal animals. Analysis of the immunoglobulin class and IgG subclass profiles evoked in mice and rats by T-cell-dependent (TD), TI-1 and TI-2 antigens shows distinct characteristics for each type of antigen. This is summarised in table I.

The classification of antigens based on rodent studies appears to be reflected in antibody responses in man. For example, the capacity to mount humoral immune responses to many bacterial capsular polysaccharides, which are TI-2 antigens, postdates the capacity to respond to either TD or TI-1 antigens by several months [8, 9].

Microenvironments Associated with B Cell Activation

Analysis of the cellular basis for B cell activation, by the three types of antigen described above, identifies 4 microenvironments where B cells are activated in vivo. Of these, two are associated with TD antibody responses [10, 11], the others with TI responses [12].

T-Cell-Dependent B Cell Activation

TD antibody responses appear to involve two distinct microenvironments where B cell activation occurs at different stages in these responses. These stages are: (a) during the few days which immediately follow exposure to antigen, be it primary or secondary exposure, and (b) throughout the established phase of TD antibody responses which may persist for many months. These two microenvironments are within secondary lymphoid organs; one is outside follicles, the other within follicles themselves.

Extrafollicular B Cell Activation. B cell activation, in periods when there has been recent exposure to antigen, seems likely to occur in secondary lymphoid organs, in extrafollicular sites rich in T cells, B cells and interdigitating cells. This stage in the response is associated with activation of both virgin B cells recently produced in the bone marrow and B cells of the recirculating peripheral pool [10]. (Virgin B cells are cells which have never been induced to proliferate by antigen or an agent mimicking antigen. Memory B cells have been formed following antigen-driven B cell proliferation.) This double recruitment has been demonstrated in immune responses in chimaeras constructed between rats differing in κ-immunoglobulin light chain allotype [11]. The donor and recipient origin of transferred B cells and the antibody secreted by plasma cells derived from these can be determined using this system. In these experiments, non-immunised recipient rats were depleted of mature peripheral B cells but their primary B lymphopoietic capacity was retained. They were reconstituted with congenic thoracic duct lymphocytes containing mature recirculating T and B but lacking haemopoietic stem cells. If donor cells were taken from rats primed and boosted with a TD antigen, chimaeras produced antibody of both donor and recipient allotypes in the early phase after challenge with the same antigen. During this period the isotype profile of antibody produced by donor and recipient cells included IgM as well as IgG and IgA [11]; i.e. in the period immediately following antigen administration newly produced virgin B cells (inevitably of host origin) were activated in competition with highly educated donor B cells. Also both the memory and virgin B cells produced IgM as well as other immunoglobulin classes. Analysis of the location of antibody-producing cells in this early stage suggests that this is mainly in the lymphoid organ where B cell activation has taken place [13]. Plasma cells at this stage in the response have a life-span of less than 3 days [14]. The features of extrafollicular B cell activation by TD antigens is summarised in table I.

Follicular B Cell Activation. In the established phase of TD antibody responses the same experimental system has shown that the response is maintained by continued reactivation of memory B cells. Very little recruitment of virgin B cells occurs during this period and memory clones remain dominant, at least for many months [11]. It is during this phase of TD antibody responses that affinity maturation of the antibody response occurs as a result of somatic mutation in active B cell clones [10]. This is not seen in association with B cell activation in other sites. IgM production is no longer a feature of the antibody response during this phase and antibody production has shifted from local to distant sites; mainly the bone marrow and intestinal lamina propria [13]. The life-span of the plasma cells is now in excess of 3 weeks [14]. It is possible to show by transfer experiments that B cell activation in the established response is dependent upon the continued presence of antigen. The most obvious source of long-term antigen is that localised on the follicular dendritic cells in B cell follicles [15, 16]. The features of this established phase of TD antibody responses are set out in table I.

T-Cell-Independent Antibody Responses

B Cell Activation by TI-1 Antigens. Many but not all antigens which fall into this class are based upon bacterial lipopolysaccharides. They can be shown to activate B cells in vitro from foetal liver and from bone marrow [17]. Analysis of these responses have shown that B cell activation by lipopolysaccharides requires signals derived from accessory cells [18]. These can be derived from macrophages, which also have receptors for lipopolysaccharide, but T-cell-derived B cell growth factors may also be effective co-factors in some situations. Lipopolysaccharide receptors are only found on a proportion of B cells and the level of expression of these receptors is subject to considerable genetic variation [19]. The features of TI-1 activation of B cells are summarised in table I.

B Cell Activation by TI-2 Antigens

While it is plausible that TI-1 antigens are bypassing the requirement for T cell help, this seems an unlikely explanation for the mechanism of activation by TI-2 antigens. For in some situations where TD B cell activation can be achieved TI-2 responses are not elicited. This applies both in CBA/N mice and in human infants during the first months of life. It seems reasonable to postulate under these circumstances that: either the B cells responding to TI-2 antigens differ from those responding to TD antigens, or that a distinct accessory signal is required which can only be evoked at a relatively late stage in ontogeny. Available evidence suggests that both of these may apply.

The best candidate accessory cell in TI-2 responses is a dendritic cell found in the marginal zone of the spleen which selectively localises neutral polysaccharides [20]. Analysis of responses to TI-2 antigens suggests that it is likely that the B cells responding to these antigens are located in the marginal zones of the spleen and equivalent sites in other secondary lymphoid organs [12, 21]. While much of the evidence for this is indirect, recent studies from our laboratory show it is most unlikely that either recirculating follicular B cells or newly produced virgin B cells are participating in these responses [12].

Although neither recirculating follicular B cells nor newly produced virgin B cells seem to respond to TI-2 antigens, analysis of the origins of marginal zone B cells show that these are derived from recirculating B cells which in turn are derived from newly produced virgin B cells [22]; i.e. a single B cell can pass through a phase when it has the potential to be activated by TD antigens before it changes phenotype to become a cell which can respond to TI-2 antigens. Recently, we have shown that memory B cells generated in TD responses can become marginal zone B cells. This finding is particularly relevant to a report from Insel and Anderson [23], showing that immunisation of infants with the polyribosyl phosphate of *Haemophilus influenzae* type b conjugated to diphtheria toxoid (now a TD antigen) resulted subsequently in an enhanced response to the polyribosyl phosphate alone. The features of TI-2 activation of B cells in the marginal zones of the spleen are summarised in table I.

Suppression of IgG Production in TI Responses

Early descriptions of antibody responses to TI antigens suggested these were mainly confined to the IgM [5]. This is patently incorrect [24–26]. However, in some strains of mice certain TI antigens give rise only to an IgM response. An example of this is the response to $\alpha(1\rightarrow 6)$ Dextran in C57BL/6 mice. However, in congenitally athymic C57BL/6 nu/nu mice good IgG responses are obtained [27]. In this situation T cells are resulting in suppression of the IgG response. Similar effects have been seen in other strains of mice with other TI antigens [28].

Conclusions

This survey indicates considerable heterogeneity in the way in which B cells are activated to proliferate and differentiate to plasma cells in vivo. This heterogeneity reflects the type of antigen, the microenvironment in which activation occurs, as well as the stage in the immune response. Monoclonal antibodies against human B cells have now identified many of the B cell surface molecules which act as receptors through which B cells are activated [29]. The receptors on B cells found in different microenvironments vary. Also B cells can be activated through more than one pathway in the same microenvironment. We do not know the precise defects which operate in the dysgammaglobulinaemias. However, it is possible now to identify which B cells, accessory cells and microenvironments are likely to be involved in particular deficiencies.

References

1   Oxelius, V.-A.; Laurell, A.B.; Lundquist, B.; Gollebowska, H.; Axelsson, A.; Björkander, J.; Hanson, L.Å.: IgG subclasses in selective IgA deficiency: importance of IgG2-IgA deficiency. New Engl. J. Med. *304:* 1476 (1981).
2   Lane, P.J.L.; Mac Lennan, I.C.M.: Impaired IgG2 antipneumococcal antibody responses in patients with recurrent infection and normal IgG2 levels but no IgA. Clin. exp. Immunol. *65:* 427 (1986).
3   Ambrosino, D.M.; Siber, G.R.; Chilmonczyk, M.D.; Jernberg, J.B.; Finberg, R.W.: An immunodeficiency characterised by impaired antibody responses to polysaccharides. New Engl. J. Med. *316:* 790 (1987).
4   Briles, D.E.; Claflin, J.L.; Schroer, K.; Forman, C.: Mouse IgG3 antibodies are highly protective against intravenous infection with type 3 *Streptococcus pneumoniae.* Nature *294:* 88 (1981).
5   Basten, A.; Howard, J.E.: Thymus independence; in Davies, Carter, Contemporary topics in immunobiology, vol. 2, p. 265 (Plenum Press, New York 1973).
6   Mosier, D.E.; Zitron, I.M.; Mond, J.J.; Ahmed, A.; Scher, I.; Paul, W.E.: Surface immunoglobulin D as a functional receptor for a subclass of B lymphocytes. Immunol. Rev. *37:* 89 (1977).
7   Mosier, D.E.; Subbarao, B.: Thymus-independent antigens: complexity of B lymphocyte activation revealed. Immunol. Today *3:* 217 (1982).
8   Anderson, P.; Smith, D.H.; Ingram, D.L.; Wilkins, J.; Wehrle, P.F.; Howie, V.M.: Antibody to polyribophosphate of *Haemophilus influenzae* type b in infants and children: effect of immunisation with polyribophosphate. J. infect. Dis. *S36:* 357 (1977).

9 Cowan, M.J.; Amman, A.J.; Wara, D.W.; Howie, V.M.; Schultz, L.; Doyle, N.; Kaplan, M.: Pneumococcal polysaccharide immunisation in infants and children. Pediatrics 62: 721 (1978).
10 Mac Lennan, I.C.M.; Gray, D.: Antigen-driven selection of virgin and memory B cells. Immunol. Rev. 91: 61 (1986).
11 Gray, D.; Mac Lennan, I.C.M.; Lane, P.J.L.: Virgin B cell recruitment and the lifespan of memory clones during antibody responses to DNP-Hemocyanin. Eur. J. Immunol. 16: 641 (1986).
12 Lane, P.J.L.; Gray, D.; Mac Lennan, I.C.M.: Differences in recruitment of virgin B cells into antibody responses to thymus-dependent and thymus-independent type-2 antigens. Eur. J. Immunol. 16: 1569 (1986).
13 Benner, R.; Hijmans, W.; Haaijman, J.J.: The bone marrow: the major source of serum immunoglobulins, but still a neglected site of antibody formation. Clin. exp. Immunol. 46: 1 (1981).
14 Ho, F.; Lortan, J.E.; Mac Lennan, I.C.M.; Khan, M.: Distinct short-lived and long-lived antibody-producing cell populations. Eur. J. Immunol. 16: 1297 (1986).
15 Tew, J.G.; Mandel, T.E.: The maintenance and regulation of serum antibody levels: evidence indicating a role for antigen retained in lymphoid follicles. J. Immun. 120: 1063 (1978).
16 Tew, J.G.; Mandel. T.E.: Prolonged antigen half life in the lymphoid follicles of specifically immunised mice. Immunology 37: 69 (1979).
17 Kearney, J.F.; Lawton, A.R.: B lymphocyte differentiation induced by lipopolysaccharide. II. Response of fetal lymphocytes. J. Immun. 115: 677 (1975).
18 Corbel, C.; Melchers, F.: Requirement for macrophages or T cell-derived factors in the mitogenic stimulation of murine B cells by LPS. Eur. J. Immunol. 13: 528 (1983).
19 Glode, M.L.; Rosenstreich, D.L.: Genetic control of B cell activation by bacterial lipopolysaccharide is mediated by multiple distinct genes or alleles. J. Immun. 117: 2061 (1976).
20 Humphrey, J.H.; Grennan, D.: Different macrophage populations distinguished by means of fluorescent polysaccharides. Recognition and properties of marginal zone macrophages. Eur. J. Immunol. 11: 212 (1981).
21 Mac Lennan, I.C.M.; Gray, D.; Kumararatne, D.S.; Bazin, H.: The lymphocytes of the splenic marginal zones: a distinct B cell lineage. Immunol. Today 3: 305 (1982).
22 Kumararatne, D.S.; Mac Lennan, I.C.M.: Cells of the marginal zone of the spleen are lymphocytes derived from recirculating precursors. Eur. J. Immunol. 11: 865 (1981).
23 Insel, R.A.; Anderson, P.W.: Oligosaccharide-protein conjugate vaccines induce and prime for oligoclonal IgG antibody responses to the *Haemophilus influenzae* b capsular polysaccharide in human infants. J. exp. Med. 163: 262 (1986).
24 Slack, J.; Der Balian, G.P.; Nahm, M.; Davie, J.M.: Subclass restriction of murine antibodies. II. The IgG plaque forming cell response to thymus-independent type 1 and type 2 antigens in normal mice and mice expressing an X-linked immunodeficiency. J. exp. Med. 151: 853 (1980).
25 Gray, D.; Chassoux, D.; Mac Lennan, I.C.M.; Bazin, H.: Selective depression of thymus-independent anti-DNP antibody responses induced by adult but not neonatal splenectomy. Clin. exp. Med. 60: 78 (1985).

26 Oldfield, S.; Jenkins, S.; Yeoman, H.; Gray, D.; Mac Lennan, I.C.M.: Class and subclass anti-pneumococcal antibody responses in splenectomised patients. Clin. exp. Immunol. *61:* 664 (1985).
27 Struckmann, K.; Schuler, W.; Kolsch, E.: Regulation of isotype expression in the immune response to type-2 thymus-independent dextran antigens. Adv. exp. Biol. Med. *186:* 739 (1985).
28 Schuler, W.; Lehle, G.; Weiler, E.; Kolsch, E.: Immune response against the T-independent antigen α (1→3) dextran. 1. Demonstration of an unexpected IgG response in athymic and germ-free-raised enthymic BALB/c mice. Eur. J. Immunol. *12:* 120 (1982).
29 Ling, N.R.; Mac Lennan, I.C.M.; Mason, D.Y.: Analysis of the B cell and plasma cell panels; in McMichael et al., Leukocyte typing. III. White cell differentiation antigens (Oxford University Press, Oxford 1987).
30 Lowe, J.; Bird, P.; Hardie, D.; Jefferis, R.; Ling, N.R.: Monoclonal antibodies to determinants on human gamma chains: properties of antibodies showing subclass restriction or subclass specificity. Immunology *47:* 329 (1982).

I.C.M. Mac Lennan, MD, Department of Immunology, University of Birmingham Medical School, Birmingham, B15 2TJ (England)

Serum IgG Subclasses in Secondary Immunodeficiencies[1]

J.L. Preud'homme[a], *P. Aucouturier*[a], *A. Barra*[a], *F. Duarte*[a], *L. Intrator*[b], *C. Cordonnier*[c], *J.P. Vernant*[c], *D. Schulz*[d], *L.H. Noël*[e], *P. Lesavre*[e]

[a]Laboratory of Immunology and Immunopathology, CNRS UA 1172, University Hospital, Poitiers; [b]Laboratory of Hematology and Immunology, CHU Henri Mondor, Creteil; [c]Unit of Bone Marrow Transplantation, CHU Henri Mondor, Creteil; [d]Institut Merieux, Marcy l'Etoile; [e]Department of Nephrology and INSERM U 25, Necker Hospital, Paris, France

IgG subclass imbalance is the most frequent immunoglobulin (Ig) abnormality in primary immunodeficiency (ID) states. Subclass deficiencies predominantly affect IgG2 and IgG4. They may be observed as apparently selective deficiencies [1–6] or in various characterized ID syndromes: ataxia telangiectasia [7–10], 'selective' IgA deficiency [4, 11–15], Di George's syndrome, severe combined immunodeficiency syndrome (SCID) with abnormal expression of HLA class II antigens, SCID with present serum Ig, 'selective' IgM deficiency, chronic mucocutaneous candidiasis [4; and unpublished results]. The existence of subclass imbalances in hypoimmunoglobulinemic patients with common varied ID (CVID) has been long reported also [16]. In fact, in our experience in more than 50 CVID cases [4; and unpublished], subclass imbalance is the rule, with predominant deficiency of either IgG2 and IgG4 or, more rarely, IgG1 and IgG3.

In view of such a high incidence in primary ID, subclass deficiencies may be expected to occur in secondary ID also. We have indeed observed IgG2-IgG4 deficiency in HTLV-I positive T cell lymphoma and in the X-linked lymphoproliferative (Purtilo's) syndrome [4; and unpublished]. We also studied sera from 61 HIV-infected adult patients (lymphadenopathy syndrome [LAS], 46 cases, and acquired im-

---

[1] This work was supported in part by Ministère de l'Education Nationale (Direction de la Recherche) and by Fondation pour la Recherche Médicale.

mune deficiency syndrome [AIDS], 15 cases) and from 13 children. These data will not be discussed in length since they have been published recently [17]. Briefly, in spite of considerable variations from patient to patient, which were partly due to the occurrence of monoclonal IgG, it is clear that the IgG increase (much more marked in LAS than in AIDS and in Africans and Haitians than in Caucasians) mostly corresponded to an increase in IgG1 and IgG3. There was a significant negative correlation between IgG1 and IgG2 levels. Mean IgG2 and IgG4 levels were low, with a number of sera displaying levels of these two isotypes in the range of deficiencies observed in primary ID disorders. Subclass imbalance was especially striking in LAS patients with lymphoid interstitial pneumonitis. Some patients presented with recurrent pyogenic infections with no clear correlation with subclass levels.

We then investigated two other situations, namely glomerulonephritis and bone marrow transplantation. We have examined the subclass distribution of glomerular deposits of patients with idiopathic membranous nephropathy (MN) and antiglomerular basement membrane (a-GBM) nephritis [18]. By immunofluorescence with subclass specific monoclonal antibodies (Mab), a striking subclass restriction was observed in idiopathic MN, with glomerular deposits predominantly containing IgG4 (81% of the studied biopsies) and IgG1 (75%). In de novo MN, occuring after transplantation, the restriction was markedly different, with a predominance of IgG1 (100%) and IgG2 (69%). In a-GBM nephritis, the restriction was considerable also with deposits containing almost exclusively IgG1 (91%) and IgG4 (73%). The same restriction was observed for circulating anti-GBM antibodies detected by an indirect immunofluorescent assay on normal kidney sections. By contrast, IgG1, IgG2 and IgG3 deposits were identified in lupus proliferative glomerulonephritis. The finding of such striking subclass restrictions of the deposits led us to study serum levels.

As for bone marrow transplantation (BMT), it is well known that a combined cellular and humoral immunodeficiency affects patients after BMT, particularly those suffering from graft-versus-host disease (GVHD), and infections represent the most frequent cause of death in the early (<6 months) post-transplant period. Reconstitution is slow and a fair percentage of long-term survivors suffer severe and/or recurrent infections also. Serum Ig classes may be long depressed, for about one year for IgG and IgM and even longer for IgA. It appears to be a correlation between infections, Ig class deficiency and chronic GVHD [19, 20]. A frequent pathogen in patients with primary subclass deficiency is *Haemophilus influenzae* [3, 5, 6], whose major antigen is the capsular polysaccharide polyribosylribitolphosphate (PRP) in the case of *Haemophilus influenzae* type b (Hib) [21]. This is not surprising since IgG2 appears to be the predominant subclass of antibacterial carbohydrate antibodies [22-24]. The observation of a relatively high incidence of Hib pneumonia in our transplanted patients [25] led us to study serum IgG subclass and anti-PRP antibody levels in transplanted patients affected with Hib pneumonia. Sera from transplanted patients with other infections or without infections were studied as controls.

Patients and Methods

Patients

This study includes sera from 20 patients affected with idiopathic form of MN and 9 patients with a-GBM nephritis. These patients were selected on the basis of the absence of conditions known to be associated with MN, unequivocal clinicopathological conditions and clear-cut glomerular deposits.

The retrospective study of BMT deals with 96 sera collected before transplant and after BMT (follow-up 4-25 months, mean 13.2 months) from 31 patients who received a BMT (allogeneic in every case but one patient who had a syngeneic BMT) for the therapy of acute leukemia or chronic myeloid leukemia. These patients were classified according to the nature of their infections: (group I) 7 patients infected with extracellular bacteria, mostly Hib (compatible with impaired humoral immunity); (group II) 10 patients with viral and/or intracellular bacterial infections (suggestive of cellular immune defect); two further patients who suffered from pneumonia of unknown origin were included in this group because these infections are more likely to be caused by viruses; (group III) 5 patients with both types of infections, including Hib pneumonia in 2 cases, and (group IV) 7 patients free of infections. Chemotherapy regimens preceding the graft varied according to the type and staging of the leukemias and to the number of relapses. The conditioning regimen uniformly consisted of cyclophosphamide and total body irradiation. GVHD was diagnosed and graded according to usual criteria. Acute and chronic GVHD were observed in 4 and 4 cases in group I, 4 and 5 cases in group II and 2 and 3 cases in group III, respectively. Not a single patient in group IV suffered GVHD. In contrast, patients with repeated infections were affected with severe chronic GVHD.

Measurement of Immunoglobulin Class and Subclass Levels

Ig class levels were measured by laser nephelometry. IgG subclass levels were determined in coded samples by a competitive indirect immunoassay (ELISA) with Mab, as previously described [26, 27]. Normal adult values were established in a study of

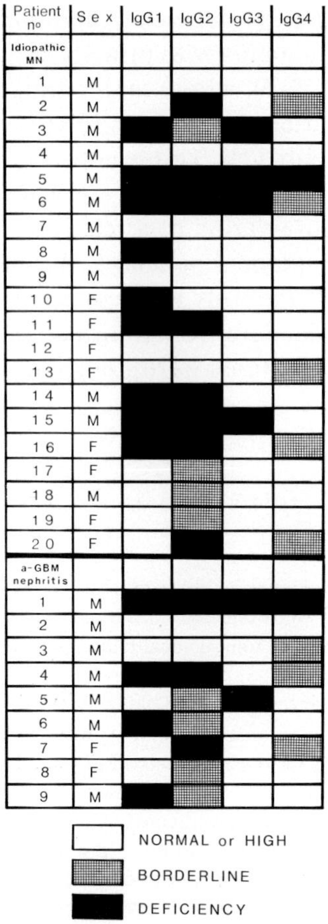

Fig. 1. IgG subclass levels in idiopathic MN and anti-GBM nephritis.

129–186 sera from normal blood donors aged 20–50 years. Values below or at the lower limit of the 95 percentile range of normal sera (i.e. 4.0, 0.6 and 0.18 mg/ml for IgG1, IgG2 and IgG3, respectively) will be mentioned below as subclass deficiencies. For IgG4, whose level differs according to sex, a 95 percentile range limit can be defined in men only (0.03 mg/ml). IgG2 and IgG4 display very heterogeneous distributions in healthy subjects and low normal values are likely to include deficiencies [27]. Borderline levels (<0.95 mg/ml for IgG2 and <0.01 mg/ml in both sexes for IgG4) will therefore be considered in the analysis.

Table I. Serum IgG subclass levels in glomerulonephritis (mean ± SD, mg/ml)

	Number	IgG1	IgG2	IgG3	IgG4
Idiopathic MN	20	5.17 ± 2.84	1.19 ± 0.92	0.32 ± 0.16	0.25 ± 0.25
a-GBM nephritis	9	4.52 ± 2.25	0.95 ± 0.66	0.41 ± 0.21	0.19 ± 0.22
Controls	129–186	6.43 ± 1.50	2.64 ± 1.36	0.42 ± 0.17	0.38 ± 0.39

Determination of Anti-PRP Antibody Levels

Anti-PRP antibodies (Ab) were measured in 79 sera from 28 BMT patients (mean follow-up 14.3 months) by ELISA using purified PRP [28] coupled to tyramine [29] (100 μl per well of PRP-tyramine [5 μg/ml of PRP] in phosphate-buffered saline [PBS]. After overnight incubation and washings, the plates were saturated for 1 h at 37 °C with 1% bovine serum albumin (BSA) in PBS containing 0.05% Tween 20. One half of every plate was treated identically except that PRP was replaced by PBS (blanks). Sera diluted ½₀ in 0.5% BSA containing PBS-Tween were incubated in triplicates in the PRP-coated and control wells. The plates were washed 6 times in PBS-Tween and revealed with class specific peroxidase-tagged goat antisera. Each ELISA plate contained standard positive and negative sera and, as a reproducibility test, 3 further known positive sera (interassay coefficients of variation were 9.8% for IgG Ab, 7.8% for IgA Ab and 11.3% for IgM Ab). For every sample, the experiment was repeated on the same plate with serum previously incubated for 45 min with high concentration (500 μg/ml) PRP. Results were expressed in arbitrary units calculated from specific (inhibited by PRP) OD in PRP-coated wells after deducting results on uncoated wells by comparison with the same data with the positive and negative standard sera.

Due to lack of material, the subclass distribution of IgG anti-PRP Ab could be studied in 4 patients only. These experiments were performed by a procedure similar to that described above except that bound anti-PRP Ab were revealed by subclass-specific Mab followed by peroxidase-coupled rabbit IgG antimouse IgG extensively absorbed with human IgG, as described in detail previously [30].

Results

Glomerulonephritis

As shown in figure 1, the predominant subclass decrease affected IgG2 (19 of 29 patients), and mean IgG2 levels in the two patient groups was significantly lower than in controls (p < 0.01, table I). Likely because of the nephrotic syndrome, 15 patients (every patient with low IgG1 levels and the a-GBM nephritis patients 5 and 7) had low total IgG levels. It is therefore interesting to consider the relative proportion of each subclass. By comparison with the distribution in normal subjects, clear-cut subclass imbalances made of significantly decreased proportions of IgG2 and of significant increase in the proportions of IgG1 and IgG3 were found in 10 patients. That these subclass imbalances could not be due to urinary loss is evidenced by their identical incidence in patients with (5 of 15 cases) and without (5 of 14 cases) hypogammaglobulinemia.

Long-Term Survivors after Bone Marrow Transplantation

Before transplant, several patients had low or borderline IgG2 (6 cases) and/or IgG4 (7 cases) levels. IgA and IgG3 were rarely depressed (2 and 1 case, respectively) whereas abnormally low IgM levels were noticed in 5 patients. None of these patients had any past history of abnormal infections. After BMT, we observed a strong tendency for certain isotypes to vary together: IgG1 and IgG3 showed a roughly parallel evolution in 68% of cases, IgG1 and IgM in 48% and IgG3 and IgM in 45%. On the other hand, roughly parallel evolution curves were observed for IgG2 and IgG4 (61% of cases), IgG2 and IgA (52%) and IgG4 and IgA (48%). In contrast, IgG1 and IgG2 varied in the opposite way in 61% of cases. Consequently, IgG2 and IgG4 levels were not rarely lower in late (more than one year after transplant) than in early samples. Subclass deficiencies or borderline levels at the end of follow-up predominantly affected IgG2 and IgG4, together with low or borderline IgA levels in 78% of cases (fig. 2). Quite unexpectedly, IgG2 levels at the end of the study appeared to be related to those before transplant: (1) all patients with low or borderline IgG2 before BMT had long-term IgG2 abnormalities; (2) all patients with normal IgG2 levels in the last studied sample also had normal IgG2 before transplant. However, certain patients with normal IgG2 levels before BMT had late IgG2 deficiency. The same tendency was observed for IgG4, although not as clear cut.

Study of the last studied samples (fig. 2) revealed long-term subclass deficiencies in the 3 groups of infected patients and not in noninfected patients except for IgG4 in one case. Every patient with an infection pattern compatible with both cellular and humoral immunodeficiency was subclass-deficient, with a maximum follow-up of 25 months. Borderline levels were observed in all patients groups, including noninfected subjects, in whom the incidence of complete recovery was the highest. Mean IgG1 and IgG3 levels were higher and IgG2

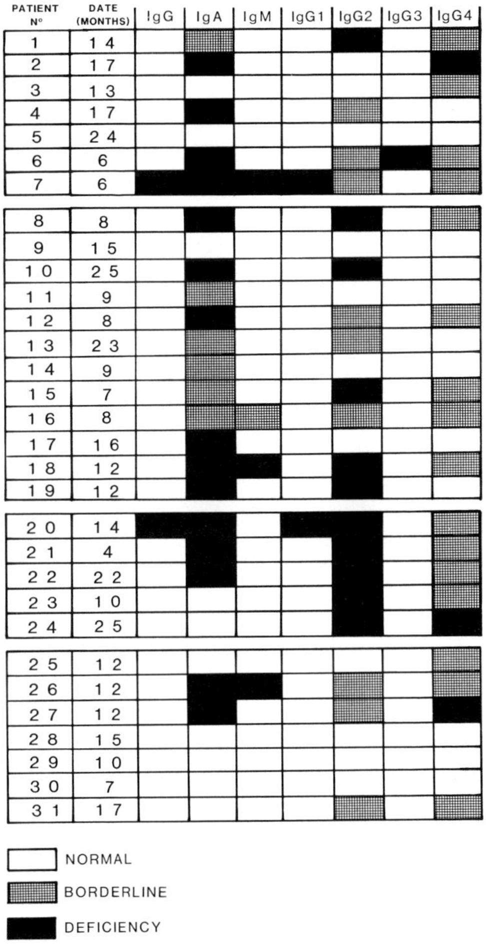

Serum IgG Subclasses in Secondary Immunodeficiencies

Fig. 2. Ig class and subclass levels in long-term survivors after BMT.

Table II. Serum IgG subclass levels in BMT patients[1] and controls (means ± SD, mg/ml)

	n	IgG1	IgG2	IgG3	IgG4
All patients					
Before graft	25	9.24 ± 3.63	2.12 ± 1.33	0.66 ± 0.59	0.39 ± 0.56
Last sample	31	11.49 ± 7.19	1.01 ± 0.77	0.58 ± 0.33	0.12 ± 0.12
Group I					
Before graft	7	7.21 ± 2.19	1.61 ± 1.05	0.37 ± 0.19	0.10 ± 0.08
Last sample	7	15.73 ± 11.77	0.98 ± 0.59	0.33 ± 0.14	0.08 ± 0.14
Group II					
Before graft	8	9.51 ± 3.08	2.70 ± 1.67	0.63 ± 0.35	0.78 ± 0.78
Last sample	12	10.63 ± 3.09	1.00 ± 0.80	0.58 ± 0.30	0.18 ± 0.16
Group III					
Before graft	3	13.60 ± 3.62	2.35 ± 1.24	1.29 ± 1.00	0.30 ± 0.20
Last sample	5	12.39 ± 7.07	0.33 ± 0.24	0.57 ± 0.21	0.06 ± 0.02
Group IV					
Before graft	7	9.07 ± 3.68	1.86 ± 0.77	0.73 ± 0.63	0.25 ± 0.35
Last sample	7	8.09 ± 2.63	1.54 ± 0.74	0.83 ± 0.38	0.08 ± 0.06
Normal adults	129–186	6.43 ± 1.50	2.64 ± 1.36	0.42 ± 0.17	0.46 ± 0.37 (men) 0.29 ± 0.40 (women)

[1] In the last studied sample, mean 13.2 months after transplant.

and IgG4 lower than in normal subjects, the lowest values for the two latter isotypes being in group III and the highest in group IV (table II). Serum collected close to infectious episodes was available in certain patients. Comparison with subclass levels in the sera from noninfected patients showed an incidence of subclass deficiency possibly but not significantly higher during infections. However, low and borderline subclass levels were found in noninfected patients also. Hence, the finding of subclass deficiency is not predictive of the occurrence of infection in individual cases. In accordance with previous studies, class deficiencies occurring late after BMT were observed predominantly in patients with chronic GVHD. In contrast, the incidence of subclass deficiency did not differ according to the presence or absence of acute or chronic GVHD. However, the patient who received a syngeneic graft is one of the only 2 patients in whom every isotype was at normal or high levels throughout the study.

Table III. Anti-PRP Ab levels in BMT patients and controls (units, means and ranges)

	n	IgG	n	IgA	n	IgM
BMT						
All patients						
Before graft	17	42.4 (4–131)	18	25.8 (3–70)	19	20.7 (3–77)
Last sample	27	17.0 (0–175)	25	11.6 (0–114)	25	9.1 (0–30)
H. influenzae						
Before graft[1]	6	39.8 (15–70)	6	29.2 (5–63)	7	23.6 (3–77)
Last sample	8	14.2 (2–34)	7	23.3 (0–114)	8	15.9 (1–30)
Other infections						
Before graft[1]	5	62.3 (13–131)	5	21.8 (3–64)	5	16.4 (4–34)
Last sample	12	21.3 (0–175)	11	4.2 (0–11)	11	5.2 (0–10)
No infection						
Before graft[1]	6	28.5 (4–56)	7	25.9 (3–70)	7	20.9 (7–51)
Last sample	7	13.0 (0–45)	7	11.6 (0–51)	7	7.1 (0–18)
N1 children						
12–25 months old	10	2.6 (0–10)	10	2.4 (0–12)	10	7.6 (2–15)
NHS pool[2]	1	60	1	21	1	21
Normal adults						
Before	5	34.8 (0–69)	5	31.8 (10–71)	3	29.0 (29–35)
3 weeks after vaccination	5	113.0 (36–235)	5	168.8 (39–323)	5	73.4 (44–100)

[1] Patients with IgG2 deficiency excluded.
[2] Normal human sera from 60 adult blood donors.

Six of 9 patients affected with Hib pneumonia had abnormally low or borderline serum IgG2 levels, an incidence which is not different from that observed in the other cases. Before transplant, two of these patients who had low IgG2 also had low anti-PRP Ab levels, but mean Ab levels before graft, calculated excluding patients with IgG2 deficiency, were similar in the different patients groups and comparable to those in normal adults (table III). We studied anti-PRP Ab at the moment of Hib pneumonia in only one patient and their levels were low although IgG2 was in the normal range. After Hib infection, IgG anti-PRP Ab remained low or kept decreasing except in 2 patients in whom (in spite of low IgG2 levels) they reached levels comparable to those in normal subjects without known Hib infection. Therefore, mean IgG anti-PRP Ab level is not higher in patients infected with Hib than in the other patients (table III). Subclass distribution of the Ab after Hib pneumonia was examined in a serum containing subthreshold levels of IgG2 and low but detectable IgG anti-PRP Ab. Two thirds of these Ab belonged to the IgG1 subclass and one third to IgG2. A moderate increase in IgM and IgA Ab was observed just after the pneumonia in 4 and 3 cases, respectively. A strong IgA response featured one case. Consequently, mean IgM and IgA Ab levels after Hib infection were similar to normal subject levels (table III).

Most patients without known Hib infection had low anti-PRP Ab of the three classes, the latest samples studied often showing the lowest values. A number of sera collected after one year contained no detectable Ab or levels similar to those in young children (table III), with some exceptions. A patient had high Ab levels before transplant and one year later in spite of a very low IgG2 level. However, anti-PRP Ab in this serum were restricted to IgG2 (95% of the Ab). Two other sera with fair Ab and low IgG2 levels were studied for subclass distribution and the Ab were equally distributed in the IgG1 and IgG2 isotypes. The correlation between IgG2 and anti-PRP Ab in the whole study, although significant ($p < 0.05$), was weak ($r = 0.23$)

Discussion

IgG subclass imbalance is a very common feature of primary ID states. The present study clearly shows that the same patterns of subclass abnormalities (predominantly IgG2-IgG4 deficiency) are frequently encountered in secondary ID since it was observed in virus (HTLV-I and EBV)-induced lymphoproliferations, in AIDS and related disorders, and in treated leukemic patients as a probable consequence of chemotherapy (it was often associated with IgM deficiency which is well known to be induced by chemotherapy), in glomerulonephritis and in long-term survivors after BMT. In the latter situation, IgG2-IgG4 deficiencies, often associated with low IgA levels, frequently developed late after transplant, while IgM, IgG1 and IgG3 and total IgG had reached normal or high levels. Indeed, IgG2, IgG4 and IgA often showed a parallel evolution whereas IgG1, IgG3 and

IgM tended to vary together in the opposite way. This, together with the evolution of subclass levels in childhood, the results in primary ID mentioned above, the well-known differences with respect to Ab specificity and with studies of in vitro B cell maturation [31–33], is compatible with the hypothesis of different regulation of IgG1-IgG3 and IgG2-IgG4 expression. Experimental work in the mouse [34, 35] favors the hypothesis that the expression of the isotypes whose genes are located downstream in the C_H locus (as IgG2 and IgG4 do in man) requires more T cell help than does control of upstream isotypes. The finding of IgG2-IgG4 deficiency in ID syndromes featuring impaired T-B cell cooperation is in keeping with this hypothesis [4]. Although bacterial polysaccharides are T-independent antigens, antipolysaccharide Ab production is highly dependent on T cell regulation [36]. It is therefore likely that both subclass and anti-PRP Ab deficiencies in BMT result from abnormal T cell function. Cells from five of the present patients were studied for in vitro suppressor activity and there was no correlation between excessive suppressor activity and the present findings. Impaired helper function is therefore likely to play a major role. GVHD is a significant factor in the occurrence of infections and of Ig class deficiency. In contrast, we observed an incidence of subclass deficiency similar in patients with and without GVHD. However, the finding of fully normal Ig levels throughout the study was exceptional and concerned virtually only the patient who received a syngeneic transplant. Therefore, that clinically undetectable GVHD might play a role in the pathogenesis of subclass deficiencies can be envisaged. Although both the mean subclass levels and incidence of subclass deficiencies differed according to the infection patterns, certain patients free of infections had low or borderline subclass levels, whereas some infected patients had normal levels at the period of infectious episodes. The explanation of the occurrence of infections is therefore more complex than a mere subclass deficiency, even in patients with Hib pneumonia. Anti-PRP Ab defect might play a role since we observed low levels just before pneumonia in a patient with normal IgG2 level and since there was a very poor IgG Ab response after pneumonia. The situation after BMT can be compared to that in IgA deficiency and ataxia telangiectasia where recent work using Mab [4, 10, 15, 37] failed to confirm the correlation between subclass deficiency and infections previously reported in studies of subclass levels performed with polyclonal Ab and where impaired Ab response to bacterial polysaccharides was demonstrated in infected patients with normal subclass levels [38]. Humoral immunodeficiency thus probably plays a role in the genesis of infections observed in BMT recipients and substitutive or prophylactic IgG therapy could possibly be indicated. On the other hand, the high incidence of Hib pneumonia in our series and the defective anti-PRP Ab response raise the questions of the indication and timing of vaccination in transplanted patients. In such a case, a protein-conjugate PRP vaccine should be used since it is effective in IgG2-deficient patients who do not respond to PRP alone [39].

In glomerulonephritis, the subclass restriction of glomerular deposits led us to measure serum subclass levels. We observed mean low IgG2 levels, with a pattern of selective IgG2 deficiency in certain patients and clear imbalance (low IgG2 and high IgG1-IgG3 proportions) in 10 cases. Such subclass imbalances could not be due to urinary loss since they were present both in normo- and in hypoimmunoglobulinemic patients, and since it has been shown that in most proteinuric patients IgG subclasses appeared in the urine in proportions similar to their relative concentrations in the serum [40]. The low IgG2 level may be related to a certain state of immune defect as already observed in vitro in patients with idiopathic MN [41]. Such a defect might be primary or secondary to the glomerular disease. In the first hypothesis, it is conceivable that low IgG2 levels might indicate a proneness to bacterial infections that might play a role in the occurrence of idiopathic MN and a-GBM nephritis.

References

1 Schur, P.H.; Borel, H.; Gelfand, E.D.; Alper, C.A.; Rosen, F.S.: Selective gammaglobulin deficiencies in patients with recurrent pyogenic infections. New Engl. J. Med. *283:* 631 (1970).
2 Oxelius, V.A.: Chronic infections in a family with hereditary deficiency of IgG2 and IgG4. Clin. exp. Immunol. *17:* 19 (1974).
3 Oxelius, V.A.: IgG subclasses and human disease. Am. J. Med. *76:* 7 (1984).
4 Aucouturier, P.; Bremard-Oury, C.; Clauvel, J.P.; Debré, M.; Griscelli, C.; Seligmann, M.; Preud'homme, J.L.: Serum IgG subclass levels in primary and acquired immunodeficiency; in Hanson, Söderström, Oxelius, Immunoglobulin subclass deficiencies. Monogr. Allergy, vol. 20, p. 62 (Karger, Basel 1986).
5 Bremard-Oury, C.; Aucouturier, P.; Debré, M.; Preud'homme, J.L.; Griscelli, C.: Immunoglobulin G subclasses in patients with immunodeficiencies; in Hanson,

Söderström, Oxelius, Immunoglobulin subclass deficiencies. Monogr. Allergy, vol. 20, p. 75 (Karger, Basel 1986).

6   Shackelford, P.G.; Polmar, S.H.; Mayus, J.L.; Johnson, W.L.; Corry, J.M.; Nahm, M.H.: Spectrum of IgG2 subclass deficiency in children with recurrent infections: prospective study. J. Pediat. *108:* 647 (1986).

7   Rivat-Peran, L.; Buriot, D.; Salier, J.P.; Rivat, C.; Dumitresco, S.M.; Griscelli, C.: Immunoglobulins in ataxia-telangiectasia: evidence for IgG4 and IgA2 subclass deficiencies. Clin. Immunol. Immunopathol. *20:* 99 (1981).

8   Oxelius, V.A.; Berkel, A.I.; Hanson, L.A.: IgG2 deficiency in ataxia telangiectasia. New Engl. J. Med. *306:* 515 (1982).

9   Berkel, A.I.: Studies of IgG subclasses in ataxia telangiectasia patients; in Hanson, Söderström, Oxelius, Immunoglobulin subclass deficiencies. Monogr. Allergy, vol. 20, p. 100 (Karger, Basel 1986).

10 Aucouturier, P.; Brémard-Oury, C.; Griscelli, C.; Berthier, M.; Preud'homme, J.L.: Serum IgG subclass deficiency in ataxia telangiectasia. Clin. exp. Immunol. *68:* 392 (1987).

11 Oxelius, V.A.; Laurell, A.B.; Lindquist, B.; Golebiowska, H.; Axelsson, U.; Björkander, J.; Hanson, L.Å.: IgG subclass in selective IgA deficiency. New Engl. J. Med. *304:* 1476 (1981).

12 Ugazio, A.G.; Out, T.A.; Plebani, A.; Duse, M.; Monafo, V.; Nespoli, L.; Burgio, G.R.: Recurrent infections in children with 'selective' IgA deficiency: association with IgG2 and IgG4 deficiency; in Wedgwood, Rosen, Paul, Primary immunodeficiency disease, Birth Defects, Orig. Article Ser., No. 19, p. 169 (Liss, New York 1983).

13 Cunningham-Rundles, C.; Oxelius, V.A.; Good, R.A.: IgG2 and IgG3 subclass deficiencies in selective IgA deficiency in the United States; in Wedgwood, Rosen, Paul, Primary immunodeficiency diseases. Birth Defects, Orig. Article Ser., No. 19, p. 173 (Liss, New York 1983).

14 Skvaril, F.; Scherz, R.: IgG subclasses in IgA deficient patients with anti-IgA antibodies; in Hanson, Söderström, Oxelius, Immunoglobulin subclass deficiencies. Monogr. Allergy, vol. 20, p. 164 (Karger, Basel 1986).

15 Plebani, A.; Monafo, V.; Avanzini, A.A.; Ugazio, G.; Burgio, R.: Relationship between IgA and IgG subclass deficiencies: a reappraisal; in Hanson, Söderström, Oxelius, Immunoglobulin subclass deficiencies. Monogr. Allergy, vol. 20, p. 171 (Karger, Basel 1986).

16 Yount, W.J.; Hong, R.; Seligmann, M.; Good, R.A.; Kunkel, H.J.: Imbalances of gammaglobulin subgroups and gene defects in patients with primary hypogammaglobulinaemia. J. clin. Invest. *49:* 1957 (1970).

17 Aucouturier, P.; Couderc, L.J.; Gouet, D.; Danon, F.; Gombert, J.; Matheron, S.; Saimot, A.G.; Clauvel, J.P.; Preud'homme, J.L.: Serum immunoglobulin G subclass dysbalances in the lymphadenopathy syndrome and acquired immune deficiency syndrome. Clin. exp. Immunol. *63:* 234 (1986).

18 Noël, L.H.; Aucouturier, P.; Monteiro, R.C.; Preud'homme, J.L.; Lesavre, P.: Glomerular and serum immunoglobulin G subclasses in membranous nephropathy and anti-glomerular basement membrane nephritis. Clin. Immunobiol. Immunopathol. (in press).

19 Storb, R.; Thomas, E.D.: Allogeneic bone marrow transplantation. Immunol. Rev. *71:* 77 (1983).

20 Witherspoon, R.P.; Lum, L.G.; Storb, R.: Immunologic reconstitution after human marrow grafting. Semin. Hematol. *21:*2 (1984).
21 Lagergard, T.; Nylen, O.; Sandberg, T.; Trollfors, B.: Antibody responses to capsular polysaccharide, lipopolysaccharide, and outer membrane in adults infected with *Haemophilus influenzae* type b. J. clin. Microbiol. *20:*1154 (1984).
22 Yount, W.J.; Dorner, N.M.; Kunkel, H.G.; Kabat, E.A.: Studies on human antibodies. IV. Selective variations in subgroup composition and genetic markers. J. exp. Med. *127:*633 (1968).
23 Siber, G.R.; Schur, P.H.; Aisenberg, A.C.; Weitzman, S.A.; Schiffman, G.: Correlation between serum IgG2 concentration and the antibody response to bacterial polysaccharide antigens. New Engl. J. Med. *303:*178 (1980).
24 Bird, P.; Lowe, J.; Stokes, R.P.; Bird, A.G.; Ling, N.R.; Jefferis, R.: The separation of human serum IgG into subclass fractions by immunoaffinity chromatography and assessment of specific antibody activity. J. immunol. Methods *71:*91 (1984).
25 Cordonnier, G.; Bernaudin, J.F.; Bierling, P.; Huet, Y.; Vernant, J.P.: Pulmonary complications occurring after allogeneic bone marrow transplantation. A study of 130 consecutive transplanted patients. Cancer *58:*1047 (1986).
26 Aucouturier, P.; Danon, F.; Daveau, M.; Guillou, B.; Sabbah, A.; Besson, J.; Preud'homme, J.L.: Measurement of serum IgG4 levels by a competitive immunoenzymatic assay with monoclonal antibodies. J. immunol. Methods *74:*151 (1984).
27 Aucouturier, P.; Mounir, S.; Preud'homme, J.L.: Distribution of IgG subclass levels in normal adult sera as determined by a competitive enzyme immunoassay using monoclonal antibodies. Diagn. Immunol. *3:*191 (1985).
28 Anderson, P.; Smith, D.H.: Isolation of the capsular polysaccharide from culture supernatant of *Haemophilus influenzae* type b. Infect. Immunity *15:*472 (1977).
29 Anthony, B.F.; Concepcion, N.F.; McGeary, S.A.; Ward, J.I.; Heiner, D.C.; Shapshak, P.; Insel, R.A.: Immunospecificity and quantitation of an enzyme-linked immunosorbent assay for group B streptococcal antibody. J. clin. Microbiol. *16:*350 (1982).
30 Barra, A.; Aucouturier, P.; Preud'homme, J.L.: Isotypic distribution of human anti-thyroglobulin IgG antibodies: methodological difficulties. Diagn. Immunol. *4:*228 (1986).
31 Mayumi, M.; Kuritani, T.; Kubagawa, H.; Cooper, M.D.: IgG subclass expression by human lymphocytes and plasma cells: B lymphocyte precommitted to IgG subclass can be preferentially induced by polyclonal mitogens with T cell help. J. Immun. *130:*671 (1983).
32 Walker, L.; Johnson, G.D.; MacLennan, I.C.M.: The IgG subclass response of human lymphocytes to B-cell activators. Immunology *50:*269 (1983).
33 Le Thi Bich-Thuy, Revillard, J.P.: Modulation of polyclonally activated human peripheral B cells by aggregated IgG and IgG-binding factors: differential effect on IgG subclass synthesis. J. Immun. *133:*544 (1984).
34 Martinez-Alonso, C.; Couthino, A.; Andrei, A.A.: Immunoglobulin C-gene expression. 1. The commitment of IgG subclass of secretory cells is determined by the quality of the nonspecific stimuli. Eur. J. Immunol. *10:*698 (1980).
35 Mongini, P.K.A.; Paul, W.E.; Metcalf, E.S.: T cell regulation of immunoglobulin class expression in the antibody response to trinitrophenyl-Ficoll. Evidence for T cell enhancement of the immunoglobulin class switch. J. exp. Med. *155:*884 (1982).

36 Khater, M.; Macai, I.; Genyea, C.; Kaplan, J.: Natural killer cell regulation of age-related and type-specific variations in antibody responses to pneumococcal polysaccharides. J. exp. Med. *164:* 1505 (1986).
37 Out, T.A.; Van Munster, P.J.J.; De Graeff, P.A.; The, T.H.; Vossen, J.M.; Zegers, B.J.M.: Immunological investigations in individuals with selective IgA deficiency. Clin. exp. Immunol. *64:* 510 (1986).
38 Lane, P.J.L.; MacLennan, I.C.M.: Impaired IgG2 anti-pneumococcal antibody responses in patients with recurrent infection and normal IgG2 levels but no IgA. Clin. exp. Immunol. *65:* 427 (1986).
39 Insel, R.A.; Anderson, P.W.: Response to oligosaccharide-protein conjugate vaccine against *Hemophilus influenzae* in two patients with IgG2 deficiency unresponsive to capsular polysaccharide vaccine. New Engl. J. Med. *315:* 499 (1986).
40 Shakib, F.; Hardwicke, J.; Stanworth, D.R.; White, R.H.R.: Asymetric depression in the serum levels of IgG subclasses in patients with nephrotic syndrome. Clin. exp. Immunol. *28:* 506 (1977).
41 Ooi, B.S.; Ooi, Y.M.; Hsu, A.; Hurtubise, P.E.: Diminished synthesis of immunoglobulin by peripheral lymphocytes of patients with idiopathic membranous glomerulopathy. J. clin. Invest. *65:* 789 (1980).

J.L. Preud'homme, MD, Laboratory of Immunology and Immunopathology, CNRS UA 1172, Poitiers University Hospital, F-86021 Poitiers (France)

IgG Subclass Distribution of Antibody Induced by Immunization with the Isolated and Protein-Conjugated Polysaccharide of *H. influenzae* b and G2m(n) Distribution of Serum IgG2 in Man[1]

Richard A. Insel, Porter W. Anderson

Departments of Pediatrics and Microbiology, University of Rochester School of Medicine and Dentistry, Rochester, N.Y., USA

Introduction

Haemophilus influenzae b (Hib) is the most common cause of meningitis and an important cause of childhood systemic infections in the USA. The major virulence determinant of the bacteria is its capsular polysaccharide (CP), and antibody to the CP is the major specificity of antibody protective against this bacterial infection. The purified isolated CP is immunogenic in adults, but is poorly immunogenic in children until about 2 years of age, and fails to induce antibody in older children to a titer attained in adults until age 4–5 [1]. To accelerate maturation of antibody responsiveness to the CP in infants, we have prepared protein-conjugated CP vaccines in which oligosaccharides prepared from the CP are covalently linked by reductive amination to diphtheria toxoid or mutant forms of diphtheria toxin [2, 3]. These conjugate vaccines induce antibody to the CP, booster responses with repetitive immunization, and a predominant IgG antibody response [2–4]. In addition, immunization of the young infant with conjugate vaccine accelerates maturation of antibody responsiveness to immunization with the isolated CP [3, 4]. The antibody induced by these conjugates in the young infant has in vitro functional activity against the

---

[1] Supported by grants AI 17217 and AI 17938 from the National Institute of Allergy and Infectious Diseases. The authors are indebted to Ann Kittelberger and Elides Marin for technical assistance, and to Pam Iadarola for secretarial assistance.

bacteria that suggests that it would confer protection against systemic Hib disease.

The CP is a repetitive polymer of ribosyl-ribitol phosphate in which the two sugars are in a 1-1 linkage. We have shown that antibody induced by immunization with this CP in the healthy adult is of high, but variable, magnitude, reaching a geometric mean postimmunization antibody titer of 33 µg/ml, predominately of the IgG isotype, and persists at over 50% of the peak postimmunization titer for at least 2 years after immunization [5]. The antibody response is highly restricted in diversity. Most, but not all, individuals have antibody with predominantly or exclusively κ light chain type [5]. Second, the IgG antibody repertoire has a highly restricted analytical isoelectric focusing profile. Most individuals express only 2–3 antibody clonotypes or spectrotypes [6]. Dominant clonotypes observed at one month after immunization persist as the dominant clonotype for years after immunization. In addition, genetically unrelated individuals share identical clonotypes [6]. These findings suggest that only a few germ-line immunoglobulin variable region genes code for this antibody in a single individual as well as in the population. The conjugated CP induces a higher magnitude total and IgG antibody response in both adults and children, but the IgG antibody repertoire remains approximately as restricted as that induced by the isolated CP [4, 6]. The booster antibody responses that occur in the infant with repetitive conjugate immunization is primarily due to the augmented expression of clonotypes induced by earlier immunization and less commonly from expression of new clonotypes [4].

IgG Subclass Distribution of Antibody

The existence of two forms of this CP, isolated and protein-conjugated, that can be safely injected into man and that induce a restricted antibody response provides an excellent system to study human IgG subclass expression. In several species, polysaccharides induce a unique IgG subclass response – IgG3 in the mouse [7], IgG2c in the rat [8] and, putatively, IgG2 in man [9]. The previous statement is somewhat controversial because several exceptions have been described. A major contribution from IgG1 has been observed in human antibody responses to several polysaccharides. We have analyzed the IgG subclass distribution of antibody induced by the isolated CP and the protein-conjugated CP in adults and the young infant to determine whether differences in IgG subclass expression can be attributed to the form of a polysaccharide or the age of the immunized subject.

IgG subclass antibody to the type b CP was quantified by enzyme-linked immunosorbent assay (ELISA) using derivatized antigen [10], and monoclonal antibody NL16 and HP6014 to IgG1 and IgG2, respectively, as described [11]. Monoclonal antibody was detected with a labelled goat antimouse antibody without human reactivity. The assay was standardized by comparing the binding of homologous subclass-specific monoclonal antibody or IgG-isotype-specific monoclonal antibody to human hybridoma antibodies of different IgG subclass produced in our laboratory [11–13]. Cord serum with maternal postimmunization antibody of only the IgG1 and IgG2 subclass [14] was used to quantify the assay by assigning an antibody value based on comparison to the USFDA serum standard in a radioantigen binding assay, and determining its relative IgG1 and IgG2 distribution by ELISA based on the relative activity of the monoclonal antibodies as determined above.

Children immunized at approximately 2, 4, and 6 months of age with the *H. influenzae* CP conjugate vaccines produce a predominate IgG isotype antibody response [15]. This response is apparent in most children after the second immunization and in most of the nonresponders after the third immunization. Booster IgG antibody responses are seen in most repetitively immunized children that are accompanied primarily by augmentation of clonotypes that were expressed after the primary injection and secondarily by expression of new clonotypes [4]. The IgG subclass distribution of antibody induced at this age with conjugates is predominately, and in many children exclusively, the IgG1 subclass (IgG1/IgG2 ratio of 9.4; table I) [16]. Two separate immunizations with conjugate of children at 12–14 months of age or one immunization at 16–23 months of age also induces an IgG1-predominant subclass antibody response (table I) [16]. The 16- to 23-month-old children immunized produce a higher magnitude IgG1 response with an IgG1/IgG2 ratio of 45. The IgG and IgG1 antibody response in the older children is induced with fewer injections and is accompanied by a higher IgG1/IgG2 ratio. None of the 46 children immunized at different ages with conjugates show an IgG2 predominant antibody response.

Table I. IgG subclass distribution of antibody to the *H. influenzae* b capsular polysaccharide induced by protein-conjugated polysaccharide (Conj.) priming and reimmunization with the isolated polysaccharide (PRP)

Conj. priming							PRP						
months	n	antibody (µg/ml), GM ± 1 SD			IgG1/IgG2	%IgG2, >IgG1	months	n	antibody (µg/ml), GM ± 1 SD			IgG1/IgG2	%IgG2, >IgG1
		IgG1	IgG2						IgG1	IgG2			
2–7	19	3.2 (0.81–13)	0.34 (0.16–0.74)		9.4	0	12–13	10	6.7 (1.7–25)	1.8 (0.30–11)		3.7	25
12–14	12	16 (2.4–100)	1.2 (0.36–3.9)		13	0	24–26	12	58 (28–120)	17 (5.2–54)		3.4	25
	–	–	–		–	–	24–26	17	4.1 (0.67–25)	1.1 (0.26–4.7)		3.7	12
	–	–	–		–	–	adults	52	11.05 (2.8–44)	12.75 (2.7–60)		0.88	42
16–23	15	27 (5.8–124)	0.59 (0.12–2.8)		45	0							

As discussed above, the children primed with conjugate vaccine acquire the ability to respond to immunization with the isolated CP at a young age [2, 4]. We have shown that the booster antibody responses to the CP are accompanied by reexpression of all the clonotypes that were originally stimulated and detected after conjugate immunization [4]. In addition, new clonotypes in the acidic region of the gel are preferentially restimulated or newly appear in some subjects with the booster response to polyribosylribitolphosphate (PRP) immunization [4, 16]. IgG2 subclass antibodies usually have lower isoelectric points than IgG1 antibodies. The IgG subclass distribution of the antibody induced by PRP immunization at 12–13 months of age or at 24–26 months of age in children primed with conjugates at 2–7 months or 12–14 months of age, respectively, has an IgG1/IgG2 ratio approximately 1/4 the level and an IgG2 antibody response 5- to 14-fold higher in magnitude than observed for conjugate-induced antibody (table I). Individuals that failed to produce an IgG2 subclass antibody response after conjugate immunization produce IgG2 antibody after CP immunization. Children immunized with the isolated CP at 24–26 months of age without priming show a similar IgG1/IgG2 ratio but markedly lower antibody levels than children of the same age reimmunized with the CP after conjugate priming. Thus, conjugate priming augments the magnitude of the antibody titer induced by CP immunization without skewing the IgG subclass distribution toward that observed after conjugate immunization and without changing it to be different from that observed without conjugate priming. These findings suggest that the memory cells present at 5–12 months after conjugate immunization that are polysaccharide responsive are not precommitted in their isotype switching, and that the isolated CP preferentially induces switching or selects precommitted cells specific for the IgG2 subclass. In contrast, the protein-conjugated CP induces or selects an IgG1 subclass response. Comparison of the responses of unprimed children immunized with polysaccharide to that of 16- to 23-month-old children immunized with conjugates (IgG1/IgG2 of 3.7 vs 45) illustrates this difference independent of the contribution of age.

Age, however, effects the magnitude of the IgG2 antibody responce and the subclass distribution induced by CP immunization. Adults immunized with the CP show a mean IgG1/IgG2 ratio of 0.88 (table I). A total of 42% of individuals show IgG2 predominance and 79% have a ratio greater than 0.3, corresponding to the ratio of normal serum. Thus, an increased total and IgG2 antibody response is observed with age with the IgG2 antibody titer increasing in the adult approximately 12-fold over the level in the infant. Although there is a mean IgG2 predominance of 0.88, the IgG1/IgG2 ratio has a range of over 300 among adults. This increased IgG2 response to the CP with age observed with the *H. influenzae* CP has been described previously with responses to other CP [17].

Differences in either the affinity or functional activity of IgG1 and IgG2 subclass antibodies are under investigation. Whether different immunoglobulin-variable region genes coding for this antibody preferentially associate with different IgG subclasses is not known at this time. It should be noted, however, that the expressed antibody repertoire is usually highly restricted in diversity, even in individuals with both IgG1 and IgG2 subclass expression, and even more restricted than the potential repertoire [6]. In addition, as described above, conjugate-primed cells of infants have accelerated maturation of responsiveness to the isolated CP and, yet, the responses to the CP show a different IgG subclass distribution than to the conjugate. This linear developmental pathway of B cell responsiveness [4] suggests that it is likely that the same V-regions are used for the responses to the two forms of the CP and are associated with either IgG1 or IgG2 constant region genes.

One difference in IgG1 and IgG2 subclass antibodies is in their relative ability to cross the placenta to the neonate. Postimmunization antibody clonotypes in mothers show differences in their relative distribution compared to their offspring [6]. Neonatal cord serum has more IgG1 and less IgG2 antibody than the corresponding maternal serum. Over a 2-fold difference is observed in transplacental passage of IgG1 and IgG2 subclass antibody in that the cord serum level is 128 and 56% of the maternal serum IgG1 and IgG2 levels, respectively.

IgG Subclass Antibody Responses in Immunodeficiency Disease

We have observed poor antibody responses to immunization with the Hib CP in patients with low levels of IgG2 with or without concomitant IgG4 and IgA deficiency [11]. In addition, we have observed low responses in patients with isolated IgA deficiency, the Wiskott-Aldrich syndrome, congenital AIDS and in patients with normal immunoglobulin levels that have recurrent pyogenic infections or who failed to be protected against Hib infection in spite of immunization [18].

Patients with IgG2 subclass deficiency that fail to respond to the isolated CP of Hib and the pneumococcus can produce antibody to the Hib CP when immunized with a protein-conjugated CP [11]. Booster responses are seen with reimmunization. Although IgG1 antibody predominates in the response, IgG2 antibody can be detected after conjugate immunization in some of these patients. In contrast to results in infants primed with conjugates, these patients after priming with conjugates fail to respond to reimmunization with the isolated CP. Thus, although CP unresponsiveness can be bypassed by an alternative form of antigen presentation in these patients, defective responses to the isolated CP are not corrected. In addition, these results demonstrate that CP unresponsiveness in IgG subclass deficiency is not a fixed defect but is an association without a direct causal relationship. In fact, it is possible that the association is due to the existence of low IgG2 levels as a result of poor antibody responses to polysaccharides.

We have also successfully immunized patients unresponsive to the Hib CP that have normal IgG subclass levels with Hib conjugate vaccines [18]. They illustrate two differences from the group of patients with CP unresponsiveness and IgG2 subclass deficiency. First, their antibody response to conjugates can include a prominent IgG2 subclass component and, second, some of these patients acquire the ability to respond to the isolated CP after priming with conjugates. Thus, some of these patients may have a different separate defect that involves an inability of environmental antigens to activate the B cell to become polysaccharide-responsive.

IgG2m(n) Allotype Expression

The enhanced IgG2 antibody response to the isolated Hib CP of adults in comparison to children as well as the basis for individual differences in the IgG subclass distribution of antibody in adults (table I) is not understood. Analysis of serum antibody clonotypes over time demonstrates that new IgG2 clonotypes appear at 7–9 months after immunization that were not apparent at 1 month after immunization [6]. Ambrosino et al. [19] have demonstrated an association of expression of the G2m(n) allotype marker with high total and

IgG responses to CP. We have quantified expression of this allotype marker on serum IgG2 of heterozygous obligate individuals at the genotype level for this marker to determine whether there is potential allotype inclusion/exclusion expressed on serum IgG2 subclass immunoglobulins. This would answer the question whether there is stochastic use of the allotype marker or preferential use of the marker due to some form of immunoregulation. Finding the latter for total serum IgG2 (as opposed to with only a specific antibody response) would provide strong evidence for the generalization of preferential allotypic inclusion. Obligate heterozygous individuals were defined as G2m(n)-positive parents with G2m(n)-negative offspring, or G2m(n)-positive offspring with one G2m(n)-negative parent. IgG2 subclass antibody was captured with the monoclonal antibody HP 6014 and the G2m(n) marker detected with monoclonal antibody SH21 and total IgG2 with HP 6017 [20]. Serum IgG2 of G2m(n)-negative individuals did not bind the allotype specific monoclonal antibody. Obligate heterozygous individuals not only express the allotype marker on over half their IgG2 but can express the allotype marker on all their serum IgG2, similar in magnitude to homozygous individuals. Thus, the G2m(n) allotype-positive molecules are preferentially included in total serum IgG2 in obligate heterozygous individuals. This means that there is preferential use of the allotype marker on the total serum IgG2 and strongly suggests that there is regulation of IgG2 through recognition of this marker. The level at which regulation of G2m(n) expression occurs is unknown at this time but is actively being investigated. One possibility includes regulation by allotype-specific T cells. Another would be an indirect regulation through association of this allotype marker with specific idiotypes found on antibodies. This finding and the described association of G2m(n) expression with high responses to CP [19] suggests that one of several explanations for individual differences in IgG2 subclass expression on CP antibody responses may be related to differences in regulation at the level of this genetic marker.

Conclusions

The IgG subclass distribution of human antibody to this CP is affected by: (a) the structural form of the antigen (isolated vs protein conjugated) – increased IgG2 responses observed with the isolated polysaccharide; (b) the age of the individual immunized – increased IgG2 responses observed in older individuals immunized with the isolated polysaccharide; increase IgG1 responses in older children immunized with conjugates; (c) the nature and timing of priming prior to immunization with the isolated polysaccharide – the isolated polysaccharide augments clonotypes induced by the conjugate vaccine and preferentially stimulates IgG2 clonotypes. Thus, this is a linear developmental pathway of antibody responsiveness that requires priming with a protein-conjugated polysaccharide to induce responsiveness to the isolated polysaccharide, but isotype responses to the isolated polysaccharide are not precommitted by conjugate priming, but are induced or selected by the form of the reimmunizing polysaccharide. Patients with defective antibody responses to polysaccharides, with or without IgG2 subclass deficiency, can produce antibody responses to protein-conjugated polysaccharides, which can include an IgG2 component. Lastly, the IgG2 allotype marker G2m(n) or (23) is preferentially expressed on total serum IgG2 in individuals genetically heterozygous for this marker, which strongly suggests immunoregulation occurs through recognition of this marker.

References

1 Smith, D.H.; Peter, G.; Ingram, D.L.; et al.: Children immunized against *Hemophilus influenzae* type b. Pediatrics *52:* 637 (1973).
2 Anderson, P.; Pichichero, M.E.; Insel, R.A.: Immunogens consisting of oligosaccharides from the capsule of *Haemophilus influenzae* type b coupled to diphtheria toxoid or the toxin protein CRM 197. J. clin. Invest. *76:* 52–59 (1985).
3 Anderson, P.; Pichichero, M.E.; Insel, R.A.: Immunization of two-month-old infants with protein coupled oligosaccharides derived from the capsule of *Haemophilus influenzae* type b. J. Pediat. *107:* 346–351 (1985).
4 Insel, R.A.; Anderson, P.W.: Oligosaccharide-protein conjugate vaccines induce and prime for oligoclonal IgG antibody responses to the *Haemophilus influenzae* b capsular polysaccharide in human infants. J. exp. Med. *163:* 262–269 (1986).
5 Insel, R.A.; Anderson, P.; Pichichero, M.E.; Schuster, S.; Amstey, M.S.; Ekborg, G.; Lewin, E.B.; Smith, D.H.: Anticapsular antibody to *Haemophilus influenzae*; in Sell, Wright, *Hemophilus influenzae*, pp. 155–168 (Elsevier/Biomedical Press, New York 1982).
6 Insel, R.A.; Kittelberger, A.; Anderson, P.: Isoelectric focusing of human antibody to the *Haemophilus influenzae* b capsular polysaccharide: restricted and identical spectrotypes in adults. J. Immun. *135:* 2810–2816 (1985).

7 Perlmutter, R.M.; Hansburg, D.; Briles, D.E.; Nicolotti, R.A.; Davie, J.M.: Subclass restriction of murine anticarbohydrate antibodies. J. Immun. *121:* 566 (1978).
8 derBalian, G.P.; Slack, J.; Clevinger, B.L.; Bazin, H.; Davie, J.M.: Subclass restriction of murine antibodies. III. Antigens that stimulate IgG$_3$ in mice stimulate IgG$_{2c}$ in rats. J. exp. Med. *152:* 209 (1980).
9 Yount, W.T.; Dorner, M.M.; Kunkel, H.G.; Kabat, E.A.: Studies on human antibodies. VI selective variations in subgroup composition and genetic markers. J. exp. Med. *127:* 633 (1968).
10 Insel, R.A.; Anderson, P.W.: *Haemophilus influenzae* type b: assays for the capsular polysaccharide and for anti-polysaccharide antibody; in Rose, Friedman, Fahey, Manual of clinical laboratory immunology; 3rd ed., pp. 379–384 (1986).
11 Insel, R.A.; Anderson, P.: Response to oligosaccharide-protein conjugate vaccines against *Hemophilus influenzae* b in two patients with IgG2 deficiency unresponsive to capsular polysaccharide vaccine. New Engl. J. Med. *315:* 499–503 (1986).
12 Gigliotti, F.; Insel, R.A.: Protection from *Haemophilus influenzae* type b by monoclonal antibody to the capsule. J. infect. Dis. *146:* 249–254 (1982).
13 Seppala, I.J.T.; Routonen, N.; Sarnesto, A.; Mattila, P.A.; Makela, O.: The percentages of six immunoglobulin isotypes in human antibodies to tetanus toxoid: standardization of isotype-specific second antibodies in solid-phase assay. Eur. J. Immunol. *14:* 868–875 (1984).
14 Amstey, M.S.; Insel, R.A.; Pichichero, M.E.: Neonatal passive immunization by maternal vaccination. Obstet. Gynec. N.Y. *63:* 105–109 (1984).
15 Anderson, P.; Pichichero, M.; Edwards, K.; Porch, C.R.; Insel, R.: Priming and induction of *Haemophilus influenzae* type b capsular antibodies in early infancy by Dpo20, an oligosaccharide-protein conjugate vaccine. J. Pediat. *111* (1987).
16 Insel, R.; Anderson, P.; Pichichero, M.: The IgG subclass distribution of antibody induced by immunization with isolated and protein-conjugated *H. influenzae* b capsular polysaccharide (submitted).
17 Frejid, A.; Hammarstrom, L.A.; Persson, M.A.A.; Smith, C.I.E.: Plasma antipneumococcal antibody activity of the IgG subclass in otitis-prone children. Clin. exp. Immunol. *56:* 233–238 (1984).
18 Insel, R.A.; Gellin, B.; Broome, C.; Smith, D.: IgG$_2$ subclass deficiency presenting as *H. influenzae* b (Hib) disease after immunization with Hib vaccine. Pediat. Res. *21:* 312A (1987).
19 Ambrosino, D.M.; Schiffman, G.; Gotschlich, E.; Schur, P.; Rosenberg, G.; DeLange, G.G.; Loghem, E. van; Siber, G.R.: Correlation between G2m(n) immunoglobulin allotype and human antibody response and susceptibility to polysaccharide encapsulated bacteria. J. clin. Invest. *75:* 1935 (1985).
20 Jefferies, R.; Reimer, C.; Skvaril, I.; et al.: Evaluation of monoclonal antibodies having specificity for human IgG subclasses. Results of an IUIS/WHO collaborative study. Immunol. Lett. *10:* 223 (1985).

Richard A. Insel, MD, Departments of Pediatrics and Microbiology, University of Rochester, School of Medicine and Dentistry, Rochester, NY 14642 (USA)

IgG Subclasses and Neonatal Infections with Group B Streptococci[1]

K.K. Christensen, P. Christensen

Research Unit, Dermaci, Science Park, Ideon, Lund, Sweden

Introduction

Group B streptococci (GBS) cause infections in the mother as well as in the infant (table I). In the early-onset form of septicemia, the infant contracts the bacteria from the birth channel, whereas the source of infection in the late-onset form might be nosocomial [17]. Pneumonia without septicemia occurs within 24 h as a result of acquisition of GBS from the maternal vagina [5]. Osteomyelitis, finally, is a complication to late-onset septicemia/meningitis [17].

In the mother, GBS may cause endometritis and/or septicemia especially following cesarean section [18].

It appears that the panorama of GBS infections is heterogenous with respect of the route of infection and the pathogenic mechanism. Furthermore, it should also be noted that 10–20% of the pregnant women are carriers of GBS in the urogenital tract at delivery, and the majority gives birth to healthy infants. However, discussing the pathogenesis, it is important to separate one infection pattern from the other.

Factors Predisposing to GBS Septicemia in the Infant (table II)

In Chicago [4] as well as in Stockholm [16] approximately 80% of the infants with GBS septicemia of the early-onset form belong to one of the risk categories premature (gestation age < 37 weeks) and rupture of fetal membranes (more than 12 h). This fact has now made

---

[1] Supported by the Medical Research Council, grant No. B87-16X-06559-05.

Table I. Infections caused by GBS in mothers and infants

Diseases in the infant
    Sepsis/meningitis early-onset
                           late-onset
    Intrauterine fetal death
    Pneumonia
    Osteomyelitis
Diseases in the mother
    Endometritis
    Sepsis following cesarean section
    Urinary tract infection

Table II. Factors predisposing to GBS septicemia in the infant

Prematurity
Prolonged rupture of fetal membranes
Maternal fever
Degree of colonization of the birth channel (bacteriuria with GBS?)
Maternal immunological status

prevention possible; by combined screening a selective administration of antibiotics [4].

An important point in this connection is the question whether prematurity and prolonged rupture of membranes is a consequence of GBS infection or vice versa. In one study [16] 22 of 39 infants with early-onset GBS septicemia were premature; nevertheless, the mothers showed the same low levels of IgG against GBS as mothers of term infants. There is also evidence that GBS bacteriuria in the mother during early pregnancy – probably a sign of heavy colonization – is associated with prematurity, abortions and stillbirth [Thomsen, personal communication]. Furthermore, the patients in the Stockholm study who gave birth to GBS-infected infants were treated with penicillin if GBS-positive during their next pregnancy, and the frequency of premature delivery dropped significantly [16]. All these findings might indicate that at least prematurity and possibly prolonged rupture of membranes might be caused by GBS colonization rather than being independent factors contributing to the development of septicemia. However, these questions await further investigation.

Table III. Types of GBS

Type	Carbohydrate antigen	Protein antigens that might be present
Ia	Ia	c[1]
Ib	Ib	c
II	II	c, R
III	III	c, R
IV	IV	?
V	V	?

[1] Ia/c was previously designated Ic.

The Antigenic Structure of GBS

GBS are divided into types, dependent of surface carbohydrate antigens (table III). A type is designated with both carbohydrate and protein antigens, e.g. a type III strain that carries both c and R as III/c, R [20]. Other antigens present in GBS are the group-specific carbohydrates, peptidoglycan and lipoteichoic acid [21].

Type-specific antigens of GBS extracted with hot HCl all contain galactose, glucose and 2-acetamido-2-deoxyglucose as exclusive sugars. All component sugars are present in the *D*-form in Ia, Ib, II and III. These acid-extracted antigens are immunologically incomplete and form a core to the native antigens, which all contain additional terminal acid-labile sialic residues [21].

Although all investigators attribute virulence and protective antibodies to the type-specific carbohydrate antigens, there is also evidence that the c protein [22] and the R protein [6] are virulence factors. The exact chemical structure of these proteins is so far unknown.

Antibodies to the group-specific antigen and peptidoglycan do not seem to be protective [21]. The role of lipoteichoic acid, for example in bacterial attachment to human cells and the possible prevention of attachment to these cells by secretory antibodies, is so far not yet fully elucidated.

Opsonization of GBS in vitro

Deficient complement alternative pathway activity in newborn sera for pathogens other than GBS and deficient classical pathway function for opsonization of Ia GBS has been shown in some normal neonates [15]. Properdin-deficient serum was shown to opsonize some strains less effectively for phagocytic killing [31]. Thus, since both pathways are important opsonins, and since neonates have low levels of components of both pathways [13], it is possible that the accentuation of these physiological deficiencies may be one factor predisposing certain neonates to the development of GBS septicemia [15].

Antibody Levels against GBS in Infants with GBS Septicemia and Their Mothers

After the original discovery of Baker and Kasper [1] of a correlation of maternal antibody deficiency against GBS type III with susceptibility to neonatal septicemia with this type, a large number of publications has confirmed the finding and extended it to other serotypes [2]. However, a few sera ($< 5\%$) still show 'normal' levels. These sera may be from mothers of preterm infants [9]. Antibody levels in infants to GBS antigens are positively correlated to gestational age, i.e. significantly lowered in preterm infants [8]. Further exceptions to the rule of low IgG levels to GBS might be explained by an increased dose of GBS, by direct injection of GBS in the blood stream [9] or by an infant born during extremely bad conditions after an instrumental delivery.

Studies of antibodies to protein antigens in mothers of GBS-infected infants are scarce. Studies using commercial human IgG batches demonstrated an association between protection in mice and antibodies to the c and R proteins [7]. In one study, mothers of infants infected with type II/R and type III/R strains showed significantly lower levels of IgG antibodies to the R protein than parturients who were urogenital carriers of the same strains but gave birth to healthy infants [6].

There are several possibilities explaining low IgG levels against GBS antigens in the infant (table IV). We know very little about GBS infections in infants of mothers who show clinical signs of increased frequency of bacterial infection due to hypo- or agammaglobulinemia or IgG subclass deficiencies. The impression is that mothers of infants

Table IV. Theoretical mechanisms leading to low IgG levels against GBS in the infant

Hypo- or agammaglobulinemia in the mother
IgG subclass deficiencies in the mother
Primary acquisition of a GBS type in late pregnancy not leading to sufficient IgG response at delivery
Maternal deficient B cell switch from IgM to IgG production against bacterial carbohydrate antigens?
Decreased IgG production in a few individuals due to the immunosuppressive effect of pregnancy?
Prematurity
Impaired placental transport of IgG
Others?

with GBS septicemia generally do not complain of increased numbers of infections or severity of infections. However, this question should be elucidated by thorough and systematic interviews. Moreover, prospective analyses are desirable, since the mothers might develop symptoms years after the delivery.

Theoretically, the primary acquisition of a GBS type in late pregnancy might give rise to an IgM response, but the IgG response might be too delayed to protect the infant. However, Boyer and Gotoff [3] demonstrated that 14 of 16 infants with GBS sepsis had mothers who were early prenatally colonized with the homologous GBS serotype. Thus, while prenatal cultures are not infallible in view of occasional third-trimester acquisitions, the group of women with carriage of GBS at prenatal visits appears to include most of the women whose infants will develop early-onset GBS septicemia.

It is not known whether the immunosuppressive effect of pregnancy per se might affect the B cell function in a few individuals or if there exists a selective impaired placental transport of IgG.

Thus, the background to low levels of IgG in the infant might very well be heterogenous. Furthermore, complement functions, i.e. inherited deficiency of certain factors, maternal colonization as well as GBS strain-specific virulence factors, may be other important possible contributors to the development of septicemia. Therefore, it is important to realize that early-onset GBS septicemia might have a heterogenous pathological basis. To complete the heterogenous picture of GBS diseases, GBS pneumonia without septicemia does not seem to be correlated to low maternal IgG levels.

Immunological Characterization of Mothers to Infants with GBS Septicemia

On a background of the heterogenous pathogenesis to GBS septicemia discussed above, it is only to be expected that general immunological deviations are not found in every single woman who gives birth to an infant with this disease. However, it is possible to detect some statistically significant differences when comparing these women to normals. These differences might reflect the presence of a major or a minor subpopulation of immunological deficiencies within the entire population of mothers giving birth to infants with GBS septicemia.

In one study, antibody levels to Salmonella, Yersinia and pneumococcal carbohydrate antigens were measured in a study group consisting of 16 mothers to GBS-infected infants (septicemia) and a control group of 29 GBS carriers giving birth to healthy infants. Significantly more individuals in the study group showed IgG levels below selected limits against all antigens except for one of five pneumococcal antigens. In contrast, more mothers of GBS-infected infants had IgM levels above a selected limit against Salmonella DO [10]. The latter finding was corroborated by the finding of total serum IgM levels above 2.4 g/l in 22 of 84 (27%) mothers to GBS-infected infants, in contrast to 12 of 91 (13%) controls similar to those used above ($p = 0.02$) [29]. Moreover, an increased IgM/IgG ratio in specific antibodies was detected in such mothers versus controls upon immunization with a multivalent pneumococcal vaccine [11].

The Gm allotypes of the IgG class in mothers of infants with GBS septicemia also differ. In a Swedish study the frequency of G1m(I) was 38.2%, in contrast to 57.7% in the Swedish population and the phenotype Gm(1,5) was found in 21.2% of the mothers, contrasting with the expected 45.5% [19].

Seven of 8 mothers of infants with GBS infections (intrauterine death or early-onset septicemia) were vaginal carriers of the same serotype of GBS up to 38 months after their pregnancy. In contrast, only 34 of 88 GBS carriers, who had given birth to healthy infants, harbored the same serotype at a 34 months' follow-up [14].

These findings might indicate the existence of a subpopulation within mothers giving birth to infants with GBS septicemia. These mothers might be characterized by prolonged carriage of GBS, and an impaired capacity to switch from IgM to IgG production of antibodies to bacterial carbohydrate antigens, probably on a genetical background. The fact that only few mothers complain spontaneously of recurrent infections might possibly be ascribed to their higher IgM levels.

IgG Subclasses in Mothers of Infants with GBS Septicemia

Several reports have demonstrated that IgG antibodies against carbohydrate antigens mainly belong to the IgG2 subclass [24, 28, 30]. Studies with respect to GBS carbohydrate antigens are scarce.

In a recent study, Quinti et al. [27] measured IgG class and subclass antibodies against GBS-type Ia in 12 patients with IgG2 subclass deficiency. Compared to 12 normal controls, the deficiency group showed significantly reduced antibody levels. The responders in the population studies showed IgG2 and IgG4 antibodies to the GBS-type Ia polysaccharide. However, in one mother-baby pair the specific antibody response was restricted to IgG1, although the total serum levels of IgG2 were within the normal range.

In another study [25], serum IgG subclasses were studied in 19 mothers of infants with serious infections caused by GBS and compared with a control group of 20 mothers of healthy infants. 13 of 19 mothers to GBS-infected infants showed decreased subclass levels: 10 of 19 low IgG2, 9 of 19 low IgG1 and 4 of 19 low IgG3. The levels of IgG1, IgG2 and IgG3 were significantly lower in these mothers than among the controls. Low total serum IgG levels were found only in 7 of 19 sera, all of these with low IgG1. The IgA levels were normal.

In a recent investigation, high doses (24g IgG at each of 5 consecutive days) of intravenous immunoglobulin were given to 7 women in pregnancy weeks 27–36 who were at risk of preterm delivery. Substantial transplacental passage could be observed in 5 patients where delivery occurred at the 34th week or later. After the 36th week of gestation, all 4 IgG subclasses and antibody concentrations against GBS, pneumococci and tetanus toxoid were increased up to the levels in maternal serum [23].

We would like to emphasize that commercial IgG preparations given to newborns might result in lowering of protective antibodies [12]. This effect was also shown for antibodies to pneumococci given to children with recurrent otitis media [26].

Conclusion

Many aspects of the relation between IgG subclass deficiencies and neonatal GBS septicemia are still unresolved. In the future, a number of different pathological mechanisms will have to be elucidated in order to define more homogenous groups of mothers to infants with GBS septicemia. We do not know the role of antibodies of GBS protein antigens or their possible IgG subclass, although antibodies to carbohydrate antigens are of major importance. These points are all crucial for the designation of vaccine programs, passive immunoprophylaxis or therapy as well as the possible pre-delivery detection of risk mothers using immunological tests.

References

1. Baker, C.J.; Kasper, D.L.: Correlation of maternal antibody deficiency with susceptibility to neonatal group B streptococcal infection. New Engl. J. Med. *294:*753 (1976).
2. Baker, C.J.; Kasper, D.L.: Vaccination as a measure for prevention of neonatal GBS infection; in Christensen, Christensen, Ferrieri, Neonatal group B streptococcal infections. Antibiot. Chemother., vol. 35, p. 281 (Karger, Basel 1985).
3. Boyer, K.M.; Gotoff, S.P.: Strategies for chemoprophylaxis of GBS early-onset infections; in Christensen, Christensen, Ferrieri, Neonatal group B streptococcal infections. Antibiot. Chemother., vol. 35, p. 267 (Karger, Basel 1985).
4. Boyer, K.M.; Gotoff, S.P.: Prevention of early-onset neonatal group B streptococcal disease with selective intrapartum chemoprophylaxis. New Engl. J. Med. *314:* 1665 (1986).
5. Christensen, K.K.; Christensen, P.; Dahlander, K.; Linden, V.; Lindroth, M.; Svenningsen, N.: The significance of group B streptococci in neonatal pneumonia. Eur. J. Pediat. *140:* 118 (1983).
6. Christensen, K.K.; Christensen, P.: The R-proteins; in Christensen, Christensen, Ferrieri, Neonatal group B streptococcal infections. Antibiot. Chemother., vol. 35, p. 114 (Karger, Basel 1985).
7. Christensen, K.K.; Christensen, P.; Duc, G.; Hitzig, W.H.; Linden, V.; Müller, B.; Seger, R.A.: Human IgG antibodies to carbohydrate and protein antigens in mouse protection tests with group B streptococci. Pediat. Res. *18:* 478 (1984).
8. Christensen, K.K.; Christensen, P.; Duc, G.; Höger, P.; Matsunaga, T.; Müller, B.; Seger, R.A.: Correlation between serum antibody-levels against group B streptococci and gestational age in newborns. Eur. J. Pediat. *142:* 86 (1984).
9. Christensen, K.K.; Dahlander, K.; Linden, V.; Svenningsen, N.; Christensen, P.: Obstetrical care in future pregnancies after fetal loss in group B streptococcal septicemia. Eur. J. Obstet. Gynec. reprod. Biol. *12:* 143 (1981).
10. Christensen, K.K.; Christensen, P.; Lindberg, A.; Linden, V.: Mothers of infants with neonatal group B streptococcal septicemia are poor responders to bacterial carbohydrate antigens. Int. Archs Allergy appl. Immun. *67:* 7 (1982).

11 Christensen, K.K.; Christensen, P.; Faxelius, G.; Henrichsen, J.; Pedersen, J.K.: Immune response to pneumococcal vaccine in mothers to infants with group B streptococcal septicemia: evidence for a divergent IgM/IgG ratio. Int. Archs Allergy appl. Immun. 76: 369 (1985).
12 Christensen, K.K.; Christensen, P.: Intravenous gamma globulin in the treatment of neonatal sepsis with special reference to group B streptococci and pharmacokinetics. Pediat. infect. Dis. 3: 189 (1986).
13 Davies, C.A.; Vallota, E.H.; Forristal, J.: Serum complement levels in infancy; age related changes. Pediat. Res. 13: 1043 (1979).
14 Dykes, A.-K.; Christensen, K.K.; Christensen, P.: Chronic carrier state in mothers of infants with group b streptococcal infections. Obstate. Gynec., N.Y. 66: 84 (1985).
15 Edwards, M.S.; Kasper, D.L.; Nicholson-Weller, A.; Baker, C.J.: The role of complement in opsonization of GBS; in Christensen, Christensen, Ferrieri, Neonatal group B streptococcal infections. Antibiot. Chemother., vol. 35, p. 170 (Karger, Basel 1985).
16 Faxelius, G.; Bremme, K.; Christensen, K.K.; Christensen, P.; Ringertz, S.: Abstr. Meet. on Infections in Obstetrics and Gynecology (Swedish Medical Association, Stockholm 1987).
17 Ferrieri, P.: GBS infections in the newborn infant: diagnosis and treatment; in Christensen, Christensen, Ferrieri, Neonatal group B streptococcal infections. Antibiot. Chemother., vol. 35, p. 211 (Karger, Basel 1985).
18 Gray, B.M.; Dillon, H.C, Jr.: GBS infections in mothers and their infants; in Christensen, Christensen, Ferrieri, Neonatal group B streptococcal infections. Antibiot. Chemother., vol. 35, p. 225 (Karger, Basel 1985).
19 Grubb, R.; Christensen, K.K.; Christensen, P.; Linden, V.: Association between maternal Gm allotype and neonatal septicaemia with group B streptococci. J. Immunogenet. 9: 143 (1982).
20 Henrichsen, J.: Nomenclature of GBS antigens; in Christensen, Christensen, Ferrieri, Neonatal group B streptococcal infections. Antibiot. Chemother., vol. 35, p. 303 (Karger, Basel 1985).
21 Kasper, D.L.; Baker, C.J.; Jennings, H.J.: Cell structure and antigenic composition of GBS; in Christensen, Christensen, Ferrieri, Neonatal group B streptococcal infections. Antibiot. Chemother., vol. 35, p. 90 (Karger, Basel 1985).
22 Lancefield, R.C.; McCarthy, M.; Everly, W.M.: Multiple mouse-protective antibodies directed against group B streptococci: special reference to antibodies effective against protein antigens. J. exp. med. 142: 165 (1975).
23 Morell, A.; Sidiropoulos, D.; Christensen, K.K.; Christensen, P.; Prellner, K.; Fey, H.; Skvaril, F.: IgG subclasses and antibodies to group B streptococci, pneumococci, and tetanus toxoid in preterm neonates after intravenous infusion of immunoglobulin to the mothers. Pediat. Res. 20: 933 (1986).
24 Oxelius, V.-A.: Chronic infections in a family with hereditary deficiency of IgG2 and IgG4 subclasses. Clin. exp. Immunol. 17: 19 (1974).
25 Oxelius, V.-A.; Linden, V.; Christensen, K.K.; Christensen, P.: Deficiency of IgG subclasses in mothers of infants with group B streptococcal septicemia. Int. Archs Allergy appl. Immun. 72: 249 (1983).
26 Prellner, K.; Christensen, P.; Kalm, O.; Offenbartl, K.: The effect of serial intravenous immunoglobulin infusion on type-specific anti-pneumococcal antibodies in children. Acta pathol. microbiol. scand., C, Immunol. 94: 207 (1986).

27 Quinti, I.; Papetti, C.; Hunolstein, C. von; Orefici, G.; Aiuti, F.: Int. Symp. on Biotechnology in Clinical Medicine, Rome 1987, abstr.
28 Riesen, W.F.; Skvaril, F.; Braun, D.G.: Natural infection of man with group A streptococci: levels, restriction in class, subclass and type, and clonal appearance of poly-saccharide group-specific antibodies. Scand. J. Immunol. *5:* 383 (1976).
29 Rundgren, Å.K.; Christensen, K.K.; Christensen, P.: Increased frequency of high serum IgM among mothers to infants with neonatal group B streptococci septicemia. Int. Archs Allergy appl. Immun. *77:* 372 (1985).
30 Siber, G.R.; Schur, P.H.; Aisenberg, A.C.; Weitzman, S.A.; Schiffman, G.: Correlation between IgG2 concentrations and the antibody response och bacterial polysaccharide antigens. New Engl. J. Med. *303:* 178 (1980).
31 Söderström, C.; Braconier, J.H.; Christensen, K.K.; Christensen, P.; Sjöholm, A.G.: Opsonization of group B streptococci in properdin deficient serum. Acta path. microbiol. scand., C, Immunol. (in press).

K.K. Christensen, MD, Research Unit, Dermaci,
Science Park, Ideon, S–223 70 Lund (Sweden)

IgG Subclasses to Group B Streptococci in Normals, Colonized Woman and IgG2 Subclass-Deficient Patients

I. Quinti[a], C. Papetti[a], C. von Hunolstein[b], G. Orefici[b], F. Aiuti[a]

[a] Department of Allergy and Clinical Immunology, University of Rome 'La Sapienza';
[b] Laboratory of Microbiology, Istituto Superiore di Sanità, Rome, Italy

Introduction

Streptococci of Lancefield group B (GBS) are a major cause of serious perinatal infections, sepsis, pneumonia, and meningitis [1]. Clinical and microbiological data strongly support the hypothesis of a pathogenesis involving an amniotic infection [2]. In animals, it has been demonstrated that specific serum antibodies protect against the infection with GBS of the corresponding serotype [3]. Low levels of serum antibodies to the type-specific polysaccharide antigen of GBS have been demonstrated in sera of colonized mothers who gave birth to infected children, but only few data on the type and protective levels of these antibodies have been reported [4, 5]. Intrapartum chemoprophylaxis, active or passive immunization of mothers could be used to prevent the neonatal group B streptococcal disease [6–8]. In particular, the possibility to vaccinate women in the last trimester of pregnancy could be considered a safe choice to achieve specific immunity in mothers and passive protection in neonates. However, vaccine research should take into account the peculiarity of response, in humans, to polysaccharide antigens, and in particular, the observation that mothers of infants with GBS septicemia are poor responders to bacterial carbohydrate antigens [9], and may have a deficiency of IgG subclasses [10]. We now report our results on the class and subclass of specific antibodies to GBS of colonized women, infected neonates, patients with IgG2 deficiency, and normals.

Materials and Methods

Study Population. Sera from 12 colonized women, 3 mothers and their infants who contracted GBS neonatal sepsis, 9 patients with IgG2 subclass deficiency and 17 normal controls were examined. Three infants contracted their infection within the first 48 h of birth, and GBS were isolated at a sterile autopsy from all inner organs. Vaginal specimens for culture were obtained, using a selective method, from all the women in the study. The 3 mothers were urogenital carriers of the strain infecting their children.

Microbiologic Studies. The cultures of specimens from colonized sites were processed with an enrichment procedure, as previously described [11]. GBS isolated were grouped and typed as described [12].

Antigen Preparation. GBS type Ia polysaccharide antigen was extracted according to Wilkinson procedure [13] and purified by WGA affinity chromatography [14].

Type-Specific GBS Antibodies
Type-Specific IgG. Type-specific IgG were measured by a 3-step enzyme-linked immunosorbent assay (ELISA). Briefly: (1) polyvinyl microtiter plates were coated with 1 µg/ml of purified antigen in 0.1 M carbonate-bicarbonate buffer, pH 9.6, overnight at room temperature. Plates were then washed with PBS-Tween and blocked with 0.1% gelatin for 2 h; (2) after 3 washes with PBS-Tween sera were added at different dilutions, and incubated for 18 h at room temperature; (3) after washes, 100 µl of a goat antihuman IgG affinity-purified, alkaline-phosphatase-conjugated, antiserum (Zymed, McLean, USA) diluted 1:1,000 was added and plates incubated for 1 h at 37 °C. After 3 washes with PBS-Tween and 1 with 0.05 M Tris HCl, 100 µl of 1 mg/ml of paranitrophenylphosphate diluted in 1 M Tris HCl was added and the optical density (OD, at 405 nm) was read after 30 min using a Titertek multiscan.

Type-specific IgG subclasses were measured by a 4-step ELISA. Steps 1 and 2 were the same as described above; (3) after washes, 100 µl of monoclonal antibody specific for human IgG1 (SG-16), IgG2 (GOM-2), IgG3 (HP5060), IgG4 (SK-40) (Bio-Yeda, Israel) was added and plates incubated for 2 h at 37 °C; (4) after washes, 100 µl of a goat antimouse Ig alkaline-phosphatase conjugated was added and plates incubated for 1 h at 37 °C. After 3 washes with PBS-Tween and 1 with 0.05 M Tris HCl, 100 µl of 1 mg/ml of paranitrophenylphosphate was added and the OD was read after 30 min. Results were expressed as delta OD, calculated for each IgG subclass in each sample subtracting the appropriate controls' OD to the samples' OD.

Results

Serum Antibodies against GBS-Type Ia Antigen. Specific IgG to type Ia GBS were measured in the sera of: (1) colonized women; (2) colonized mothers who gave birth to infants with GBS sepsis and their

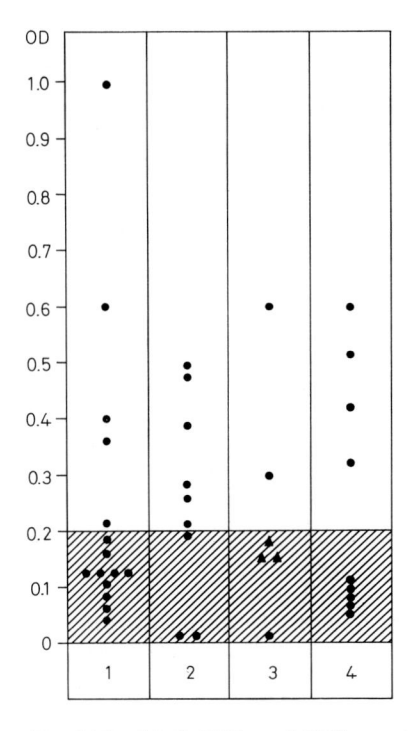

Fig. 1. Total IgG (OD) anti-GBS type Ia polysaccharide measured by ELISA in sera of: (1) normal adults; (2) vaginally colonized women; (3) septic neonates (▲) and their mothers (●); (4) patients with IgG2 subclass deficiency.

infants; (3) patients with IgG2 subclass deficiency; (4) normal controls. No significant differences were demonstrated in the specific IgG levels between colonized women, colonized mothers, infected infants and normal controls. A significant difference has been observed between the IgG2 subclass deficiency group and controls. In all groups, independently of the clinical evidence of a GBS-type Ia colonization, it has been possible to distinguish between a seropositive and a seronegative population (fig. 1). When we analyzed the distribution of specific antibodies among IgG subclasses again we could not demostrate any significant difference in the behavior of serum antibody levels in the different groups, except for the IgG2-deficient group who showed decresed levels of specific IgG1 ($p < 0.001$), IgG2 ($p < 0.001$), IgG3 ($p < 0.05$), and IgG4 ($p < 0.05$) (fig. 2). Moreover, we

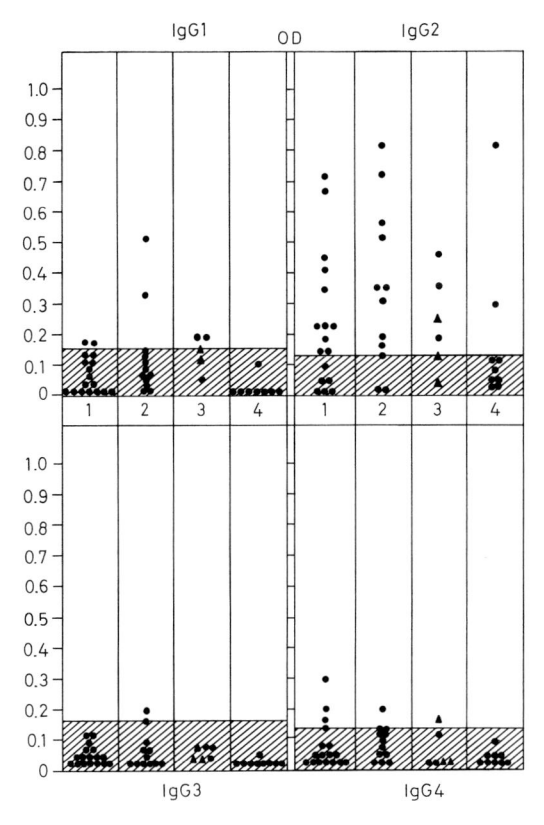

Fig. 2. Serum levels of IgG subclasses (OD) anti-GBS type Ia polysaccharide in group: (1) normal adults; (2) vaginally colonized women; (3) septic neonates (▲) and their mothers (●); (4) patients with IgG2 deficiency.

demonstrated that the seropositive normals or colonized women showed significant differences in comparison to the seronegative in the specific IgG2 (p<0.0001) and IgG4 (p<0.001), while no significant differences were found in the specific IgG1 and IgG3 levels. This prevalence of the GBS-type Ia IgG2 antibody response is similar to that already described for specific responses to other capsular polysaccharide antigens. Furthermore, all maternal specific IgG subclasses were transferred across the placenta, because we found comparable levels in the mothers and their infants. Interestingly, in a baby who died of sepsis, the specific antibody response was restricted to the IgG1 antibody, although his serum total level of IgG2 was within the normal range. In the group of patients with IgG2 deficiency, we found no correlation between levels of total and GBS-specific IgG2 antibodies.

Discussion

The results of this study demonstrate that the IgG2 subclass is the predominant antibody in the response to the GBS-type Ia capsular polysaccharide antigen. We could demonstrate a defective response only in a small group of GBS-colonized women and mothers and only in one infant who died of sepsis. Most of the normal controls showed serum antibodies to the GBS, even if they did not have any sign of bacterial colonization at the time of the test. 50% of patients with IgG2 subclass deficiency had specific IgG and IgG2 antibodies.

Neonatal group B streptococcal disease with early onset is associated with maternal GBS colonization. The frequent occurrence of primary rupture of the membranes suggests an ascending infection [2]. Animal models have been used to demonstrate that serum antibody protects against the GBS infection of the corresponding serotype. The biological importance of serum antibodies to the native GBS polysaccharide antigen is also reinforced by the demonstration of their interaction with the surface of the organism during opsonization and killing [15]. It has been demonstrated that mothers of GBS-infected infants have a deficiency of serum IgG subclasses and are poor responders to bacterial carbohydrate antigens [9, 10]; another study showed that women delivering infants with invasive GBS infection have the immune response to native GBS vaccine and to the pneumococcus polysaccharide vaccine similar to those of women matched for age and preimmunization levels [16]. No data were available on the presence of a deficiency in specific subclass response to the homologous GBS serotype polysaccharide antigen. Our results show a not significant difference in the specific antibody levels between groups studied, also due to the wide ranges observed. These data are similar to those found by others [17], and illustrate the inadequacy of our understanding of normal and susceptible populations. Normals with serum levels of GBS-specific IgG could have been previously infected by

GBS or other bacteria before the test, while colonized women without specific antibodies to GBS could only have a local immune response, or a non-IgG–mediated response. Alternatively, they could be a nonresponder group with a selective deficiency in the response to GBS polysaccharide antigen. It is noteworthy that all colonized women with low anti-GBS-specific serum titers have normal serum levels of total IgG2. The finding that the IgG2 subclass is the predominant antibody in the response to the GBS type Ia polysaccharide, as demonstrated for other polysaccharide antigens, suggests that in a vaccination program for colonized women with low levels of specific antibodies it is important to take into account the peculiar response to polysaccharides in man.

Vaccines to GBS significantly increase the levels of antibody in the nonimmune adult, and these levels persist for up to 2 years [18], but no booster effect has been observed, as for other polysaccharide vaccines. Nonresponders do not develop specific antibodies even with repeated antigenic stimulus. Screening of candidates for prophylaxis assumes a great importance for prenatal care. IgG2-deficient patients are poor responders to polysaccharide antigens, and our data suggest that a group of these patients do not respond to GBS antigen. Other IgG2-deficient patients show GBS-specific serum IgG2 antibodies. This observation and the demonstration that there is no correlation between total and specific IgG2 levels suggest that this humoral immunodeficiency is heterogeneous. Even if these patients have only a slight increase in the levels of specific antibodies after immunization with polysaccharide, they could be considered possible candidates for vaccination in order to increase their antibody levels to a protective level [19]. Also the group of colonized women where we could not detect specific antibodies might be considered as candidates for vaccination, in the last trimester of the pregnancy, to achieve protective levels of GBS-specific IgG. These antibodies, which are known to be transferred across the placenta [8], will passively immunize the fetus and decrease the incidence of GBS perinatal sepsis.

References

1   Baker, C.J.; Edwards, M.S.: Group B streptococcal infections; in Remington, Klein, Infectious diseases of the foetus and newborn infant, p. 820 (Saunders, Philadelphia 1983).

2   Bernirschke, K.: Routes and types of infection in the fetus and the newborn. Am. J. Dis. Child. *99:* 714 (1960).
3   Fleming, D.O.: Mouse protection assay for group B streptococcus type III. Infect. Immunity *35:* 240 (1982).
4   Klegerman, M.E.; Boyer, K.M.; Papierniak, C.K.; Gotoff, S.P.: Estimation of the protective level of human IgG antibody to the type specific polysaccharide of group B streptococcus type Ia. J. infect. Dis. *148:* 648 (1983).
5   Gotoff, S.P.; Odell, C.; Papierniak, C.K.; Klegerman, M.E.; Boyer, K.M.: Human IgG antibody to group B streptococcus type III: comparison of protective levels in a murine model with levels in infected human neonates. J. infect. Dis. *153:* 511 (1986).
6   Boyer, K.M.; Gotoff, S.P.: Prevention of early-onset neonatal group B streptococcal disease with selective intrapartum chemoprophylaxis. New Engl. J. Med. *314:* 1665 (1986).
7   Morell, A.; Sidiropulos, D.; Herrman, U.; Christensen, K.K.; Christensen, P.; Prellner, K.; Skvaril, F.: IgG subclasses and antibodies to group B streptococci in preterm neonates after intravenous infusion of immunoglobulin to the mothers. Pediat. infect. Dis. *5:* 195 (1986).
8   Boyer, K.M.; Papiernak, C.K.; Gadzala, R.N.: Transplacental passage of IgG antibody of group B streptococcus type Ia. J. Pediat. *104:* 618 (1984).
9   Christensen, K.K.; Christensen, P.; Lindberg, A.; Linden, V.: Mothers of infants with neonatal group B streptococcal septicemia are poor responders to bacterial carbohydrate antigens. Int. Archs Allergy appl. Immun. *67:* 7 (1982).
10 Oxelius, V.A.; Linden, V.; Christensen, K.K.; Christensen, P.: Deficiency of IgG subclasses in mothers of infants with group B streptococcal septicemia. Int. Archs Allergy appl. Immun. *72:* 249 (1983).
11 Boyer, K.M.; Gadzala, C.A.; Kelly, P.D.; Burd, L.I.; Gotoff, S.P.: Selective intrapartum chemoprophylaxis of neonatal group B streptococcal early-onset disease. II. Predictive value of prenatal cultures. J. infect. Dis. *148:* 802 (1983).
12 Christensen, K.K.; Christensen, P.; Dahlander, K.; Faxelius, G.; Jacobson, B.; Svenningsen, N.: Quantitation of serum antibodies to surface antigens of group B streptococci types Ia, Ib and III: low antibody levels in mothers of neonatally infected infants. Scand. J. infect. Dis. *12:* 105 (1980).
13 Wilkinson, H.W.; Jones, W.J.: Radioimmunoassay for measuring antibodies specific for group B streptococcal type Ia, Ib, Ic, II and III. J. clin. Microbiol. *3:* 480 (1976).
14 Gray, B.M.; Dillon, H.C.; Pritchard, D.G.: Interaction of group B streptococcal type-specific polysaccharides with wheat germ agglutinin and other lectins. J. immunol Methods *72:* 269 (1984).
15 Edwards, M.S.; Nicholson-Weller, A.; Baker, C.J.; Kasper, D.L.: The role of specific antibody in alternative complement pathway-mediated opsonophagocytosis of type III, group B streptococcus. J. exp. Med. *151:* 1275 (1980).
16 Fisher, G.; Horton, R.E.; Edelman, R.: Summary of the National Institutes of Health Workshop on group B streptococcal infection. J. infect. Dis. *148:* 163 (1983).
17 Baker, C.J.; Kasper, D.L.: Group B streptococcal vaccines. Rev. infect. Dis. *7:* 458 (1985).

18 Baker, C.J.; Edwards, M.S.; Kasper, D.L.: Immunogenicity of polysaccharides from type III, group B streptococcus. J. clin. Invest. *61:* 1107 (1978).
19 Umetsu, D.T.; Ambrosino, D.M.; Quinti, I.; Siber, G.R.; Geha, R.S.: Recurrent sinopulmonary infection and impaired antibody response to bacterial capsular polysaccharide antigen in children with selective IgG-subclass deficiency. New Engl. J. Med. *313:* 1247 (1985).

I. Quinti, MD, Department of Allergy and Clinical Immunology, University of Rome 'La Sapienza', I-00185 Rome (Italy)

Concentrations and Production of IgG Subclasses in Preterm and Small-for-Gestation Low Birth Weight Infants

Ranjit Kumar Chandra

Departments of Pediatrics, Medicine and Biochemistry, Memorial University of Newfoundland, St. John's, Newfoundland, Canada

Introduction

Approximately 12% of all infants born in industrialized affluent countries have a birth weight less than 2,500 g. Of these, about 3% are small-for-gestational age (SGA) and 9% are appropriate-for-gestational age (AGA). The incidence of low birth weight (LBW) is very high in underprivileged populations; the figure may be as high as 40% in some countries in Africa [9]. Intrauterine growth retardation is associated with a high prevalence of neurodevelopmental handicaps, visceral hemorrhage, and infection.

Observations

Morbidity data showed that about one third of SGA LBW infants (group 1) suffered from almost three-fold greater incidence of common infections such as upper respiratory tract congestion, otitis media and diarrhea (18.6 ± 2.4 illness days/100 child-days), compared with the remaining two thirds (group 2) (6.9 ± 0.9 illness days/100 child-days) and full-term infants with birth weights above 2,500 g (5.8 ± 1.7 illness days/100 child-days). The difference is highly significant ($p < 0.01$).

Cell-mediated immunity was impaired in the majority of infants in group 1 (table I). This was assessed by enumerating rosette-forming T lymphocytes, Leu3 + helper cells, and Leu2 + suppressor cells. Serum thymic hormone activity estimated by a bioassay was increased in cord

Table I. Immunologic findings in small-for-gestation low birth weight infants and healthy full-term infants

Immune response	Small-for-gestation		Healthy full-term
	group 1[1] (n = 21)	group 2 (n = 40)	(n = 50)
Lymphocyte number			
T cells, %	46 ± 3	64 ± 5	74 ± 4
Helper T cells, %	29 ± 3	40 ± 3	48 ±
Suppressor T cells, %	16 ± 2	18 ± 2	21 ± 3
Median serum thymic hormone activity (log$_{-2}$)			
Cord blood	8.5	8.0	6.0
Age > 4 weeks	4.0	4.5	6.5
Fetal:maternal ratio			
IgG1	0.62 ± 0.12	0.56 ± 0.09	1.23 ± 0.20
IgG2	0.38 ± 0.09	0.51 ± 0.11	0.73 ± 0.14
Antibody-producing cells/10^6 lymphocytes			
G1	2,240 ± 463	2,941 ± 984	3,456 ± 812
G2	678 ± 165	1,226 ± 564	1,835 ± 503

Data are shown as means ± SEM.
[1] SGA LBW infants were divided into groups based on morbidity experience (see text).

blood samples but decreased in serum samples obtained from SGA infants older than 4 weeks. In earlier studies, we found impaired delayed cutaneous hypersensitivity reactions to 2,4-dinitrochlorobenzene [2]. The depression of cell-mediated immunity in SGA LBW persists for several months to years [4, 6–8]. In contrast, AGA infants show a return to normal immunocompetence by 12 weeks of age [4]. The prolonged depression of immune responses in intrauterine growth retardation has been confirmed in laboratory animals [3].

Immunoglobulin G subclass levels were quantitated by radial immunodiffusion in agar using commercial antisera (Seward). The fetal: maternal ratio of IgG1 was lower in both groups of SGA LBW infants compared with full-term infants (table I) and that of IgG2 was lower in group 1 than in group 2, both of which were lower than healthy full-term infants [1]. The production of IgG subclasses in vitro was studied by the reverse hemolytic plaque assay. The number of IgG1 antibody-producing cells was slightly recovered in group 1 infants. IgG2-producing plaques were reduced significantly in group 1 infants and to a lesser extent in group 2, compared with healthy controls (table I).

Conclusions

LBW infants demonstrate impaired immunocompetence. Immunologic abnormalities including impaired cell-mediated immunity and reduced levels and production of IgG subclasses are more prominent in SGA infants, particularly among those who show a higher incidence of common infectious illnesses in the first year of life. It is possible that immunologic dysfunction is causally linked to the susceptibility of young infants to infection.

References

1 Chandra, R.K.: Levels of IgG subclasses, IgA, IgM and tetanus antitoxin in paired maternal and foetal sera; findings in healthy pregnancy and placental insufficiency; in Hemmings, Maternofoetal transmission of immunoglobulins, pp. 77–90 (Cambridge University Press, London 1975).
2 Chandra, R.K.: Fetal malnutrition and postnatal immunocompetence. Am. J. Dis. Child. *129:* 450–455 (1975).
3 Chandra, R.K.: Antibody formation in first and second generation offspring of nutritionally deprived rats. Science *190:* 189–190 (1975).
4 Chandra, R.K.: Serum thymic hormone activity and cell-mediated immunity in healthy neonates, preterm infants and small-for-gestation age infants. Pediatrics, Springfield *67:* 407–411 (1981).
5 Chandra, R.K.: Serum levels and synthesis of IgG subclasses in small-for-gestation low birth weight infants and patients with selective IgA deficiency. Monogr. Allergy, vol. 20, pp. 90–99 (Karger, Basel 1986).
6 Chandra, R.K.; Matsumura, T.: Ontogenetic development of immune system and effects of fetal growth retardation. J. perinatal Med. *7:* 279–287 (1979).

7 Dutz, W.; Rossipal, E.; Ghavami, H.; Vessel, K.; Kohout, E.; Post, G.: Persistent cell-mediated immune deficiency following infantile stress during the first 6 months of life. Eur. J. Pediat. *122:* 117–129 (1976).
8 Moscatelli, P.; Bricarelli, F.C.; Piccinini, A.; Tomatis, C.; Dufour, M.A.: Defective immunocompetence in foetal undernutrition. Helv. paediat. Acta *31:* 241–247 (1976).
9 WHO Scientific Group: Low birth weight infant (WHO, Genève 1975).

R.K. Chandra, MD, FRCP(C), Janeway Child Health Centre,
St. John's Newfoundland A1A 1R8 (Canada)

# IVIG Replacement Therapy in IgG Subclass Deficiency States

Immunoglobulin Treatment of Patients with Selective IgG Subclass and IgA Deficiency States

Janne Björkander[a], Vivi-Anne Oxelius[b], Ruzena Söderström[a], Lars Å. Hanson[c]

[a] Asthma and Allergy Research Centre, University of Göteborg, Göteborg;
[b] Department of Pediatrics, University of Lund, Lund; [c] Department of Clinical Immunology, University of Göteborg, Göteborg, Sweden

Risks from and Requirements of Immunoglobulin Prophylaxis

Intravenous Ig (IVIG) treatment of patients with common varied immunodeficiency (CVID) or X-linked agammaglobulinaemia (XLA) have proven to have a definite place in the therapeutic arsenal [1, 2]. IVIG offers certain advantages over the intramuscular (i.m.) or subcutaneous (s.c.) route of administration, but has also shown to be connected with the transmission of non-A, non-B hepatitis (NANBH) in some instances [3-6].

Because the intramuscular Ig (IMIG) was known to be safe since the 1960s, also the IVIG was considered to be safe against virus contamination. The reports from England, USA and Sweden about NANBH caused by unmodified IVIG preparations were therefore totally unexpected and no obvious explanation has been offered why these preparations caused hepatitis. There are minor differences, however, in the last steps of the processing of fraction II to prepare IMIG and IVIG, which might affect the infectivity of the final product [7]. It is clearly unacceptable that Ig products can transmit infections and biological products must be secured in the future so that they cannot contain infective material such as viruses.

IVIG should also not cause adverse reactions on infusion. Earlier preparations often had an unacceptable frequency of adverse reactions, most probably due to the presence of IgG polymers in the products. There appears to be a relation between the percentage of aggregated IgG and the frequency of side effects [8, 9]. In order to diminish the amounts of IgG aggregates, different preparation techniques have been tried with various chemical and/or enzymatic changes of the IgG molecule to minimize the formation of IgG aggregates. These procedures influence considerably the amount of monomeric, dimeric and polymeric IgG appearing [10, 11].

However, the modification steps to decrease the formation of IgG aggregates also effect the biological function of the Ig molecules. This has been illustrated for Fc-mediated functions on thrombocytes [12] and recently on monocytes [13]. Full biological efficacy both of the antibody binding (Fab) and the receptor binding part (Fc) of the molecule should preferably remain.

There should also be a representative content of the different subclasses in the IVIG [10, 14]. Some preparation procedures affect the proportion between different subclasses, especially by decreasing IgG3 and IgG4. The possible clinical significance of that is still unknown. A normal proportion of the IgG subclasses, as in serum, should be approached.

It may also be desirable to decrease the levels of IgA in Ig preparations because of the risk of induction of anti-IgA antibodies on injection with the consequent risk of adverse reactions on infusion (for review see Björkander et al. [15]). These adverse reactions have been rare using IVIG, but they can be severe. We have found anti-IgA antibodies quite commonly in individuals with selective IgA deficiency (29%) or IgA-IgG2 deficiency (60%) and even in patients with CVID or XLA (22%) [15]. Using IVIG low in IgA patients with anti-IgA antibodies do not usually react. Only in one instance out of seven did we note a severe anaphylactoid reaction on infusion of IVIG. This patient who had reacted severely previously to plasma infusions and to undefined Ig had received six infusions with the same preparation uneventfully. This preparation (Gammonativ, KabiVitrum, Stockholm, Sweden) was very low in IgA (<0.004 g/L). However, the anti-IgA of this patient increased continuously during these six infusions and he reacted fiercely at the seventh infusion. By prospectively following anti-IgA levels noting increases, such reactions can presumably be prevented. It has been suggested that the anti-IgA of this patient was of the IgE class but we have not been able to confirm that [15, 16].

Table I. Clinical characteristics of 14 patients with combined IgG subclass and IgA deficiency

Patient No	Age years	IgG subclass levels, g/l 1	2	3	4	Anti-IgA	Impaired lung function	URTI	Chronic sinusitis	Recurrent pneumonia	Chronic bronchitis	Bronchiectasis	Gastrointestinal involvement	HA or ITP	Additional diseases
1	31	8.87	3.30	0.37*	0.88	–	X	X	–	–	X	–	–	–	tuberculosis, prurigo Besnier
2	24	1.57	0.38	0.38	0.07	–	–	X	–	–	–	–	X	–	rhinoconjunctivitis
3	50	31.11	6.45	0.27	0.01	1:8	–	X	–	X	–	–	X	–	gastroduodenitis, epilepsia anemia, rheumatoid arthritis, hypothyreosis Sjögren's disease, celiac disease
4	66	10.51	2.65	0.21	0.43	1:8	X	–	–	X	X	–	X	–	psoriasis, emphysema
5	64	10.54	<0.01	1.99	md	1:2	X	–	X	X	X	X	X	X	salmonella, celiac disease, achylia, warts, tuberculosis, G-I candidiasis, alopecia, vitiligo antibodies against basophil and eosinophilic cells
6	48	9.69	0.20	2.29	0.08	–	X	X	X	X	X	X	–	–	hepatitis
7	34	3.13	2.06	0.19	md	–	–	–	X	X	X	X	X	–	prurigo Besnier, warts
8	60	4.15	0.80	0.53	md	–	X	X	–	X	X	X	X	–	angioneurotic edema, recurrent sinusitis, arthralgia

Table I. (cont.)

9	43	*3.40*	0.73	*0.08*	md	–	–	–	X	X	–	–	–	prurigo Besnier
10	27	*13.04*	0.52	0.44	0.13	1:128	X	X	–	X	–	–	X	von Willebrand's disease
11	29	*10.54*	0.73	*1.97*	md	1:512	X	X	X	X	X	–	–	non-A, non-B hepatitis, drug abuse
12	39	*1.62*	0.23	*1.39*	md	–	X	–	X	X	X	–	–	meningitis with abscess
13	39	4.42	0.87	0.31	<0.01	1:4	–	X	–	X	–	–	–	hypothyreosis
14	21	*0.72*	*0.08*	*1.75*	md	–	X	X	–	X	–	–	X	conjunctivitis
Normal range		4.22–12.92	1.17–7.47	0.41–1.29	<0.01–2.91									

URTI = Upper respiratory tract infection: HA = hemolytic anemia; ITP = idiopatic thrombocytopenic purpura; md = missing data.
* cursiv = pathological value.

Indications for Ig Prophylaxis in Primary Immunodeficiency

The indications for giving immunoprophylaxis to patients with primary immunodeficiencies should be based on the diagnosis of manifest antibody deficiency, a functional inability to respond to antigenic stimulation with one or a few relevant pathogens. Selective IgA deficiency has not yet been shown to be an indication for Ig prophylaxis. However, some of them have severe infectious problems, and recently it has been shown that some patients with IgA deficiency but normal IgG and IgG subclasses are still deficient in their serum responsiveness to certain vaccines [17].

Combined IgA Deficiency and Low Levels of IgG Subclasses

Patients with IgA deficiency seem to be low in one or more of the IgG subclasses in 10–20% [18, 19]. Among patients with IgG subclass deficiency IgA deficiency is also commonly seen [20, 21]. The combined deficiency brings with it an increased risk of impaired lung function [19].

We have noticed combined IgA and IgG subclass deficiency in altogether 14 patients with increased frequency of respiratory tract infections (table I). Patient Nos. 1–4, were all infectious prone and two had signs of an impaired lung function. One of the patients had celiac disease, Sjögren syndrome and rheumatoid arthritis. They have not yet been given Ig prophylaxis.

Patient Nos. 5–10 had recieved IMIG with a mean dose of 35 mg/ kg/week for altogether 72 years. Retrospective investigation of patient records showed that these 6 patients had all been helped by the IMIG and only patient No. 5 had to remain on antibiotic prophylaxis continuously. These patients were more heavily infected than patient Nos. 1–4 and 4 out of the 6 patients had bronchiectasis. Patient No. 5 with a very low IgG2 level had a remarkable number of autoimmune-associated diseases.

Patient Nos. 11–14 have all been on IMIG and IVIG except patient No. 11 who only had received IVIG. All patients but No. 13 have improved with fewer days of infection and less consumption of antibiotics. Two of the 3 patients with IgG2 deficiency had bronchiectasis and severely impaired lung function. Patient No. 14 had only had low

IgG levels for 4 years and still had signs of lung fibrosis. No side effects occurred during the Ig prophylaxis and the levels of anti-IgA antibodies did not increase in the 3 patients, Nos. 10, 11 and 13, with detectable levels.

Conclusion

These preliminary observations suggest that several of these patients with IgA deficiency and low levels of IgG subclasses may be helped by Ig prophylaxis. It can already be said at this stage that using an Ig preparation low in IgA seems to be safe. Only one case reacted via increasing levels of anti-IgA. This could presumably have been prevented by continuous monitoring of the serum IgA stopping the infusions when the increase was noticed. A controlled study is required, however, to define whether or not the patients with combined deficiency of one or more of the IgG subclasses and of IgA are protected from recurrent infections by Ig prophylaxis. Such prophylaxis, if successful, could be expected to prevent the appearance of chronic lung function impairment for which patients with this combined deficiency show an increased risk.

Acknowledgements

Our colleagues at the Asthma and Allergy Research Centre, Göteborg, and Dr. Tönnes Eilard at the Department of Infectious Diseases in Karlstad are thanked for stimulating cooperation. This work was supported by grants from the Swedish National Society against Allergy (RmA), Göteborg, the Swedish Medical Research Council (No. 215), the Ellen, Walter and Lennart Hesselman Foundation for Medical Research, the Medical Faculty of the University of Göteborg, Sweden, the Göteborg Medical Society and AB KabiVitrum, Stockholm, Sweden.

References

1 Bruton, O.C.: Agammaglobulinaemia. Pediatrics *9:* 722–728 (1952).
2 British Medical Research Council: Hypogammaglobulinaemia in the United Kingdom. Spec. Rep. Ser. No. 310 (HMSO, London 1971).
3 Lane, R.S: Non-A, non-B hepatitis from intravenous immunoglobulin. Lancet *ii:* 974–975 (1983).

4 Lever, A.M.L.; Brown, D.; Webster, A.D.B.; Thomas, H.C.: Non-A, non-B hepatitis and intravenous immunoglobulin. Lancet *ii:* 1062–1064 (1984).
5 Ochs, H.D.; Fischer, S.H.; Virant, F.S.; Lee, M.L.; Kingdon, H.S.; Wedgwood, R.J.: Non-A, non-B hepatitis and intravenous immunoglobulin. Lancet *i:* 404–405 (1985).
6 Björkander, J.; Cunningham-Rundles, C.; Lundin, P.; Olsson, R.; Söderström, R.; Hanson, L.Å.: Intravenous immunoglobulin prophylaxis and non-A, non-B hepatitis in antibody-deficient patients; in Vossen, Griscelli, Progress in immunodeficiency research and therapy, vol. II, pp. 177–182 (Excerpta Medica, Amsterdam 1986).
7 Lane, R.S.: Important parameters in plasma fractionation. Vox Sang. *51:* suppl. 1, pp. 49–51 (1986).
8 Barandun, S.: Die Gammaglobulin-Therapie. Chemische, immunologische und klinische Grundlagen. Bibliotheca haemat., No. 17 (Karger, Basel 1964).
9 Björkander, J.: Antibody deficiency syndromes; thesis, Göteborg (1985).
10 Römer, J.; Morgenthaler, J.J.; Scherz, R.; Skvaril, F.: Characterization of various immunoglobulin preparations for intravenous application. I. Protein composition and antibody content. Vox Sang. *42:* 62–73 (1982).
11 Björkander, J.; Wadsworth, C.; Hanson, L.Å.: 1040 prophylactic infusions with an unmodified intravenous immunoglobulin product causing few side-effects in patients with antibody deficiency syndromes. Infection *13:* 102–110 (1985).
12 Gross, B.; Haessig, A.; Luescher, E.F.; Nydegger, U.E.: Monomeric IgG preparations for intravenous use inhibit platelet stimulation by polymeric IgG. Br. J. Haemat. *53:* 289–299 (1983).
13 Jungi, T.W.; Santer, M.; Lerch, P.G.; Barandun, S.: Effect of various treatments of gamma-globulin (IgG) for achieving intravenous tolerance on the capacity to interact with human monocyte fc receptors. Vox Sang. *51:* 18–26 (1986).
14 Skvaril, F.: Subclass composition of intravenous IgG preparations. Monogr. Allergy, vol. 19, pp. 266–276 (Karger, Basel 1986).
15 Björkander, J.; Hammarström, L.; Smith, E.C.I.; Buckley, R.H.; Cunningham-Rundles, C.; Hanson, L.Å.: Immunoglobulin prophylaxis in patients with antibody deficiency syndromes and anti-IgA antibodies. J. clin. Immunol. *7:* 8–15 (1987).
16 Burks, A.W.; Sampson, H.A.; Buckley, R.H.: Anaphylactic reactions after gamma globulin administration in patients with hypogammaglobulinemia. Detection of IgE antibodies to IgA. New Engl. J. Med. *314:* 560–564 (1986).
17 Björkander, J.; Griffiss, J.; Berner, M.; Söderström, T.; Hanson, L.Å.: Serological response in infectious-prone IgA deficient patients to meningococcal polysaccaride group A + C vaccine compared to healthy controls. 16th Symp. Collegium internationale allergologicum, Göteborg 1986, abstr., book 10a.
18 Oxelius, V.-A.; Laurell, A.B.; Lindquist, B.; Golebiowska, H.; Axelsson, U.; Björkander, J.; Hanson, L.Å.: IgG subclasses in selective IgA deficiency: importance of IgG2-IgA deficiency. New Engl. J. Med. *304:* 1476–1477 (1981).
19 Björkander, J.; Bake, B.; Oxelius, V.-A.; Hanson, L.Å.: Impaired lung function in patients with IgA deficiency and low levels of IgG2 or IgG3. New Engl. J. Med. *313:* 720–724 (1985).
20 Björkander, J.; Bengtsson, U.; Oxelius, V.-A.; Hanson, L.Å.: Symptoms in patients with lowered levels of IgG subclasses with or without IgA deficiency, and Effects of immunoglobulin prophylaxis. Monogr. Allergy, vol. 20, pp. 157–163 (Karger, Basel 1986).

21 Söderström, T.; Söderström, R.; Bengtsson, U.; Björkander, J.; Hellstrand, K.; Holm, J.; Hanson, L.Å.: Clinical and immunological evaluation of patients low in single or multiple IgG subclasses. Monogr. Allergy, vol. 20, pp. 135–142 (Karger, Basel 1986).

Janne Björkander, MD, Asthma and Allergy Research Centre,
University of Göteborg, S-41345 Göteborg (Sweden)

Clinical Results of a Prospective, Double-Blind, Placebo-Controlled Trial of Intravenous γ-Globulin in Children with Chronic Chest Symptoms

Thomas F. Smith[a], Marion F. Muldoon[a], Raymond P. Bain[b], Elaine L. Wells[b], Thomas L. Tiller[c], Michael H. Kutner[b], Gerald Schiffman[d], Janardan P. Pandey[e]

[a] Department of Pediatrics, Emory University, Atlanta, Ga.;
[b] Department of Biometry, Emory University, Atlanta, Ga.;
[c] Private Practice, Greenville, S.C.;
[d] Department of Microbiology/Immunology, State University of New York, Brooklyn, N.Y.;
[e] Department of Microbiology/Immunology, Medical University of South Carolina, Charleston, S.C., USA

Patients with deficiencies of one or more IgG subclasses often experience recurrent or continuous respiratory tract symptoms [1–5]. It is likely that symptoms in many of these patients result from localized mucosal infection with encapsulated bacteria [6]. The host usually is able to keep these bacteria from invading systemically yet appears unable in most instances to clear them completely and heal the mucosa. Evidence has been presented that antibody replacement therapy is beneficial to adults with IgG subclass deficiencies [7]. It also has been suggested that chronic chest symptoms in certain nonallergic children might be related to deficiency of an IgG subclass, since these children as a group have an abnormal distribution of IgG subclass levels [3].

Several problems arise in approaching the diagnosis and therapy of children with suspected IgG subclass deficiency. First, IgG subclass levels are not good predictors of antibody responses in children [8], although they appear to be in adults [9]. This suggests that some children with low levels (< 2 SD below mean for age) of an IgG subclass might have normal subclass-specific antibody responses, while others with 'normal' levels of IgG subclasses might be unable to make certain specific antibodies. It has been our experience that partial antibody deficiency, defined as the ability to respond to some but not all antigens appropriately, is common among nonallergic children with chronic chest symptoms. Second, the natural history of partial antibody deficiencies in children is not known. Many children with chronic chest symptoms will 'outgrow them' eventually, and this suggests that maturation of specific antibody responses also occurs eventually. Third, previous trials of γ-globulin therapy in children with chronic chest symptoms have been uncontrolled [10, 11] or have found no beneficial effect [12, 13]. It is not clear whether failure to demonstrate benefit was related to improper patient selection, use of subtherapeutic dosage, or that it really is not beneficial; these studies all predate concepts of IgG subclass deficiencies. Last, there has been great concern about producing 'immunologic cripples' [14] or provoking unwanted immunologic responses in children treated unnecessarily with γ-globulin [15].

In the present study, we investigated the response to therapy with intravenous γ-globulin of children recruited because of their history of chronic chest symptoms. It was our intent to assess both beneficial and adverse effects of γ-globulin therapy and to see if immunologic measurements made beforehand would predict clinical response.

Methods and Materials

We enrolled 50 subjects (30 boys) age 1–13 years (mean ± SD = 6.6 ± 3.5 years) based on physicians' and parents' history of the children having chronic chest symptoms and having had a consistent need for either antibiotics or corticosteroids as part of the management of these symptoms. On entry each child was given a complete physical examination and blood was drawn for baseline immunologic measurements, including IgG, IgA, IgM, IgG subclasses, preimmunization antibody levels, and anti-allotype antibodies. Each child was immunized with diphtheria, tetanus, and 23-valent pneumococcal vaccines; 47 children also received trivalent influenza vaccine. Each family then began keeping daily records of symptoms listed quantitatively and qualitatively and of medicine doses given. Four weeks later, each child was reexamined and blood was drawn for immunologic measurements (including postimmunization antibody levels). Therapy was then instituted using either intravenous immunoglobulin (IVIG, Sandoglobulin) 200 mg/kg every 3 weeks or an equivalent volume of 0.03% human serum albumin as placebo. Both IVIG and placebo were received in the hospital pharmacy as lyophilized preparations labelled by patient number only and were reconstituted by a pharmacist beforehand. The reconstituted materials were identical in appearance, and the identity of subject groups was blinded from all investigators and participants until after the completion of the study. Each subject received seven doses of IVIG or placebo during January through May 1985. Daily diaries were maintained until 8 weeks after the last infusion; at that time a blood sample was obtained for post-treatment immunologic measurements.

Results

Clinical Description of Subject. The children enrolled appeared to meet the general criteria of having chronic chest symptoms. Forty-eight (96%) had been diagnosed previously as having asthma, 38 (76%) as having chronic bronchitis, 26 (52%) with recurrent pneumonia, 11 (22%) with persistent pulmonary infiltrates, and 5 (10%) with bronchiectasis. All had a history of cough and all but one had a history of wheezing. Age of onset of chest symptoms was less than 2 years in 76%, including 48% of children who first experienced symptoms when less than 6 months old. Thirty-two (64%) had been experiencing chest symptoms at least weekly during the 3 months before study entry; in 14 others symptoms had been at least monthly. Forty-three (86%) reported viral respiratory infections as major triggers of their chest symptoms; other significant factors included weather changes (86%), allergy (70%), irritants such as tobacco smoke (56%), and exercise (42%). Other respiratory complaints by history included rhinitis (96%), sinusitis (86%), otitis media (82%), and pneumonia (78%). Seasonal history of symptoms by history was as follows: autumn, 98% of subjects; winter, 94%; spring, 86%; and summer, 26%. There were no statistical differences between groups in age, gender, past medical history, or symptoms or medicines during the 4-week period before treatment.

It was interesting that children in both groups did well clinically during these 4 weeks. There was little therapy with antibiotics in either

Table I. Symptoms and medicine doses

	Treatment group	
	IVIG (n = 23)	placebo (n = 24)
Total number of days		
Sick	14 ± 10	20 ± 16
With all chest symptoms	113 ± 85	130 ± 74
With any chest symptom	61 ± 40	70 ± 36
With all nasal symptoms	67 ± 39*	112 ± 65
With aly nasal symptom	51 ± 32*	76 ± 41
Total qualitative scores		
Sick	27 ± 19	37 ± 24
Runny nose	54 ± 44	79 ± 64
Nasal congestion	55 ± 49**	111 ± 70
Cough	90 ± 68	80 ± 49
Chest tightness	30 ± 30	42 ± 38
Wheezing	37 ± 54*	57 ± 47
Mucus in chest	26 ± 33	30 ± 39
Total number of medicine doses		
Bronchodilators	781 ± 578*	1,136 ± 496
Corticosteroids	121 ± 268*	161 ± 177
Antirhinitis medicines	311 ± 401	425 ± 381
Antibiotics	31 ± 28	36 ± 40

* $p < 0.05$; ** $p < 0.01$.

group. Seven children experienced essentially no chest symptoms, 3 experienced no nasal symptoms, 3 received essentially no bronchodilator therapy, 19 received no corticosteroids, and 17 received no antirhinitis medicines (antihistamines, decongestants, or intranasal therapy); these subjects were excluded from calculations of improvement (defined as a 25% decrease in symptoms or medicines). Three patients were excluded from the clinical analysis because of failure to complete the daily diaries over the course of the study.

Responses to Therapy

Summaries of medicine doses over the course of the study are displayed in table I. Children receiving IVIG experienced fewer nasal

Table II. Percent of children experiencing improvement[1]

	After 4th dose		After 7th dose	
	IVIG	placebo	IVIG	placebo
Total number of days				
All chest symptoms	60	50	80	65
Any chest symptom	55	35	75	70
All nasal symptoms	57	43	87	67
Any nasal symptom	52	30	83	55
Total number of medicine doses				
Bronchodilators	18	9	36	23
Corticosteroids	63	42	75	67
Antirhinitis medicines	50	21	69	36

[1] Improvement is defined as a 25% decrease in number over two consecutive 3-week observation periods, compared to pretreatment number.

symptoms than did those receiving placebo; they also took fewer antirhinitis medicines, although this difference did not reach statistical significance. Those treated with IVIG also received fewer doses of bronchodilators and of corticosteroids than did those receiving placebo; there was a similar indication of decreased days with chest symptoms in the treated group as well. There were few infections, little antibiotic usage, few doctor visits, few days with fever, and few days in hospital in either group.

Children in both treatment groups experienced a considerable decrease in days with symptoms and number of doses of medicines given over the course of the study (January through May), as would have been predicted from clinical history. There were clear, consistent trends indicating the children receiving IVIG experienced more improvement more rapidly than did those receiving placebo (table II). The differences did not reach statistical significance.

We found no statistically significant relationships between immunologic measurements (level of immunoglobulins, IgG subclasses, or antibodies to diphtheria, tetanus, three influenza strains, or 12 pneumococcal serotypes either before or after immunization) and total clinical symptoms, total medicine doses, or improvement in either treatment group.

Adverse Effects

There were seven reactions seen in 175 infusions of IVIG (3.4%) and 15 reactions in 166 infusions of placebo (8.4%). These included fatigue, headache, rashes (placebo only), and vomiting (placebo only). All were mild and self-limited.

Forty-five of 47 children had normal serum ALT documented before beginning the study. Interestingly, all 47 children had normal ALT at the end of the study.

We were unable to detect any adverse immunologic consequences of therapy with IVIG. There were no statistical differences between groups after treatment in any immunologic measurements, including serum level of immunoglobulins, level of antibodies before or after immunization, and incidence and titer of anti-allotype antibodies. In addition, there were no statistically significant relationships between presence of or level of anti-allotype antibodies, immunoglobulin levels, or immunization-related antibody levels.

Discussion

We studied the use of IVIG for children with chronic chest symptoms in a prospective double-blind, placebo-controlled trial. We found consistent beneficial effects of IVIG in children selected by clinical criteria. Treatment with IVIG resulted in a statistically significant decrease in nasal symptoms and use of chest medicines (bronchodilators and corticosteroids) when compared to placebo; it also appeared to decrease chest symptoms and use of antirhinitis medicines. Current understanding of the dose dependency of response suggests that greater clinical benefit might have been seen had a larger dose of IVIG been used. To our surprise, we were unable to identify any immunologic measurements which predicted a beneficial response.

It should be kept in mind that studies of this type are at risk of commiting a type II statistical error because of a small number of patients, a wide range of values for each measurement, and marked improvement seen in both treatment groups. It may be that we are underestimating the effect of IVIG and making a type II error. On the other hand, performing multiple statistical analyses also increases the risk of a type I error. In this study, this is most likely to occur when analyzing relationships between immunologic and clinical measurements. Our inability to demonstrate statistically significant relationships suggests that type I errors are unlikely.

We cannot explain the basis for the beneficial effect of IVIG in these children. We were unable to demonstrate an immunologic basis for effect. It is possible that we were providing specific antibody which individual subjects needed to prevent or clear mucosal infections. It has been speculated that exogenous γ-globulin might decrease the incidence of episodes of infectious asthma [11]. We were unable to document a difference between treatment groups in the number of infections, in part because both groups experienced few infections; thus, we believe this is a less likely explanation for its beneficial effect. IVIG has been shown to be immunomodulatory, and it may be that IVIG will benefit host defense specifically or nonspecifically, apart from provision of antibodies against infectious agents.

Children enrolled in the study were healthier during the study than would have been predicted by clinical history. It is possible that the multiple immunizations given initially were beneficial in preventing specific infections or in augmenting overall immune responsiveness. We previously have noted a dramatic clinical improvement in chest symptoms in certain children after immunization with polyvalent pneumococcal vaccine. However, it is likely that requiring parents to grade symptoms and document each medicine dose on a daily basis resulted in earlier access to medical care and increased compliance, both improving their children's health.

There was significant improvement documented in *both* treatment groups over the course of the study. It is not clear whether this relates only to seasonal variations in symptoms, as would have been predicted by history, or whether it might be the result of spontaneous improvement in immune function as well. In either event, some caution must be used before concluding that clinical responses in children with chronic chest symptoms receiving γ-globulin indicate immunodeficiency.

We documented no adverse effects of IVIG in the children studied. Although exogenous antibody will ablate endogenous formation of antibody of the same specificity, there is no evidence that it will alter concurrent responses to other antigens. In addition, our results and previous studies indicate that exogenous immunoglobulin does not adversely effect the level of immunoglobulins or antibodies or antibody-forming capacity after treatment has been stopped. It has been argued that immunoglobulin treatment of infants and small children will produce 'γ-globulin cripples' [14] who experience an increased number of infections when therapy is discontinued. Considering the clinical challenge of treating significant pulmonary disease in this aged patient, it might be to the physician's and patient's advantage to allow some lung growth and maturation before these infections occur.

We observed no instances of severe reactions to infusion of IVIG, and we identified no instances of non-A, non-B hepatitis as a result of IVIG. The incidence of either would make it unlikely that either would occur in small study sample.

Conclusion

Therapy with intravenous immunoglobulin is beneficial in children with chronic chest symptoms. Our results do not suggest an immunologic measurement which will predict response, however. We recommend that intravenous immunoglobulin be used only for those children experiencing significant morbidity in spite of optimal medical care, after an immunologic evaluation (including measuring specific antibody responses) is performed. The likelihood of spontaneous reduction in symptoms indicates that IVIG therapy should be stopped and clinical and immunologic reassessment performed on a regular basis; reinstitution of therapy should be delayed until symptoms recur.

References

1 Schur, P.H.; Borel, H.; Gelfand, E.W.; Alper, C.A.; Rosen, F.S.: Selective gamma-G globulin deficiencies in patients with recurrent pyogenic infections. New Engl. J. Med. *283:* 631–634 (1970).
2 Oxelius, V.A.: Chronic infections in a family with hereditary deficiency of IgG2 and IgG4. Clin. exp. Immunol. *17:* 19–27 (1974).
3 Smith, T.F.; Morris, E.C.; Bain, R.P.: IgG subclasses in children with chronic chest symptoms. J. Pediat. *105:* 896–900 (1984).
4 Umetsu, D.T.; Ambrosino, D.M.; Quinti, I.; Siber, G.R.; Geha, R.S.: Recurrent sinopulmonary infection and impaired antibody response to bacterial capsular polysaccharide antigen in children with selective IgG-subclass deficiency. New Engl. J. Med. *313:* 1247–1251 (1985).

5 Shackelford, P.G.; Polmar, S.H.; Mayus, J.L.; Johnson, W.L.; Corry, J.M.; Nahm, M.H.: Spectrum of IgG2 subclass deficiency in children with recurrent infections: prospective study. J. Pediat. *108:* 647–653 (1986).
6 Smith, T.F.; Ireland, T.A.; Zaatari, G.S.; Zwiren, G.T.; Andrews, H.G.: Characteristics of children with endoscopically-proven chronic bronchitis. Am. J. Dis. Child. *139:* 1039–1044 (1985).
7 Björkander, J.; Bengtsson, U.; Oxelius, V.A.; Hanson, L.A.: Symptoms in patients with lowered levels of IgG subclasses, with or without IgA deficiency, and effects of immunoglobulin prophylaxis. Monogr. Allergy, vol. 20, pp. 157–163 (Karger, Basel, 1986).
8 Smith, T.F.; Morris, E.C.; Bain, R.P.: Serum IgG2 concentration does not correlate with antibody response to pneumococcal polysaccharides in immunodeficient children. J. Allergy clin. Immunol. *75:* 189 (1985).
9 Siber, G.R.; Schur, P.H.; Aisenberg, A.C.; Weitzman, S.A.; Schiffman, G.: Correlation between serum IgG2 concentrations and the antibody response to bacterial polysaccharide antigen. New Engl. J. Med. *303:* 78–82 (1980).
10 Bowen, R.: Gammaglobulin and the asthmatic child. J. Allergy *26:* 87 (1955).
11 Brown, E.B.; Botstein, A.: The effect of gamma globulin in asthmatic children. N.Y. St. J. Med. *60:* 2539–2545 (1960).
12 Abernathy, R.S.; Strem, E.L.; Good, R.A.: Chronic asthma in childhood: double-blind controlled study of treatment with gammaglobulin. Pediatrics, Springfield *21:* 980–992 (1958).
13 Fontana, V.J.; Kuttner, A.G.; Wittig, H.J.; Moreno, F.: The treatment of infectious asthma in children with gammaglobulin. J. Pediat. *62:* 80–84 (1963).
14 Miller, M.D.: Uses and abuses of plasma therapy in the patient with recurrent infections. J. Allergy clin. Immunol. *51:* 45–56 (1973).
15 Buckley, R.H.: Immunoglobulin replacement therapy: indication and contraindication for use and variable IgG levels achieved; in Immunoglobulins: characteristics and uses of intravenous preparations, DHHS publ. No. 80-9005, pp. 3–7 (US Dept. of Health and Human Services, Washington 1979).

Thomas F. Smith, MD, Department of Pediatrics,
Emory University, Atlanta, GA 30322 (USA)

Intravenous Immune Serum Globulin Replacement in Hypogammaglobulinemia
A Comparison of High- versus Low-Dose Therapy

Erwin W. Gelfand[a], Brenda Reid[b], Chaim M. Roifman[b]

[a] Department of Pediatrics, National Jewish Center for Immunology and Respiratory Medicine, Denver, Colo. and [b] Division of Immunology and Rheumatology, The Hospital for Sick Children, Toronto, Ontario, Canada

Introduction

Since its introduction in the late 1950s, immune serum globulin (ISG) has been the treatment of choice and life saving for many patients with congenital or acquired hypogammaglobulinemia [1, 2]. Given intramuscularly on a regular basis, ISG has resulted in a significant reduction in the incidence of some bacterial infections. Although reactions to intramuscular ISG are rare, there are limitations to this form of therapy. The injections are painful and therefore limit the amount which can be administered. Since the incidence of infections and febrile episodes appears to be inversely related to the amount of immunoglobulin (Ig) administered [3], many approaches have been used to overcome the limitations of single or multiple intramuscular injections.

Regular plasma infusions offer the patient a pain-free means for Ig replacement, without major limitations concerning volume. Administration of 20 ml plasma per kg body weight results in roughly 2-fold higher levels of serum IgG when compared to intramuscular ISG at the recommended dosage of 0.6 ml(100 mg)/kg body weight on a monthly basis. However, because of the serious threat of transmission of hepatitis or other viral diseases, plasma programs have become markedly curtailed.

The ability to administer ISG intravenously provided a new opportunity for delivering increased passive antibody protection [4]. Intravenous administration may also avoid the local tissue proteolytic degradation which follows intramuscular injection of ISG.

There have been only limited studies comparing the efficacy of intramuscular versus intravenous replacement, particularly in reducing infections. At roughly comparable doses (100–200 mg/kg/month), both forms of therapy are sufficient to maintain serum IgG levels at or near 300 mg/dl [5–7]. Their effects on reducing or preventing infections were also roughly the same [8]. To date, there have been few studies determining the effects of higher doses of intravenous ISG in the prophylaxis against infection in a given group or groups of patients [9].

Recurrent and chronic sinopulmonary infections persist in a group of adults and children with hypogammaglobulinemia, despite the administration of standard doses of Ig on a regular basis. In an attempt to prevent progressive pulmonary deterioration in these individuals, we evaluated the effects of high-dose ISG replacement therapy in patients with chronic sinopulmonary disease and hypogammaglobulinemia. The amount administered every 4 weeks, 0.6 g/kg, was chosen in an attempt to provide trough levels above 500 mg/dl.

Methods

Patients

Seven patients, 4 males and 3 females, were evaluated in the initial study [10]. Five of the patients were classified as having common variable immunodeficiency disease and 2 as having X-linked agammaglobulinemia. Their ages ranged from 7 to 49 years. In the second or cross-over study [11], 4 female and 8 male patients aged 7–50 years were evaluated.

All patients were selected because of chronic sinopulmonary disease as established by clinical signs and symptoms of chronic cough, acute exacerbations of pneumonia, radiographic abnormalities of the chest and sinuses and pulmonary function tests at least 25% below predicted values.

All patients had serum IgG levels of less than 300 mg/dl at presentation and all but 3 (who were previously untreated), rarely achieved trough serum IgG levels greater than 300 mg/dl while on intramuscular ISG replacement at 0.1 g/kg every 2–4 weeks.

Protocol and Evaluation

Patients received intravenous ISG (Sandoglobulin, Sandoz, Montreal, Canada) at a dosage of 0.6 g/kg every 4 weeks in the initial study. In the cross-over trial, for the first 6 months, patients were allocated randomly to receive either 0.2 or 0.6 g/kg every 4 weeks and for the second 6 months were switched to the alternative dose.

The patients were monitored carefully for side effects, including alterations in heart rate, respiratory rate, blood pressure and temperature. Each treatment visit included a

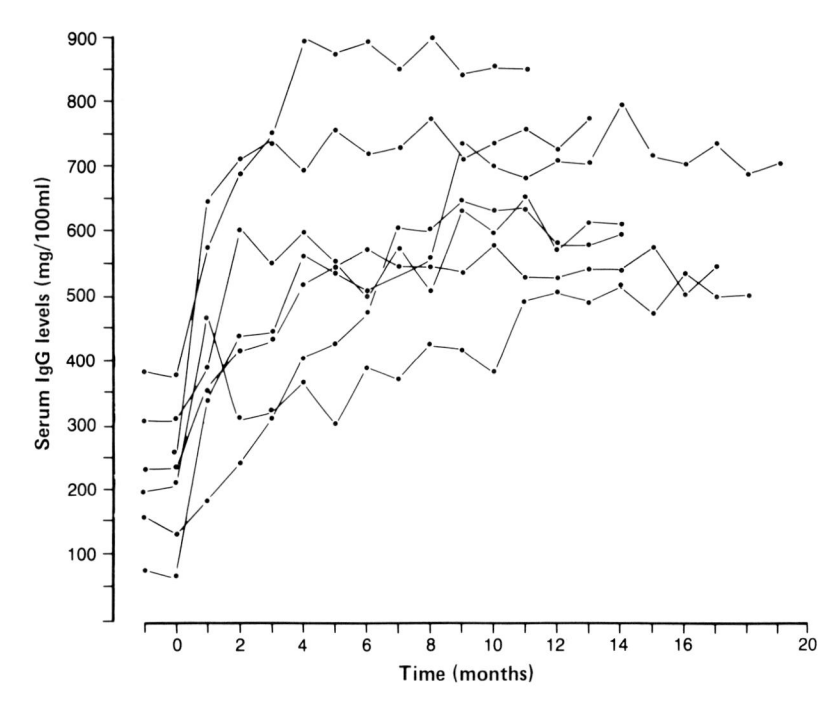

Fig. 1. Preinfusion serum IgG levels. All patients received 0.6 g/kg intravenous immune serum globulin every 4 weeks. Serum IgG levels were determined prior to each infusion.

physical examination and review of health status from patients' diaries and interviews. Sputum cultures, blood counts and quantitative Ig determinations were obtained at every visit. Chest and sinus radiographs and spirometric recordings were made before the start of the study and every 3 months thereafter.

Results

The effects of regular 4-weekly infusions of intravenous ISG in the initial 7 patients are illustrated in figure 1. At initiation of intravenous therapy, serum IgG levels in 6 of 7 patients were 300 mg/dl or less. Administration of 0.6 g/kg led to increased serum IgG levels which attained a plateau between 3 and 6 months. The 'steady-state' levels of IgG achieved and the time taken to reach plateau levels varied from patient to patient, despite their receiving a constant quantity based on

Table I. Improvement in pulmonary function testing

Patient	FEV_1, % predicted		FVC, % predicted	
	pre	post	pre	post
1	91	100	90	100
2	80	86	69	80
3	78	98	84	94
4	54	74	62	82
5	50	60	50	61
6	41	50	45	58
7	40	47	50	54

Table II. Acute infections requiring hospitalization

Infection	Number of admissions	
	intramuscular	intravenous
Pneumonitis	12	0
Sinusitis	8	3
Miscellaneous	5	1
	25	4

body weight. As shown in figure 1, this dosage of intravenous ISG achieved the goal of trough levels of a minimum of 500 mg/dl in virtually all patients. The variation of trough levels from patient to patient was attributed to individual differences in catabolic rates.

Associated with the elevated serum IgG levels, there was clinical, subjective and objective improvement. There was a marked reduction in cough, improvement or elimination of symptoms of sinusitis associated with normalization of sinus radiographs and a 10–25% improvement in pulmonary function results (table I). All 7 patients had radiographic evidence for bronchiectasis, but radiographic improvement was noted in only 2 patients.

In addition, administration of intravenous ISG in this way influenced the incidence of severe, acute infections requiring hospitalization (table II). Prior to entry in the study and for the equivalent

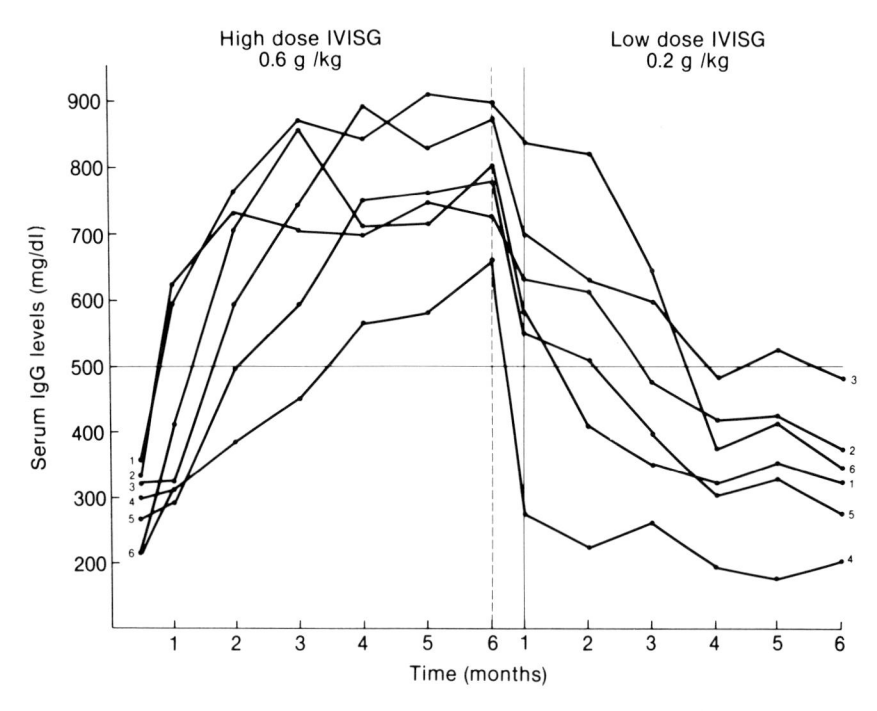

Fig. 2. Preinfusion serum IgG levels in patients begun on high-dose therapy. Patients 1–6 received 0.6 g/kg of intravenous ISG every 4 weeks for 6 months and were then switched to 0.2 g/kg for a further 6 months. Serum IgG levels were determined prior to each infusion.

number of months, there were 25 admissions compared to only 4 admissions during the intravenous program.

Based on these data, a randomized cross-over study was initiated in 12 additional patients with chronic sinopulmonary disease. In four, chronic lung disease developed despite regular intramuscular replacement therapy and, in five, there was gradual worsening of lung disease over 1–7 years of conventional IgG replacement. The remaining three had not previously been treated.

A total of 144 intravenous ISG infusions were administered to this group of patients during the study. In patients receiving 0.6 g/kg, serum IgG levels increased to 500 mg/dl (trough) or more within 2–4 months, as shown in figure 2. Decreasing the dose to 0.2 g/kg resulted in a rapid decline in serum IgG levels within the first 2–3 months in 4

Table III. Acute infections in patients

	Serum IgG < 500 mg/dl	Serum IgG > 500 mg/dl
Minor infections		
Upper respiratory tract	23	10
Otitis	4	1
Urethritis	1	0
Skin	3	1
	31	12
Major infections		
Pneumonitis	11	3
Sinusitis	4	0
Arthritis	1	0
	16	3

of 6 patients, while in the 2 other patients, a level of less than 500 mg/dl was only achieved after the third or fourth month of low-dose infusions (fig. 2).

Acute infections were divided into two categories, mild and not requiring hospitalization, and severe, requiring hospitalization. In the first group, 43 episodes were recorded, 24 episodes during the low-dose phase and 19 during the high-dose phase. When these episodes of acute infection were analyzed not by whether they were in the high- or low-dose phase but according to the serum IgG levels, the differences were much clearer. There were 31 episodes when serum IgG levels were less than 500 mg/dl (table III). In the second category of infections requiring hospitalization, the results were even more dramatic, with 16 major infections during the period when serum IgG levels were less than 500 mg/dl versus only 3 admissions during the period above 500 mg/dl (table III).

In all 6 patients switched from high-dose to low-dose ISG, pulmonary function (spirometry) values deteriorated (table IV). In contrast, in the 6 patients switched from low dose to high dose, there was a consistent improvement. Overall, the differences of the means of FVC and FEV_1 under high-dose versus low-dose replacement were highly significant ($p < 0.001$).

Table IV. Improvement in pulmonary function testing

Patient	FEV$_1$, % predicted high → low dose	Patient	FEV$_1$, % predicted low → high dose
1	100 → 80	7	82 → 92
2	90 → 75	8	80 → 98
3	80 → 70	9	68 → 72
4	70 → 62	10	63 → 88
5	68 → 48	11	52 → 60
6	51 → 42	12	42 → 54

Table V. Mycoplasma isolates from sputum of patients with hypogammaglobulinemia and chronic lung disease

Patient	Number of isolates low-dose therapy	high-dose therapy
1	3	1
2	1	0
3	0	0
4	4	1
5	3	1
6	2	0
7	4	1
8	3	2
9	1	0
10	5	3
11	2	1
12	1	0
	29	10

Adverse Effects. In approximately 20% of the infusions, there were mild side effects consisting of low grade fever, flushing, headache and back pain. These appeared related to the infusion rate and abated when the rate was slowed. In 3 patients, repeated reactions were experienced, but these could be prevented by hydrocortisone premedication as previously described [12].

Liver Function Studies. Serum aminotransferase levels were monitored regularly and remained within the normal range throughout the study.

Microbiological Studies. Patients with compromised immunity are susceptible to a variety of infections, often due to organisms considered to be of low pathogenicity. Hypogammaglobulinemia may result in a unique susceptibility to infection with mycoplasma, particularly *Ureaplasma urealyticum* (formerly known as T strain mycoplasma) [13–15]. Mycoplasmas have been regularly isolated from our patients with hypogammaglobulinemia during episodes of acute or chronic respiratory illness [16]. Improvement only followed institution of specific antibiotic therapy and elimination of the mycoplasma. In our cross-over study, the number of mycoplasma isolates from sputum of patients with chronic sinopulmonary disease was 3-fold higher during the period of low-dose replacement, compared with the 6 months on high-dose therapy (table V).

Discussion

Conventional doses (0.1–0.2 g/kg) of intramuscular or intravenous ISG have been effective in preventing infections in a large percentage of patients with antibody deficiency. Nevertheless, approximately 30% of patients with hypogammaglobulinemia develop chronic sinopulmonary disease. At the present time, it is not known whether early replacement with conventional or high-dose ISG can prevent the occurence of chronic sinopulmonary disease. Once chronic disease is established, replacement with conventional doses appears insufficient.

Treatment with high-dose intravenous ISG has been successful in controlling life-threating ECHO virus infection [17]. In our initial study, the effects of high-dose therapy were clearly demonstrated to reduce the frequency of major infections and to improve chronic lung disease [10]. A direct comparison of high-dose and low-dose regimens further emphasized the importance of achieving adequate serum IgG levels [11]. Although initial analysis comparing the effects of high-dose versus low-dose therapy on the incidence of major or minor infections was marginal, reevaluation of the data based on serum IgG levels was striking. During periods when serum levels of IgG were below 500 mg/

dl, the number of infections was significantly higher than during an equal time period when IgG levels were greater than 500 mg/dl. The most dramatic differences associated with the two regimens were in the assessments of pulmonary function.

Spirometric indices were significantly improved in all patients at the completion of the high-dose treatment period, whereas the results at the end of the low-dose period were significantly worse.

The infusions were, in general, well tolerated, with only minor reactions which responded to adjustments of rates of flow. In the 3 patients with recurrent reactions, hydrocortisone premedication eliminated these side effects [12]. Liver function studies remained within the normal range for all patients throughout the study.

These studies demonstrate the efficacy of high-dose intravenous ISG therapy in hypogammaglobulinemic patients with chronic sinopulmonary disease. Monthly infusions of 0.6 g/kg were effective in achieving trough serum IgG levels of more than 500 mg/dl within 4 months of initiation of this therapy. Individual variability in sustaining a serum IgG level was likely a reflection of differing individual catabolic rates. Attainment of trough serum IgG levels of 500 mg/dl or more appeared to provide better protection against infection and was associated with amelioration of chronic symptoms and improvement in pulmonary function. Since patients with hypogammaglobulinemia appear to be uniquely susceptible to infection with mycoplasma, it may be that serum IgG levels of 500 mg/dl are required for adequate prophylaxis against such organisms. Preliminary data have shown only low antimycoplasma antibody titers in ISG, and isolates of mycoplasma are much more infrequent when serum IgG levels are above 500 mg/dl than when they fall below this level.

References

1   Barandun, S.; Riva, G.; Spengler, G.A.: Immunologic deficiency: diagnosis, forms and current treatment. Birth Defects, Orig. Article Ser., No. 6, pp. 40–48 (1968).
2   Janeway, C.A.; Rosen, F.S.: The gammaglobulins. Therapeutic uses of gammaglobulin. New Engl. J. Med. *275:* 826–831 (1966).
3   Hypogammaglobulinemia in the United Kingdom. Medical Research Council Special Services Report. *310:* 1–319 (1971).
4   Nolte, M.T.; Pirofsky, B.; Gerritz, G.A.; Golding, B.: Intravenous immunoglobulin therapy for antibody deficiency. Clin. exp. Immunol. *36:* 237–243 (1979).

5 Pirofsky, B.; Campbell, S.M.; Montanaro, A.: Individual patient variations in the kinetics of intravenous immunoglobulin administration. J. clin. Immunol. 2: 7–14 (1982).
6 Buckley, R.H.: Long-term use of intravenous immune globulin in patients with primary immunodeficiency diseases: inadequacy of current dosage practices and approaches to the problem. J. clin. Immunol. 2: 15–21 (1982).
7 Ochs, H.D.; Fisher, S.H.; Wedgwood, R.J.: Modified immune globulin: its use in the prophylactic treatment of patients with immune deficiency. J. clin. Immunol. 2: 22–30 (1982).
8 Ammann, A.J.; Ashman, R.F.; Buckley, R.H.; Hardie, W.R.; Krantmann, H.J.; Nelson, J.; Ochs, H.; Stiehm, E.R.; Tiller, T.; Wara, D.W.; Wedgwood, R.: Use of intravenous gammaglobulins in antibody immunodeficiency: results of a multicenter controlled trial. Clin. Immunol. Immunopathol. 22: 60–67 (1982).
9 Sorensen, R.U.; Polmar, S.H.: Efficacy and safety of high-dose intravenous immune globulin therapy for antibody deficiency syndromes. Am. J. Med. 76: 83–90 (1984).
10 Roifman, C.M.; Lederman, H.M.; Lavi, S.; Stein, L.D.; Levison, H.; Gelfand, E.W.: Benefit of intravenous IgG replacement in hypogammaglobulinemic patients with chronic sinopulmonary disease. Am. J. Med. 79: 171–174 (1985).
11 Roifman, C.M.; Levison, H.; Gelfand, E.W.: High-dose versus low-dose intravenous immunoglobulin in hypogammaglobulinemia and chronic lung disease. Lancet ii: 1075–1077 (1987).
12 Lederman, H.M.; Roifman, C.M.; Lavi, S.; Gelfand, E.W.: Corticosteroids for prevention of adverse reactions to intravenous immune serum globulin infusions in hypogammaglobulinemic patients. Am. J. Med. 81: 443–446 (1986).
13 Stuckey, M.; Quinn, P.A.; Gelfand, E.W.: Identification of *Ureaplasma urealyticum* (T-strain mycoplasma) in a patient with polyarthritis. Lancet ii: 917–920 (1978).
14 Taylor-Robinson, D.; Gumpel, J.M.; Itill, A.; Swannell, A.J.: Isolation of *Mycoplasma pneumoniae* from the synovial fluid of a hypogammaglobulinemic patient in a survey of patients with inflammatory polyarthritis. Ann. rheum. Dis. 37: 180–182 (1978).
15 Webster, A.B.D.; Taylor-Robinson, D.; Furr, P.M.; Asherson, G.L.: Mycoplasma (ureaplasma) septic arthritis in hypogammaglobulinemia. Br. med. J. ii: 478–479 (1978).
16 Roifman, C.M.; Rao, C.P.; Lederman, H.M.; Lavi, S.; Quinn, P.A.; Gelfand, E.W.: Increased susceptibility to mycoplasma infection in patients with hypogammaglobulinemia. Am. J. Med. 80: 590–594 (1986).
17 Mease, P.J.; Ochs, H.D.; Wedgwood, R.J.: Successful treatment of echovirus meningoencephalitis and myositis-fasciitis with intravenous immune globulin therapy in a patient with x-linked agammaglobulinemia. New Engl. J. Med. 304: 1278–1279 (1981).

Dr. E.W. Gelfand, National Jewish Center for Immunology and Respiratory Medicine, 1400 Jackson Street, Denver, CO 80206 (USA)

Replacement Therapy in IgG4-Deficient Patients

D.C. Heiner, S.I. Lee, K. Kim, J. Schoettler

Division of Immunology and Allergy, Harbor-UCLA Medical Center, Torrance, Calif., USA

Experience in the study of sera from 400 consecutive patients referred for quantitation of IgG subclass levels because of an increased frequency of infections revealed that 26% had a deficiency of IgG4 defined as a serum level under 30 µg/ml. Of healthy age-matched controls 5.6% had levels in this range. The difference between patients and controls is highly significant. Normal values for IgG3 and IgG4 obtained in our laboratory have been published elsewhere [1]. A modified list of the ranges of normal for all IgG subclasses with rounding off of the values is given in table I. Interpolation of values is necessary for estimating the ranges at ages between those given. Values for IgG1 and IgG2 represent a composite of normal ranges taken from the literature [2-6]. We utilize the radial immunodiffusion technique for IgG1 and IgG2, but for quantitation of IgG3 and IgG4 we use radioimmunoassays.

Roughly half of the IgG4-deficient patients had a concomitant deficiency of IgG2; a few of these had IgG4 and IgG2 plus another class or subclass deficiency. Approximately one quarter of those with a low IgG4 had an isolated IgG4 deficiency, and the other quarter had normal levels of IgG2 but had IgG4 deficiency in association with IgA, IgG1, or IgG3 deficiency.

Approximately 38% of infection-prone patients had an IgG2 deficiency. Nearly half of these were isolated IgG2 deficiency but 40% were associated with IgG4 deficiency. Using the normal ranges listed in table I, IgG2 deficiency proved to be the most common IgG subclass deficiency in infection-prone subjects. IgG2 was followed by IgG4, then IgG1 and IgG3. Table II lists the findings for the 85 patients most recently studied. Just over half of all patients with unex-

Table I. Ranges of normal IgG subclasses according to age

Age (m = months, y = years)	IgG1 mg/dl	IgG2 mg/dl	IgG3 µg/ml	IgG4 µg/ml
4 m	150–390	25–150	8–1,000	9–460
6 m	190–390	40–160	13–2,000	7–600
9 m	200–500	30–200	14–3,000	5–800
1–2 y	230–700	30–300	100–2,200	15–900
3–5 y	350–800	60–350	110–2,300	30–1,000
6–8 y	350–800	70–410	110–2,500	60–1,000
9–11 y	350–1,000	100–530	110–2,800	55–1,000
12–14 y	350–1,000	130–500	90–2,100	60–1,000
15–17 y	350–1,000	120–550	100–2,300	60–1,000
18–20 y	350–1,050	130–600	130–1,850	60–1,000
21–60 y	350–1,100	120–760	150–2,500	60–1,500
Over 60 y	390–1,150	150–820	200–3,500	65–3,000

Table II. Number of subjects with a deficiency of any IgG subclass among 85 patients susceptible to infections and 85 age-matched healthy controls

Subclass	Susceptible to infections	Age-matched controls
IgG1	17	1
IgG2	33	2
IgG3	4	0
IgG4	24	1

plained susceptibility to infection had subnormal levels of one or more of the four IgG subclasses. Less than 3% of the healthy population had subnormal levels of a given subclass, and only 5% had a serum level of any subclass which was more than two standard deviations below the mean for a particular age. 19% of subjects with an increased susceptibility to infection had an elevation in one or more of the IgG subclasses. Most commonly this involved IgG1.

Sixteen (19%) of 85 recently studied patients with 'increased susceptibility' to infection had low levels of IgG antibodies to the capsular polysaccharide of *H. influenza* (polyribosylribitol phosphate,

Table III. Of 16 patients susceptible to infection who had very low ($\bar{x}$-2SD) levels of anti-*H. influenza* capsular polysaccharide, the following number had abnormal IgG subclass levels

Subclass	Deficiency	Elevation
IgG1	7	3
IgG2	5	0
IgG3	2	1
IgG4	4	0

PRP). This was defined as a value more than two standard deviations below the mean value of age-matched controls. Ten of the 16 had a deficiency of one or more IgG subclasses whereas 6 did not. Only 3 had normal levels of all four subclasses since three had an elevation of one or more subclasses. There appears to be an association between aberrations in subclass levels and an inability to produce 'normal' levels of antibodies to this particular polysaccharide, but it is not a universal phenomenon. It is of interest that subclass deficiencies seen in association with low levels of anticapsular polysaccharide were by no means limited to the IgG2 subclass. Indeed, deficiency of IgG1 was the one most commonly associated with low levels of anti-PRP (table III). Aberrations in IgG1 levels were twice as frequent as aberrations in any other subclass. Although IgG2 and IgG4 deficiencies are more common in the general population than IgG1 or IgG3 deficiencies, when an *isolated* IgG1 deficiency is seen, it may represent a more significant disorder of humoral immunity than IgG2 or IgG4 deficiency. Three of 7 such patients produce low levels of antibody to *H. influenza* PRP in response to natural exposure whereas only one of 14 patients with isolated IgG2 deficiency had low levels of antibody to the capsular polysaccharide. In the overall group of 85 patients, there was a positive correlation ($r = 0.623$, $p = 0.04$) between total IgG1 levels and total IgG anti-PRP levels. There was no significant correlation between IgG2 levels and anti-PRP. Fifty four of the 85 subjects were 15 years of age or less.

Other studies carried out in our laboratory [7-9] suggest that the effects of the different IgG subclasses are interrelated, i.e. for optimal resistance against microorganisms, it may be essential to have intact mechanisms for producing antibodies of each of the IgG subclasses. Patients with a deficiency of one subclass are generally not as prone to infection as patients who have deficiencies of two or more subclasses. At least a few subjects, perhaps more than currently suspected, have functional deficiencies of antibody production even though they have normal total levels of each subclass.

We consider IgG4 deficiency in the same light as deficiency of any of the other subclasses. When a specific deficiency is documented in a patient who has frequent or severe infections, a decision must be made concerning two aspects of treatment, namely the use of antimicrobials and the use of γ-globulin replacement therapy. Antibiotics are routinely used for acute pyogenic infections. γ-Globulin therapy, usually intravenously administered, is used when acute infections are severe. If episodes of infection are not life-threatening and occur less often on average than every 2 months, they are treated with supplemental γ-globulin if indicated clinically. If they recur more frequently but are relatively mild, we recommend a trial of continuous antibacterial prophylaxis with an agent such as trimethoprim sulfa, ampicillin, or amoxicillin. If this does not bring the infections under control or if there is chronic infection, we recommend continuous γ-globulin replacement. This can be given intramuscularly if clinically efficacious and well tolerated. Some patients clearly are treated more successfully with intravenous than with intramuscular γ-globulin. The goal is to reverse or significantly ameliorate the susceptibility to infection. A 3- to 6-month trial sufficient to bring trough levels of the deficient subclass(es) within the range of normal should be made before deciding that γ-globulin is of no value.

We have seen a number of severe, life-threatening infections associated with an isolated deficiency of IgG4 which did not respond to antibiotics until γ-globulin replacement therapy was given. Two such patients narrowly escaped death in our hospital. The first was a 9-year-old boy [10] who was admitted with septic arthritis of multiple joints, extensive osteomyelitis, and purulent pericarditis, all due to *Staphylococcus aureus*. He failed to respond to intensive antibacterial therapy for 2.5 weeks using antimicrobials to which the organism was susceptible in vitro. Only after intravenous γ-globulin therapy was instituted and IgG4 antistaphylococcal antibodies reached normal level did drainage sites and fever come under control.

An infant was recently discharged from this hospital who at 4 weeks of age had overwhelming meningococcal sepsis with extensive ecchymoses and necrosis of the skin and underlying tissues, ultimately requiring amputation of several extremities. He and his mother both had an isolated deficiency of serum IgG4. In all likelihood, he would not have survived without extensive blood and plasma transfusions. Only careful follow-up will determine whether or not the child can produce his own IgG4.

We have seen several other instances in which severe infections in neonates have been associated with an IgG subclass deficiency in the mother. Placental transfer of a full complement of immunoglobulins to the newborn infant may be critical to survival in certain instances.

The adverse effects of prematurity, congenital heart disease, bronchopulmonary dysplasia, and other disorders may be additive to those of a subclass deficiency in causing undue susceptibility to infection. Two infants with bronchopulmonary dysplasia were followed conscientiously by our housestaff for 12 months and 3 years, respectively. Both had recurrent febrile illnesses during which respiratory inadequacy became pronounced. Each finally succumbed to respiratory failure. At or near the time of death, each was found to have an isolated severe deficiency of IgG4 with compensatory increases of other subclass levels. Neither was given replacement therapy. Another infant with a similar clinical picture was recently found to have a combined IgG2-IgG4 deficiency. She is currently under treatment and hopefully will have a better outcome. A third infant with isolated deficiency of serum IgG4 recently died in our hospital [11]. She was infected with the AIDS virus and was seen by us at 21 months of age when she had severe Candida sepsis as well as thrombocytopenia and a B cell lymphoma. She received replacement therapy only when terminally ill. No one knows whether or not γ-globulin would have been of benefit if it had been given early to this child, but it has been thought to help other children with AIDS. If this infant had presented herself to us at an earlier age, she would have received regular infusions of intravenous γ-globulin sufficient to normalize his IgG4 level.

At the present time, there are no hard and fast rules to govern the use of γ-globulin replacement therapy in IgG subclass deficiencies. We believe γ-globulin can be lifesaving for those patients who have severe infection. We also believe the frequency of infections can be decreased in subclass-deficient subjects who have recurrent febrile illnesses. It can reverse or slow the progression of chronic disease in selected patients.

Double-blind placebo-controlled multicenter studies conducted under meticulous protocol are needed to determine the value of γ-globulin in subjects with subclass deficiencies who have recurrent minor infections. Specific criteria should define: (1) The patient populations to be studied including the type and number of infections required for admission to the study. (2) The frequency, amount, duration and route of γ-globulin to be administered. (3) The use of antibiotics. (4) An appropriate placebo. (5) Laboratory tests to be done at the onset and during therapy. (6) Acceptable evidences of benefit.

This would be the most efficient cost-effective method of putting to rest questions which some knowledgeable academicians have raised concerning the need for γ-globulin therapy in subclass deficiencies.

References

1 Lee, S.I.; Heiner, D.C.; Wara, D.: Development of serum IgG subclass levels in children. Monogr. Allergy, vol. 19, pp. 108–121 (Karger, Basel 1986).
2 Morell, A.; Skvaril, F.; Hitzig, W.H.; Barandun, S.: IgG subclasses: development of the serum concentrations in 'normal' infants and children. J. Pediat. 80: 960–964 (1972).
3 Giessen, M. van der; Rossouw, E.; Algra-Van Veen, T.; Loghem, E. van; Zegers, B.T.M.; Saunders, P.C.: Quantification of IgG subclasses in sera of normal adults and healthy children between 4 and 12 years of age. Clin. exp. Immunol. 21: 501–509 (1975).
4 Oxelius, V.-A.: IgG subclass levels in infancy and childhood. Acta paediat. scand. 68: 23–27 (1979).
5 Schur, P.H.; Rosen, F.; Norman, M.E.: Immunoglobulin subclasses in normal children. Pediat. Res. 13: 181–183 (1979).
6 Zegers, B.J.M.; Giessen, M. van der; Reerink-Brongers, E.E.; Stoop, J.W.: The serum IgG subclass levels in healthy infants of 13–62 weeks of age. Clinica chim. Acta 101: 265–269 (1980).
7 Dengrove, J.; Lee, E.J.; Heiner, D.C.; St. Geme, J.W., Jr.; Leake, R.; Baraff, J.; Ward, J.I.: IgG and IgG subclass specific antibody responses to diphtheria and tetanus toxoids in newborns and infants given DTP immunization. Pediat. Res. 20: 735–739 (1986).
8 Schoettler, J.J.; Kim, K.S.; Hong, J.H.; Heiner, D.C.: Protective and opsonic activity of IgG subclass antibodies (Ab) against *Haemophilus influenzae* type B (Hib). Pediat. Res. Program Issue 21: 318A (1987).

9 Kim, K.S.; Kim, J.S.; Wass, C.A.; Short, J.A.; Heiner, D.C.: A human immunoglobulin G (IgG) subclass, IgG3, is opsonic against type III group B streptococcus (GBS). Clin. Res. *35:*219A (1987).
10 Schoettler, J.J.; Heiner, D.C.: Hypercatabolism of IgG4 associated with severe staphylococcal infection. Clin. Res. *128A:*34 (1986).
11 Honda, N.S.; Heiner, D.C.; Sun, N.C.: Isolated IgG4 subclass deficiency and malignant lymphoma in a child with acquired immunodeficiency syndrome. Am. J. Dis. Child. *141:*398–399 (1987).

Douglas C. Heiner, MD, PhD, Professor of Pediatrics, Chief, Division of Immunology/Allergy, Harbor-UCLA Medical Center, 1000 West Carson, E-6, Torrance, CA 90509 (USA)

IgG Replacement Therapy in IgG Subclass-Deficient Children

Lorraine J. Beard, Antonio Ferrante[1]

Department of Paediatrics and Department of Immunology, University of Adelaide, Adelaide Children's Hospital, Adelaide, South Australia

The Significance of IgG Subclass Deficiency in Children

The incidence of IgG subclass deficiency in children is unknown although it has been reported increasingly in association with recurrent infections [1–3]. As in adults, IgG subclass deficiency is not apparently uncommon in symptomatic IgA-deficient children. In a group of 22 IgA-deficient children, we found IgG subclass deficiency to be considerably more common in those with slightly low than in those with markedly low IgA levels [4]. Others also have found a higher incidence of IgG subclass deficiencies among children with partial IgA deficiency than among those with complete IgA deficiency [5, 6].

It is difficult to clearly define IgG subclass deficiencies in children. Nevertheless, it is important to do so because the severe degrees of deficiency, which are more readily defined, probably represent only the 'tip of the iceberg' as far as clinical relevance and possible benefit from Ig replacement therapy is concerned. Difficulties in definition arise because of the wide variation in IgG subclass levels in normal children and are compounded because the few studies that have been conducted show differences particularly in defining lower limits of normal. Such differences may reflect the use of different techniques, different antisera (polyclonal or monoclonal), different ways of ex-

---

[1] We thank Prof. G.M. Maxwell, Dr. E.F. Robertson and Dr. T.S. Pouras for helpful discussion on patients. The work was supported by grants from the Channel 10 Children's Medical research Foundation of South Australia.

pressing normal ranges, inadequate numbers of subjects [7], different criteria for normality or genetically different populations.

While there may be a causal relationship between IgG subclass deficiency and recurrent infections, IgG subclass deficiencies have been found in some healthy subjects [8–10], and so the finding of such a deficiency, even in an infection-prone patient, may not explain the infection-proneness.

In deciding whether to treat symptomatic IgG subclass-deficient patients with Ig replacement, assessment of compensatory immune mechanisms including the ability to produce particular antibodies may be helpful. Antibody production can be impaired in both IgA-deficient [11, 12] and IgG subclass-deficient [2, 13–15] subjects. This may involve antibodies of not only the deficient isotype but also of other isotypes [14–16]. Assessment of subclass-specific antibody responses is yet in its infancy. IgG subclass deficiency may be an indicator of an underlying defect in antibody production [13].

For those reasons, our current practice in deciding which infection-prone children with low or borderline low IgG subclass levels to treat with Ig replacement includes assessment of ability to produce antibodies to particular antigens and assessment of various lymphocyte, neutrophil and complement functions.

The Use of Immunoglobulin Replacement in IgG Subclass-Deficient Children

Intramuscular immunoglobulin (IMIG) has been used to treat hypogammaglobulinaemia successfully for nearly 40 years. More recently intravenous immunoglobulin (IVIG) has been shown to be equally effective or in larger doses, more effective [17–19]. There appears to be wide variation in Ig levels from patient to patient even when a uniform dose of Ig has been administered at a uniform rate [19]. There have, however, been relatively few reports of the treatment of isolated IgG subclass deficiencies with Ig. Schur et al. [20] reported 2 children and an adult with different combinations of IgG subclass deficiencies and life-long susceptibility to infections who were treated with IMIG. Oxelius [21] reported a family with IgG2-IgG4 deficiency, and 4 patients with IgA-IgG2 deficiency [22] who responded well to IMIG, and a patient with systemic lupus erythematosus, recurrent pericarditis and infections, and a subclass deficiency who also improved with Ig prophylaxis [14]. Bass et al. [23] described an IgG2-deficient infant who suffered 2 episodes of meningococcal meningitis prior to being given IMIG prophylaxis which proved effective. Plebani et al. [16] reported an 11-year-old with recurrent infections and bronchiectasis who had a deficiency of IgG2 and of specific IgG and IgM antibodies who improved on 100 mg/kg/week of subcutaneous Ig. Serum IgG2 normalised and IgG tetanus toxoid antibodies rose significantly. Björkander et al. [24] described 3 IgA-IgG2-deficient patients with respiratory infections who benefited from Ig replacement therapy.

Such studies indicate that Ig replacement is probably worthwhile in symptomatic IgG subclass deficiency and that IMIG may, at times, be effective. By analogy with the situation in other hypogammaglobulinaemias, IVIG would be expected to be even more effective. IMIG is more convenient, less expensive and less likely to be associated with systemic side-effects than is IVIG, and it has not been associated with the transmission of non-A non-B hepatitis as has IVIG, albeit very rarely [25]. Some contend that IMIG is safer in IgA-deficient patients who may have IgA antibodies, but such patients may react to either form [26].

There have been several studies in patients with primary humoral immunodeficiencies seeking to establish the optimal dosage and frequency of administration of IVIG [18, 19, 26]. None of these have dealt specifically with the use of IVIG to treat symptomatic IgG subclass deficiencies. In healthy subjects IgG1, IgG2, and IgG4 have similar half-lives to IgG (about 21 days) and IgG3 has a shorter half-life (about 7 days [27]). In hypogammaglobulinaemic subjects the half-lives are often prolonged [28]. It is expected that half-lives of deficient isotypes may also be prolonged in patients with isolated IgG deficiencies but this is not known. The half-lives of IgG subclasses may vary according to the method of preparation of the Ig. Further studies are needed to determine the optimal use of Ig replacement in IgG subclass deficiencies.

Theoretical dangers of administering Ig to partially immunocompetent patients include the suppression of endogenous antibody formation to antigens not previously encountered, and the induction of antibodies to Ig alloantigens that differ from those of the recipient [26].

While many would agree that infection-prone IgG-subclass-deficient patients with impaired antibody production should be offered Ig replacement therapy, there is less agreement about how to treat patients who seem equally infection-prone, but have more borderline deficiencies.

The case reports described below illustrate some of these points in 3 very different patients with differing degrees of IgG subclass deficiency.

Materials and Methods

IgG subclasses were measured by an enzyme-linked immunosorbent assay (ELISA) using subclass specific monoclonal antibodies (Miles Scientific, Naperville, Ill.) and goat anti-mouse Ig ('catching' antibodies) used to coat microwells [29]. Human standard serum H00-02 (Central Laboratory, Netherlands Red Cross Blood Transfusion Service) was used as a standard.

Total serum IgA, IgG, IgM C3 and C4 were measured by radial immunodiffusion (RID) or by nephelometry (ICS, Beckman Instruments Inc., Calif.). CH_{50} by lysis of haemolysin-coated sheep red cells, and cellular studies included lymphocyte subpopulations and responsiveness to mitogens and neutrophil chemotaxis, iodination, bactericidal and fungicidal activities as previously described [30].

Specific antibody titres were measured by haemagglutination inhibition for tetanus toxoid and pneumococcal capsular polysaccharide, agglutination for pertussis, and ELISA for diphtheria.

Immunising agents were triple antigen (diphtheria, tetanus, pertussis-adsorbed) and tetanus toxoid (Commonwealth Serum Laboratories, CSL, Australia) and pure pneumococcal polysaccharide and pure pertussis antigen (privately supplied).

Normal immunoglobulin (human) prepared by Cohn's cold ethanol fractionation and supplied by CSL Australia was the Ig preparation used unless otherwise stated. The intravenous form was subject to incubation at low pH. Sandoglobulin (Sandoz Ltd., Basle) prepared by cold ethanol fractionation and treatment at pH 4 with a minimum amount of pepsin was used recently in one patient as described. We have found both preparations to contain physiological proportions of the IgG subclasses.

Case Report 1 (J.B.)

This girl experienced severe recurrent respiratory infections from age 4 months. She was previously reported as having a primary selective deficiency of IgM with impaired production of certain antibodies [31]. Following immunisation with a 14-valent pneumococcal vaccine, J.B. failed to produce antibody against all 14 serotypes. Infections included otitis, sinusitis, bronchitis and pneumonia, and organisms pneumococcus, haemophilus and staphylococcus. By age 19 years she had chronic sinusitis and suppurative bronchitis which was worsening despite the constant use of antibiotics and physiotherapy. Lung function tests were poor and X-rays indicated widespread pulmonary disease and chronic sinusitis. Her serum IgA, IgG and IgM were now each in the low or low normal range. Serum IgG subclasses were measured and showed low levels particularly for IgG1, IgG2 and IgG4 (table I). IVIG therapy was begun with a loading

Table I. Serum immunoglobulin levels in 3 patients receiving immunoglobulin replacement therapy

Patient	Age years	Interval since last IgG dose weeks	Serum levels, g/l IgA	IgG
J.B.	12.2	*	1.47	5.81 ↓
	19.0	*	1.16	5.60 ↓
	19.4	2	0.95	6.20 ↓
	19.5	2	0.92	6.00 ↓
	20.5	5	0.79 ↓	4.76 ↓
	20.6	5	0.74 ↓	4.25 ↓
	21.1	5	0.71 ↓	5.04 ↓
M.W.	0.9	*	<0.10 ↓	2.06 ↓
	12.1	2	0.03 ↓	2.21 ↓
	13.2	2	<0.01 ↓	1.99 ↓
	14.9	2	0.01 ↓	1.87 ↓
P.S.	0.8	*	0.18 ↓	4.12
	1.1	4	0.18 ↓	4.66
	1.4	8	0.34	5.12
	1.7	12	0.31	4.67
	3.4	*	0.54	7.41
Normal ranges	0.8–2		0.19–1.73	2.48–12.51
	3–4		0.35–2.55	4.68–14.58
	12–13		0.80–4.75	6.48–17.28
	14–15		0.86–5.18	6.48–17.28
	Adult		0.86–5.18	6.48–17.28

* = Not receiving Ig; n.d. = not done.

dose of 300 mg/kg followed by 50 mg/kg of IVIG every 2 weeks. Within 4 months her chronic productive cough had resolved and her exercise tolerance had improved. Her sinusitis showed marked improvement. She was able to take on part-time work for the first time. For J.B., however, IVIG infusions have not been problem-free. She had a fear of needles which was very difficult to overcome. Invariably she experienced malaise, chest tightness, dyspnoea and sometimes muscle pains during infusions. Very recently she was given Sandoglobulin (Sandoz, Basle) instead of normal immunoglobulin (CSL, Australia) and for the first time symptoms were minimal. The dose given was able to be increased.

Previously, because of problems with infusions, the dose of IVIG had been limited to 50 mg/kg. Variations had been made in the frequency of infusions. For the first 6 months IVIG was given 2 weekly, for the next 8 months 3 weekly and for the next 14 months 5 weekly. Trough levels of IgG subclasses did not fall consistently, but J.B. developed an episode of severe bronchitis requiring hospitalisation and since then has

Table I. (cont.)

Serum levels, g/l				
IgM	IgG1	IgG2	IgG3	IgG4
0.05 ↓	3.37	0.77 ↓	0.40	0.07 ↓
0.43 ↓	3.04 ↓	0.69 ↓	0.26 ↓	0.05 ↓
0.45 ↓	3.30 ↓	0.56 ↓	1.02	0.009 ↓
1.05 ↓	3.31 ↓	0.43 ↓	1.01	0.007 ↓
0.43 ↓	3.37 ↓	0.63 ↓	0.36	0.06 ↓
0.42 ↓	2.87 ↓	0.79 ↓	0.27 ↓	0.06 ↓
0.44 ↓	2.19 ↓	0.36 ↓	0.73	0.02 ↓
1.56	n.d.	n.d.	n.d.	n.d.
0.14 ↓	0.93 ↓	0.59 ↓	0.05 ↓	0.05
0.16 ↓	2.72 ↓	0.77 ↓	0.04 ↓	0.07
0.20 ↓	1.20 ↓	0.29 ↓	0.04 ↓	0.04 ↓
0.43	4.56	0.39	0.32	0.06
0.51	7.35	0.89	0.46	0.12
0.74	4.12	0.83	0.36	0.12
0.53	3.43	0.73	0.19	0.16
1.24	5.15	1.64	0.42	0.62
0.27–1.55	1.51–7.25	0.30–1.75	0.10–0.61	0.02–0.83
0.39–1.67	3.35–7.80	0.46–2.09	0.14–1.17	0.05–1.30
0.46–1.83	2.94–7.21	0.86–3.01	0.21–0.76	0.03–1.41
0.46–1.88	4.74–8.21	0.97–2.59	0.15–0.99	0.10–1.14
0.47–1.88	3.82–14.27	1.24–4.96	0.30–1.57	0.18–2.10

been receiving 100 mg/kg of IVIG 3 weekly. In the 2 years before commencing IVIG she spent 53 days in hospital with respiratory infections but in the 2 years after starting IVIG she has spent only 4 days in hospital. Despite subjective and clinical improvement, lung function tests have continued to show restrictive and obstructive abnormalities.

This patient, originally considered to have a primary IgM deficiency, was subsequently shown to have IgG subclass deficiency. The use of IVIG has improved the quality of her life considerably, but was started too late to prevent chronic lung damage. It appears that the side-effects of IVIG which previously limited her therapy may largely be avoided by using Sandoglobulin which has recently become available to us. Brearley and Rowbotham [32] reported that the IgG aggregate content of Sandoglobulin is considerably less than that of the CSL preparation.

Case Report 2 (M.W.)
This patient is now 15 years old. She presented at age 10 months with extensive

pneumonia and bilateral otitis media. Her serum IgA level was low, serum IgG borderline low and serum IgM borderline elevated (table I). She continued to suffer recurrent chest and ear infections. At 25 months of age, antibodies to tetanus toxoid and pertussis were undetectable although she had previously received 4 standard doses of triple antigen. Re-immunisation produced a tetanus toxoid titre of 1:32 and a pertussis titre of 1:128. Immunisation with type 3 pneumococcal capsular polysaccharide gave a very poor response. In her fourth year she had 5 episodes of pneumonia. Serum IgA and IgM were by then undetectable and IgG was very low. Ig replacement therapy was begun with IMIG, 100 mg/kg being given every 2 weeks.

M.W. improved considerably. For several years she continued to have one or two brief episodes of chest infection per year, but generally she was well whereas previously she had been chronically ill. At age 9 years, neutrophil function, lymphocyte transformation to mitogens and serum complement studies were normal. In recent years her main problem has been asthma which has been well controlled with bronchodilators. She attends school and leads a normal active life. Lung function tests have shown reversible bronchoconstriction. The persistent changes seen in her chest radiographs in her early years have disappeared almost completely.

IgG subclass levels were first measured in this patient immediately before one of her regular doses of IMIG. Trough levels have been repeated on subsequent occasions. Levels of IgG1, IgG2 and IgG3 have been low on all occasions with IgG3 levels being disproportionately lower than the others. IgG4 was low or low normal (table I).

This patient with common variable immunodeficiency and low levels of IgG1, IgG2 and IgG3 has benefited from IMIG replacement therapy. She has tolerated very large volumes of IMIG extremely well and has elected to continue with IMIG rather than to change to IVIG, largely for reasons of convenience.

Case Report 3 (P.S.)

P.S. experienced an unusually high number of respiratory infections requiring antibiotic treatment in her first year of life. At 9 months of age her serum IgA was borderline-low and IgG and IgM levels were within the age-normal range (table I). Other immune function studies were normal except for a questionaly low neutrophil bactericidal activity. Serum IgG subclass levels were measured at age 10 months and showed a low normal IgG2 level (table I). After 3 standard doses of triple antigen, P.S. had protective titres of tetanus toxoid and pertussis antibodies but not of diphtheria antitoxin (1:1,024; 1:128; < 1:4, respectively).

Concern about her infections was such that IVIG was begun without further investigation. She received 150 mg/kg IVIG at ages 11, 12, 15, 17 and 20 months. Her health improved dramatically and infections ceased to be a problem. She has remained well for the 21 months since IVIG has been discontinued. Serum Ig, including IgG subclasses, are now within normal limits.

In this patient, the indications for IVIG were not clear-cut. She had a borderline-low IgA level and a borderline-low IgG2 level and may have had impaired antibody production but this was not adequately demonstrated. Her recurrent infections were the cause of such concern that treatment was instituted. Her excellent progress both during and after her course of IVIG was gratifying and suggests that the IVIG did not depress the development of normal immune responsiveness significantly. The natural history of

IgG subclass deficiency in children is not known. Smith and Bain [33] have suggested that in some instances IVIG administration may actually accelerate spontaneous improvement in IgG subclass levels.

References

1. Smith, T.F.; Morris, M.D.; Bain, R.P.: IgG subclasses in nonallergic children with chronic chest symptoms. J. Pediat. *105:* 896–900 (1984).
2. Umetsu, D.T.; Ambrosino, D.M.; Quinti, I.; Siber, G.R.; Raif, S.G.: Recurrent sinopulmonary infection and impaired antibody response to bacterial capsular polysaccharide antigen in children with selective IgG subclass deficiency. New Engl. J. Med. *313:* 1247–1251 (1985).
3. Shackleford, P.G.; Palmar, S.H.; Mayus, J.L.; Johnson, W.L.; Corry, J.M.; Nahm, M.H.: Spectrum of IgG2 subclass deficiency in children with recurrent infections. Prospective study. J. Pediat. *108:* 647–653 (1986).
4. Beard, L.J.; Ferrante, A.; Oxelius, V.A.; Maxwell, G.M.: IgG subclass deficiency in children with IgA deficiency presenting with recurrent or severe respiratory infections. Pediat. Res. *20:* 937–942 (1986).
5. Ugazio, A.G.; Out, T.A.; Plebani, A.; Duse, M.; Monafo, V.; Nespoli, L.; Burgio, G.R.: Recurrent infections in children with 'selective' IgA deficiency: association with IgG2 and IgG4 deficiency. Birth Defects, Orig. Article Ser., No. 19, pp. 161–171 (1983).
6. Plebani, A.; Monafo, V.; Avanzini, M.A.; Ugazio, A.G.; Guiseppe, R.B.: Relationship between IgA and IgG subclass deficiencies: a reappraisal; in Hanson, Oxelius, Int. Symp. Immunoglobulin Subclass Deficiencies, Lund 1985. Monogr. Allergy, vol. 20, pp. 171–178 (Karger, Basel 1986).
7. Bird, D.; Duffy, S.; Isaacs, D.; Webster, A.D.B.: Reference ranges for IgG subclasses in preschool children. Archs Dis. Childh. *60:* 204–207 (1985).
8. LeFranc, M.P.; LeFranc, G.; Rabbitts, T.H.: Inherited deletion of immunoglobulin heavy chain constant region genes in normal human individuals. Nature, Lond. *300:* 760–762 (1982).
9. Hammarström, L.; Smith, C.I.E.: IgG2 deficiency in a healthy blood donor. Concomitant lack of IgG2, IgA and IgE immunoglobulins and specific anti-carbohydrate antibodies. Clin. exp. Immunol. *5:* 600–604 (1983).
10. Carbonara, A.O.; Demarchi, M.: IgG isotypes deficiency caused by gene deletions; in Hanson, Oxelius, Int. Symp. Immunoglobulin Subclass Deficiencies, Lund 1985. Monogr. Allergy, vol. 20, pp. 13–17 (Karger, Basel 1986).
11. Heddle, R.J.; Kwitko, A.O.; Shearman, D.J.C.: Specific IgM and IgG antibodies in IgA deficiency. Clin. exp. Immunol. *41:* 453–458 (1980).
12. Hammarström, L.; Persson, M.A.A.; Smith, C.I.E.: Immunoglobulin subclass distribution of human anti-carbohydrate antibodies: aberrant pattern in IgA-deficient donors. Immunology *54:* 821–826 (1985).
13. Siber, G.R.; Scharp, P.M.; Aisenberg, A.C.; et al.: Correlation between serum IgG2 concentrations and the antibody response to bacterial polysaccharide antigens. New Engl. J. Med. *303:* 178–182 (1980).

14 Oxelius, V.-A.: Immunoglobulin G (IgG) subclasses and human disease. Am. J. Med. 76: 7–18 (1984).
15 Hammarström, L.; Granström, M.; Mollby, R.; Oxelius, V.-A.; Persson, M.A.A.; Smith, C.I.E.: Ontogeny of IgG2 antibodies against *S. aureus* teichoic acid in normal and immunodeficient children. Acta paediat. scand. 74: 126–130 (1985).
16 Plebani, A.; Duse, M.; Monafo, V.: Recurrent infections with IgG2 deficiency. Archs. Dis. Childh. 60: 670–672 (1985).
17 Ammann, A.J.; Ashman, R.F.; Buckley, R.H.; et al.: Use of intravenous gammaglobulin in antibody immunodeficiency: results of a multi-center controlled trial. Clin. Immunol. Immunopathol. 22: 60–67 (1982).
18 Cunningham Rundles, C.; Siegal, F.; Smithwick, E.M.; et al.: Efficacy of intravenous immunoglobulin in primary humoral immunodeficiency disease. Ann. intern. Med. 101: 435–439 (1984).
19 Leen, C.L.S.; Yap, P.L.; McClelland, D.B.L.: Increase of serum immunoglobulin level into the normal range in primary hypogammaglobulinaemia by dosage individualisation of intravenous immunoglobulin. Vox Sang. 51: 278–286 (1985).
20 Schur, P.H.; Borel, H.; Erwin, W.; Gelford, M.D.; Chester, A.; Alper, M.D.; Rosen, F.S.: Selective gamma-G globulin deficiencies in patients with recurrent pyogenic infections. New Engl. J. Med. 283: 631–634 (1970).
21 Oxelius, V.-A.: Chronic infections in a family with hereditary deficiency of IgG2 and IgG4. Clin. exp. Immunol. 17: 19–27 (1974).
22 Oxelius, V.-A.; Laurell, A.B.; Lindquist, B.; Henryka, G.; Axelsson, U.; Björkander, J.; Hansen, L.A.: IgG subclasses in selective IgA deficiency. Importance of IgG2-IgA deficiency. New Engl. J. Med. 304: 1476–1477 (1981).
23 Bass, J.L.; Nuss, R.; Menta, K.A.; Morganelli, P.; Bennett, L.: Recurrent meningococcaemia associated with IgG2-subclass deficiency. New Engl. J. Med. 309: 430 (1983).
24 Björkander, J.; Bake, B.; Oxelius, V.-A.; Hanson, L.A.: Impaired lung function in patients with IgA deficiency and low levels of IgG2 or IgG3. New Engl. J. Med. 313: 720–724 (1985).
25 Lever, A.M.L.; Webster, A.D.B.; Brown, D.; Thomas, H.C.: Non-A non-B hepatitis occurring in agammaglobulinaemic patients after intravenous immunoglobulin. Lancet ii: 1062–1064 (1984).
26 Buckley, R.H.: Gamma-globulin replacement. Clinics Immunol. Allergy 5: 141–158 (1985).
27 Morell, A.; Terry, W.D.; Waldmann, T.A.: Metabolic properties of IgG subclasses in man. J. clin. Invest. 49: 673–680 (1970).
28 Ochs, H.D.; Morell, A.; Skvaril, F.; Fischer, S.H.; Wedgwood, R.J.: Survival of IgG subclasses following administration of intravenous gammaglobulin in patients with primary immunodeficiency diseases; in Morell, Nydegger, Proc. Conf. Clinical Use of Intravenous Immunoglobulins, Interlaken 1985, pp. 77–85 (Academic Press, London 1986).
29 Ferrante, A.; Rowan-Kelly, B.; Beard, L.J.; Maxwell, G.M.: An enzyme-linked immunosorbent assay for the quantitation of human IgG subclasses using monoclonal antibodies. J. immunol. Methods 93: 207–212 (1986).
30 Beard, L.J.; Maxwell, G.M.; Thong, Y.H.: Immunocompetence of children with frequent respiratory infections. Archs Dis. Childh. 56: 101–105 (1981).

31 Thong, Y.H.; Maxwell, G.M.: Primary selective deficiency of immunoglobulin M. Aust. N.Z. J. Med. *8:* 436–438 (1978).
32 Brearley, R.L.; Rowbotham, B.: High-dose gammaglobulin for idiopathic thrombocytopenic purpura. Aust. N.Z. J. Med. *14:* 67–68 (1984).
33 Smith, T.F.; Bain, R.P.: IgG subclasses in children with chronic chest symptoms; in Hanson, Söderström, Oxelius, Immunoglobulin Subclass Deficiencies. Monogr. Allergy, vol. 20, pp. 119–127 (Karger, Basel 1986).

Dr. L.J. Beard, University Department of Paediatrics, Adelaide Children's Hospital, North Adelaide 5006 (South Australia)

Intravenous γ-Globulin Therapy and Serum IgG Subclass Levels in Intractable Childhood Epilepsy

A. Plebani[a], M. Duse[b], S. Tiberti[c], M.A. Avanzini[a], V. Monafo[a], E. Menegati[c], A.G. Ugazio[b], G.R. Burgio[a, 1]

[a] Department of Pediatrics, University of Pavia, Pavia;
[b] Department of Pediatrics, University of Brescia, Brescia;
[c] Division of Neurology and Child Psychiatry, Hospital of Brescia, Brescia, Italy

Introduction

Intravenous γ-globulins (IVGG) have been used with encouraging results for the treatment of epilepsy [1–3]. Pachadre et al. [4] reported that IVGG reduced the frequency of seizures and electroencephalogram (EEG) anomalies in 10 children with severe epilepsy and other groups [5, 6] partially confirmed their observations. In these studies, measurement of Ig levels and numbers of T lymphocytes revealed no abnormalities.

In spite of its empirical nature, the treatment of epileptic patients with IVGG may be justified on the hypothesis that an immunological mechanism is involved in the pathogenesis of some epileptic events. In fact, autoimmune mechanisms have been demonstrated to play a causal role in animal models of epilepsy and in some autoimmune disorders of man, IVGG have been used with good results [7].

In a previous study, we reported the results of IVGG treatment in 12 children with intractable childhood epilepsy (ICE) [6] 6 of whom had an IgG2 subclass deficiency (3 with associated IgG4 deficiency). A striking response to 6 months of treatment was observed in 5 of the 6 children with associated IgG2 deficiency but in none of the 6 with normal IgG2 levels.

---

[1] We thank Mr. A. Ascione for his expert technical assistance. This work was partly supported by CNR, Rome, Italy.

Table I. Main clinical features in the 12 patients with ICE treated with high-dose IVGG

Patient	Sex	Age years/months	ICE duration months	Type of ICE	Neurologic abnormality	CT scan findings
1 A.A.	F	1/10	12	PEE	cerebral palsy	microcephaly
2 T.C.	F	1/3	12	West	cerebral palsy	diffuse cerebral atrophy
3 G.D.	F	3/0	33	PEE	cerebral palsy	diffuse cerebral atrophy
4 B.R.	M	1/3	11	PEE	cerebral palsy	diffuse cerebral atrophy
5 C.Mi.	M	4/0	43	West	cerebral palsy	minimal cortical atrophy
6 C.Mo.	M	4/0	35	West	dysequilibrium	minimal cortical atrophy
7 Z.L.	M	6/6	62	Lennox	cerebral palsy	diffuse cerebral atrophy
8 R.M.	M	6/9	43	Lennox	motor disability	intracerebral calcifications
9 V.C.	F	6/5	36	Lennox	cognitive disorder	negative
10 G.M.	M	4/10	11	Lennox	cerebral palsy	congenital hydrocephalus
11 G.N.	M	6/8	12	Lennox	cerebral palsy	negative
12 T.A.	F	12/0	70	Lennox	mental retardation	negative

PEE = Precocious epileptic encephalopathy.

We report here a 2-year immunological and clinical follow-up of the 12 children included in the previous study. We also report the results of IgG subclass determinations in 53 children with seizure disorders other than ICE.

Subjects and Methods

The clinical and neurological features of the subjects have been reported elsewhere [6] and are briefly summarized in table I. All subjects, followed by the Division of Neurology from diagnosis, presented a high frequency of generalized (atypical absence and atonic, tonic-clonic, tonic and myoclonic) and/or complex partial seizures refractory to treatment in accordance with the diagnostic criteria for ICE [8]. Age ranged from 1 to 12 years and duration of the convulsive disorder ranged from 11 months up to almost 6 years. The type of epilepsy, classified according to international criteria [8], neurologic abnormalities and findings of computerized cerebral tomography (CT) are summarized in table I. All patients were being treated with one or more anticonvulsant agents (phenobarbital, and/or carbamazepine, and/or a benzodiazepine) and the same medications in the same doses employed over the preceding 3 months were continued throughout the study; no patient had received steroids or adrenocorticotropic hormone

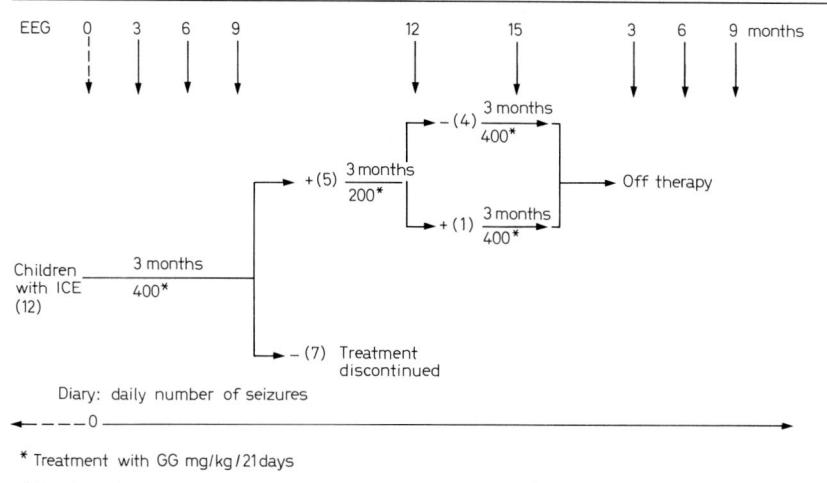

Table II. IVGG treatment schedule of the 12 children with ICE (see text)

```
EEG    0   3   6   9           12            15              3    6   9 months
       │   │   │   │            │             │              │    │   │
       ▼   ▼   ▼   ▼            ▼             ▼              ▼    ▼   ▼
                                       ┌─ −(4) 3 months ─┐
                                       │       ─────    │
                                       │        400*    │
                            ┌─ +(5) 3 months ─┤          ├──► Off therapy
                            │       ─────     │          │
                            │        200*     │          │
                            │                 └─ +(1) 3 months ─┘
                            │                         ─────
                            │                          400*
Children ___ 3 months ──────┤
with ICE     ─────
(12)          400*
                            │
                            └─ −(7) Treatment
                                    discontinued

         Diary: daily number of seizures
◄ − − − − 0 ───────────────────────────────────────────────────────────►
```

* Treatment with GG mg/kg/21 days
( ) Number of children; + = positive and − = negative response to treatment

in the 6 months prior to the study. Immunologic evaluation included determination of serum IgG, IgA, IgM and IgG subclass levels, delayed hypersensitivity skin tests, enumeration of T and B lymphocytes and in vitro lymphocyte response to mitogens. Laboratory tests for cellular immunity were carried out as previously reported [9].

Intact human IVGG (Endobulin, Immuno, Vienna, Austria) were administered intravenously in a dose of 400 mg/kg at time 0, after 15 days and then every 21 days for 9 months. At the end of this period, treatment was discontinued in the 7 children who had shown no improvement and continued at a lower dose (200 mg/kg every 21 days) for 3 more months in the 5 responders (table II). Four of the 5 responders showed worsening of the EEG associated in 2 with reappearance of seizures, so the dose was increased again to 400 mg/kg every 21 days for another 3 months. IVGG infusions were then discontinued and from that time the 5 children were followed off therapy for a period ranging from 11 to 14 months.

Serum IgG, IgA, IgM and IgG subclass levels were determined by radial immunodiffusion, the latter using monoclonal antibodies; subclass levels were considered low when below age-normal fifth percentile values for our laboratory, except IgG4 which was considered low only when undetectable (< 0.006 mg/ml), since IgG4 serum levels varied so widely in normals that reference ranges could not be determined.

During the week preceding the first infusion, patients were hospitalized for a baseline EEG in the waking state recorded over a period of 2 h and seizures were recorded in a daily diary. For evaluation of the efficacy of treatment, the daily number of seizures observed was recorded at home throughout the study by the mother and a 2-hour EEG was recorded at 3, 6, 9, 12 and 15 months of treatment and every 3 months after IVGG infusions were discontinued.

Response to treatment was assessed in each patient on the basis of the average daily number of seizures reported in the diary as well as of the number of paroxysms

Table III. IgG subclass levels in the 12 patients with ICE before treatment (A) and 21 days after (B) the second infusion of γ-globulins (400 mg/kg)

Patient		Age years/ months		Serum IgG subclass levels, mg/ml			
				G1	G2	G3	G4
1	A.A.	1/10	A	6.0	0.60	0.38	–
			B	5.8	2.10	0.25	–
2	T.C.	1/3	A	5.2	0.39	0.49	–
			B	4.2	1.76	0.21	–
3	G.D.	3/0	A	9.0	0.37 ↓	0.24	–
			B	7.2	1.95	0.25	–
4	B.R.	1/3	A	3.8	0.26 ↓	0.21	–
			B	3.8	1.96	0.19	–
5	C.Mi.	4/0	A	5.40	0.96	0.17	0.39
			B	4.32	3.20	0.20	0.38
6	C.Mo.	4/0	A	8.2	0.26 ↓	0.13	0.07
			B	6.8	1.35	0.17	0.06
7	Z.L.	6/6	A	11.0	2.15	0.24	0.49
			B	8.0	3.80	0.20	0.41
8	R.M.	6/9	A	15.8	2.55	0.52	0.06
			B	11.2	3.35	0.65	0.07
9	V.C.	6/5	A	5.0	0.54 ↓	0.30	0.12
			B	5.0	2.30	0.30	0.12
10	G.M.	4/10	A	9.4	0.44 ↓	0.26	0.06
			B	6.2	1.75	0.20	0.11
11	G.N.	6/8	A	7.7	0.21 ↓	0.26	–
			B	5.8	0.96	0.25	–
12	T.A.	12/0	A	7.6	3.80	0.25	0.43
			B	7.0	5.40	0.28	0.43

– = <0.006 mg/ml; ↓ = below age-normal 5th percentile values.

recorded in the 2-hour EEG tracings. Overall response to treatment was considered satisfactory when complete disappearance or significant reduction in the daily number of clinically apparent seizures (i.e. to less than 5 per day) was accompanied by a reduction of 75% or more in the number of paroxysms recorded on the EEG (percentage calculated considering the number of paroxysms recorded on the 2-hour baseline pretreatment EEG).

IgG subclasses were also evaluated in 53 children with various types of epilepsy other than ICE. The age of these children ranged from 2 months to 18 years; 26 were males and 27 were females. All were in treatment with carbamazepine and/or phenobarbital and/or a benzodiazepine when studied.

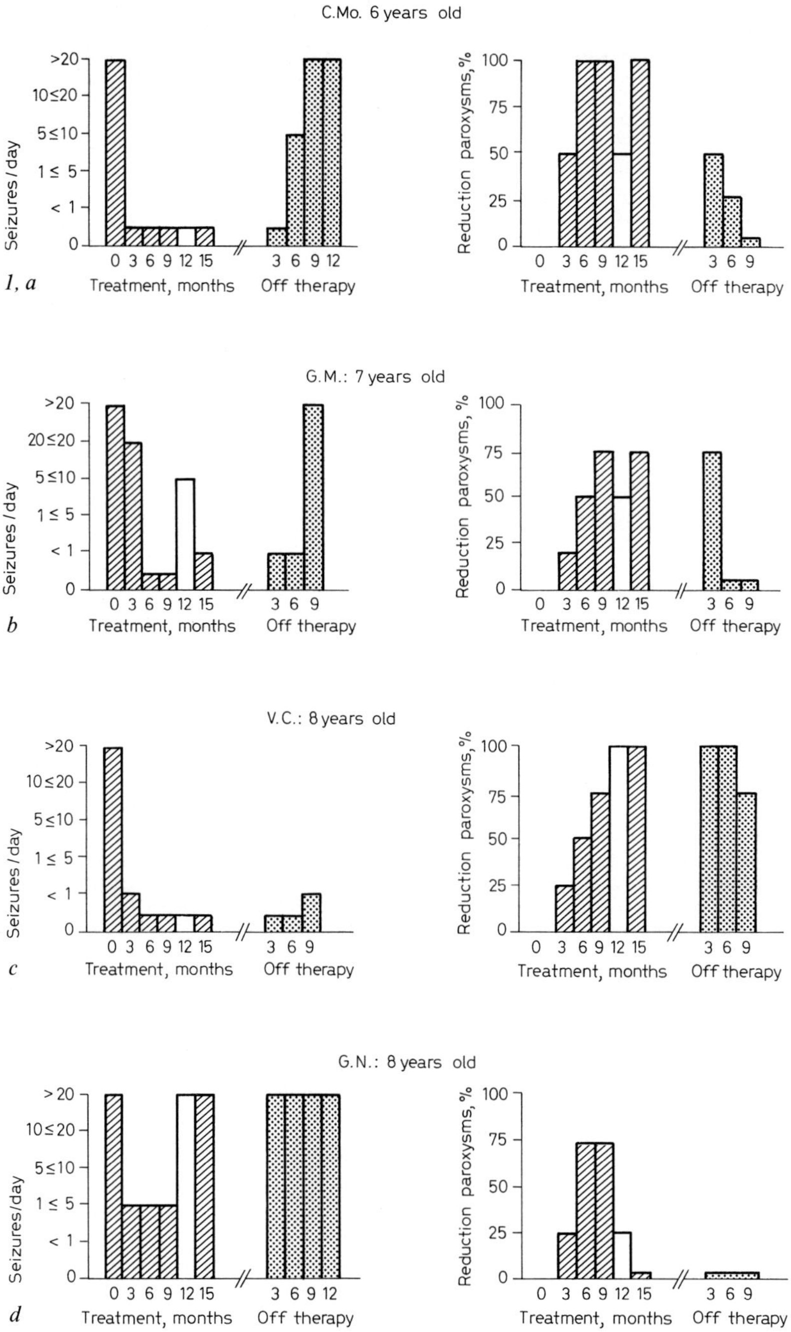
C.Mo. 6 years old
Seizures / day
>20
10≤20
5≤10
1≤ 5
< 1
0
0 3 6 9 12 15
3 6 9 12
Treatment, months
Off therapy
Reduction paroxysms, %
100
75
50
25
0
0 3 6 9 12 15
3 6 9
Treatment, months
Off therapy
1, a
G.M.: 7 years old
Seizures / day
>20
20≤20
5≤10
1≤ 5
< 1
0
0 3 6 9 12 15
3 6 9
Treatment, months
Off therapy
Reduction paroxysms, %
100
75
50
25
0
0 3 6 9 12 15
3 6 9
Treatment, months
Off therapy
b
V.C.: 8 years old
Seizures / day
>20
10≤20
5≤10
1≤ 5
< 1
0
0 3 6 9 12 15
3 6 9
Treatment, months
Off therapy
Reduction paroxysms, %
100
75
50
25
0
0 3 6 9 12 15
3 6 9
Treatment, months
Off therapy
c
G.N.: 8 years old
Seizures/day
> 20
10≤20
5≤10
1≤ 5
< 1
0
0 3 6 9 12 15
3 6 9 12
Treatment, months
Off therapy
Reduction paroxysms, %
100
75
50
25
0
0 3 6 9 12 15
3 6 9
Treatment, months
Off therapy
d

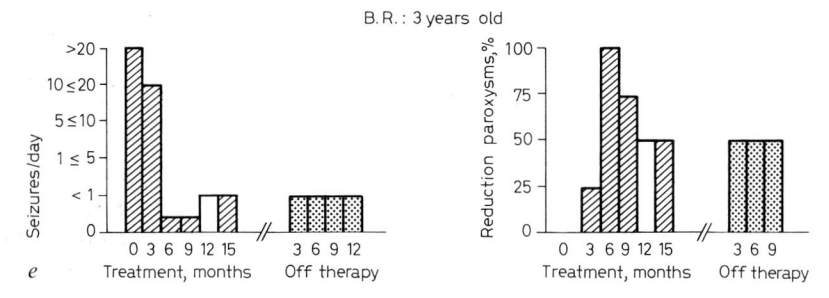

Fig. 1. *a–e* Daily number of seizures and percent reduction in the number of paroxysms during the 15 months of IVGG treatment and the 9–12 months off therapy in the 5 children with IgG2 deficiency responding to treatment. The number of paroxysms is expressed as percent of the pretreatment values (see text). Hatched columns = 400 mg/kg/21 days; plain columns = 200 mg/kg/21 days; spotted columns = off therapy.

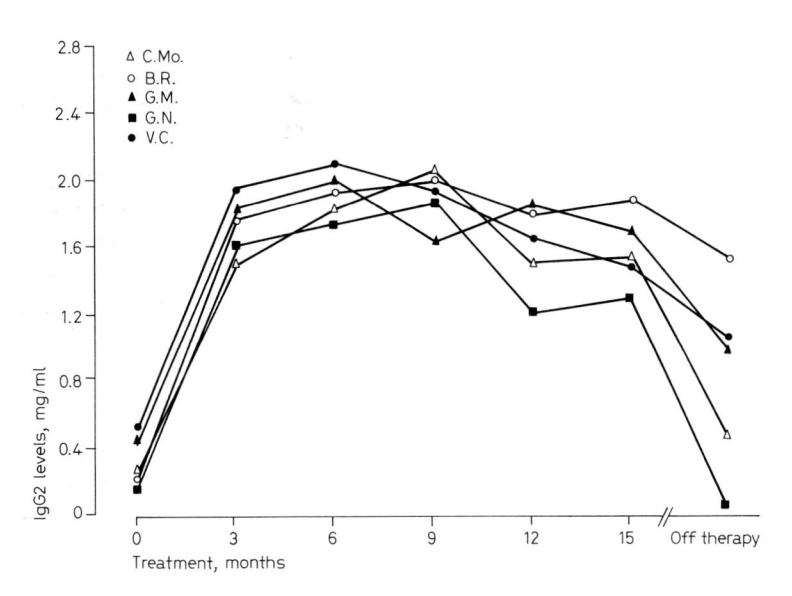

Fig. 2. IgG2 levels of the 5 patients during the 15 months of treatment with IVGG and after 11–14 months off therapy.

Results

In the 12 children with ICE, immunologic workup showed that cell-mediated immunity and serum Ig concentrations were age-normal (data not shown). IgG1 and IgG3 levels were always normal for age but deficits of the IgG2 and/or IgG4 subclasses were present in 8 children (table III). IgG2 deficiency was observed in 6 (50%) and IgG4 deficiency in 5 (42%) with a combined IgG2–IgG4 deficit in 3 patients.

After the first few IVGG infusions, IgG2 reached normal levels in all those with low IgG2 and remained normal thereafter while serum IgG4 was undetectable throughout the study in 3 patients and reached detectable levels in the other 2 during the third month of treatment.

Clinical response to treatment was first observed during the second month and confirmed in the third month in 7 patients; in 2 of them, however, improvement was slight and transient, while in the remaining 5 the seizures decreased gradually with almost complete disappearance at 6 months, persisting also at 9 months (fig. 1a–e). Slow but progressive improvement of the EEG up to 50–100% was observed by the sixth month and persisted also at 9 months in all 5 patients (fig. 1a–e). Response to treatment was therefore considered satisfactory in these 5 children all of whom had IgG2 deficiency. None of the 6 patients with normal IgG2 levels responded to treatment, while only one of the 6 with low IgG2 did not respond. After 9 months of treatment, IVGG infusion were discontinued in the 7 patients who had not shown a significant response; 6 of them had normal IgG2 levels while one had an initial IgG2 deficiency.

In the 5 patients who showed substantial improvement over the 9 months of treatment, the dose of IVGG was halved and then continued for 3 more months. After the second infusion at 200 mg/kg, a deterioration of the EEG was observed in 4 of the 5 patients, in 2 associated with an increase of the daily number of seizures, so the dose was again increased to 400 mg/kg/21 days with good results in 2 and no response in 2.

At 15 months 3 patients were in remission, i.e. one who had been well from the beginning of treatment (also at 200 mg/kg/21 days) and 2 who had experienced a second remission when the dose was again increased to 400 mg/kg/21 days. The remaining 2 patients were in relapse. Treatment was then discontinued in all 5 patients; on follow-up 2 of the 3 patients in remission relapsed from 1 to 9 months later and moderate deterioration of the EEG tracing was recorded in the third child. The other 2 children remained in relapse. Serum levels of IgG1, IgG3, IgG4 did not change significantly during treatment in the 12 patients. IgG2 levels remained in the normal range in the 6 patients with initially normal IgG2 levels, while after the first few infusions normalization of IgG2 was observed in the 6 patients with initial selective deficiency of this subclass. In the latter group, IgG2 levels remained within the normal range over the 9-month period of treatment at 400 mg/kg/21 days. In the 5 patients with a favorable reponse, IgG2 levels remained within the normal range also when IVGG dosage was reduced by half. After a period of 11–14 months off therapy, IgG2 levels dropped again to subnormal levels in 2, and remained within the normal range in the other 3 (fig. 2).

In the 53 patients with various types of epilepsy other than ICE, as shown in figure 3, IgG subclass levels were in the age-normal range. Eight of the 53 children had undetectable levels of IgG4; the data of the IgG4 levels are not shown because, as already mentioned, age-normal reference ranges could not be constructed.

Discussion

In a previous study we found that 6 of 12 children with ICE had an associated IgG2 deficiency; 5 of the 6 had a very good clinical and EEG response to treatment with high dose IVGG for 6 months. IgG2 levels normalized after the first few infusions of IVGG and remained normal thereafter over the 6-month treatment period; none of the children with normal IgG2 levels showed a clinical or EEG response to IVGG.

We update here the results of a 2-year follow-up period in these 12 children. At 9 months, IVGG infusions were discontinued in the 7 children who did not respond to treatment, 6 with normal levels of IgG2 and one with IgG2 deficiency. At this time the 5 children who had shown a good clinical response at 6 months remained clinically well with persistent EEG improvement. In these 5 children, the dose of IVGG was then halved to 200 mg/kg every 21 days, but after the second infusion, deterioration of the EEG was observed in 4 of 5, associated with seizure reappearance in 2 cases. When IVGG was again increased to the initial dose of 400 mg/kg every 21 days, 2 patients

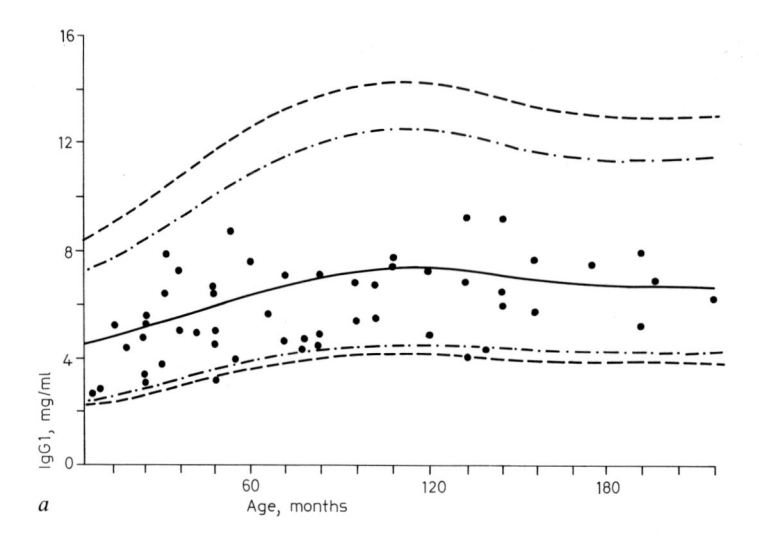

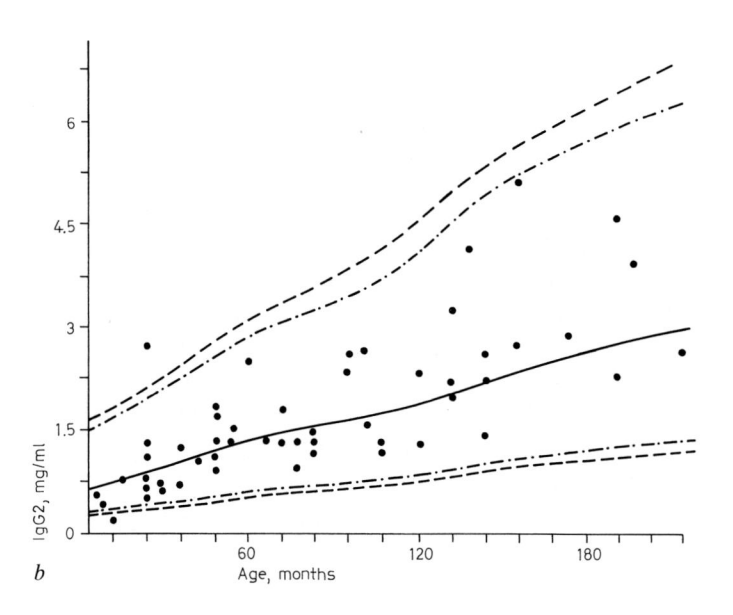

Fig. 3. a–c Serum levels of IgG1, IgG2 and IgG3 in 53 children with epilepsy other than ICE.

3, c

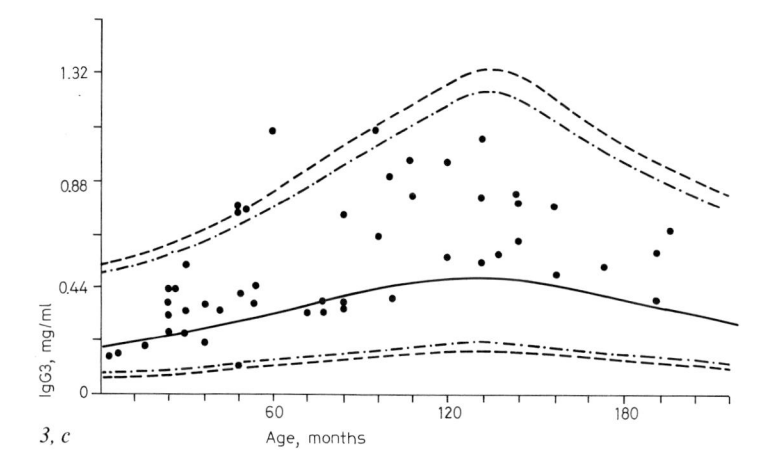

underwent a second remission. On repeated determinations, IgG2 levels remained in the normal range in spite of the lower dose of IVGG used, suggesting that EEG improvement was related to the dose of IVGG and not to the levels of IgG2 attained. To the present 5 patients have been followed off-therapy for 11–14 months; during this period 4 of the 5 patients relapsed and the EEG tracing of the fifth showed moderate deterioration.

However, evaluation of serum IgG subclass levels demonstrated that only 2 of these 5 patients had a concomitant decrease of IgG2 to subnormal levels which, on the contrary, remained in the normal range in the other 3.

Although our data demonstrate that high-dose IVGG is beneficial in some cases of ICE, the explanation for this finding and for the related observation that patients with ICE and associated IgG2 deficiency are more likely to benefit from treatment is still obscure. In fact, IVGG is being used with good results in the replacement therapy of various immunodeficiency diseases [10, 11] and in some immunologically mediated disorders such as immune thrombocytopenia purpura (ITP) [7].

Some authors have reported that selective IgG2 deficiency is quite common in immune ITP, suggesting that low levels of IgG2 may be a predisposing factor. In fact, there is evidence that low IgG2 levels are significantly associated with a good response to IVGG in ITP [14]; unfortunately, no follow-up data are available on IgG2 levels during and after treatment of ITP.

On the other hand, viral infections as well as autoimmune mechanisms [12, 13] have been suggested to play a pathogenetic role in childhood epilepsy. Therefore, the beneficial effects of IVGG could be explained by the replacement of missing IgG2 with antiviral effects. A severe form of echovirus encephalitis which responds to high-dose IVGG has been described in children with agammaglobulinemia [11]; by analogy IgG2 deficiency could also predispose to some type of viral encephalitis leading to ICE and responding to high-dose IVGG treatment. Alternatively IVGG could interfere with the immune mechanisms contributing to the pathogenesis of epilepsy.

In the present report all 5 children with associated IgG2 deficiency at the onset responded to treatment with IVGG and relapsed or worsened after IVGG was discontinued but IgG2 levels returned to subnormal pretreatment values in only 2 of them. This suggests that, at least in ICE, the relationship between response to IVGG treatment and IgG2 levels is more complicated than previously recognized; simple replacement of IgG2 is unlikely to account for the therapeutic effect of IVGG.

On the other hand, IgG2 deficiency is often transient [15], perhaps due to delayed maturation in childhood. In some cases it has been shown that IgG2 deficiency results from prolonged drug treatment [6]. Since all our patients had been treated with various drugs, we cannot rule out that the observed IgG2 deficiency was secondary to treatment and that the observed association between IgG2 deficiency and favorable response to treatment merely identified a subgroup of ICE susceptible to the immunosuppressive effect of some anticonvulsant drugs and, at the same time, to the beneficial effects of IVGG. Whatever the role of IgG2 deficiency and the long-term behavior of IgG2 levels, our results suggest that low levels of IgG2 can be used empirically in ICE as a marker predicting a good response to IVGG; this awaits confirmation from studies in larger populations.

References

1 Arizumi, N.; Shihara, H.; Hibio, S.; Ryo, S.; Baba, K.; Ogawa, K.; Suzuki, Y.; Momuki, T.: High dose gamma globulin for intractable childhood epilepsy. Lancet *ii:* 162-163 (1983).
2 Sandstedt, P.; Kostulas, V.; Larsson, L.E.: Intravenous gamma globulin for postencephalitic epilepsy. Lancet *ii:* 1154-1155 (1984).
3 Laffont, F.; Esnault, S.; Gilbert, A.; Peitour, M.A.; Cathala, H.P.; Eygonnet, J.P.: Effets des gammaglobulines sur des épilepsies rebelles. Etude préliminaire. Annls Méd. Int. *130:* 307-312 (1979).
4 Pachadre, J.C.; Sauvezie, B.; Osier, C.; Gibert, J.: Traitement d'encéphalopathies épileptiques de l'enfant par les gamma-globulines. Rev. EEG Neurophysiol. *7:* 443-447 (1977).
5 Bedini, R.; De Feo, M.R.; Orano, A.; Rocchi, L.: Effect of gamma-globulin therapy in severely epileptic children. Epilepsia *26:* 98-102 (1985).
6 Duse, M.; Tiberti, S.; Plebani, A.; Avanzini, M.A.; Gardenghi, M.; Menegati, E.; Monafo, V.; Ugazio, A.G.: IgG2 deficiency and intractable epilepsy of childhood; in Hanson, Söderström, Oxelius, Monogr. Allergy, vol. 20, pp. 128-134 (Karger, Basel 1986).
7 Warier, I.; Lusher, J.M.: Intravenous gammaglobulin treatment for chronic idiopathic thrombocytopenia purpura in children. Am. J. Med. *76:* 193-198 (1984).
8 Commission on classification and terminology of the International League against Epilepsy: Proposal for an international classification of the epilepsies. Epilepsia *11:* 117-128 (1970).
9 Ugazio, A.G.; Altamura, D.; Girandi, V.; Mingrat, G.; Belloni, C.; Burgio, G.R.: Peripheral blood T lymphocyte subpopulations in newborns. Boll. Ist. sieroter. milan. *55:* 451-459 (1976).
10 Ochs, H.D.; Fischer, S.H.; Wedgwood, R.S.: Modified immuneglobuolin: its use in the prophylactic treatment of patients with immune deficiency. J. clin. Immunol. *2:* 22-29 (1982).
11 Meeting report: Primary immunodeficiency disease. Report prepared for the WHO by a scientific group on immunodeficiency. Clin. Immunol. Immunopathol. *28:* 450-475 (1983).
12 Rasmussen, T.: Further observations on the syndrome of chronic encephalitis and epilepsy. Appl. Neurophysiol. *41:* 1-12 (1978).
13 Aarli, J.A.; Fontana, A.: Immunological aspects of epilepsy. Epilepsia *21:* 451-459 (1980).
14 Bussel, J.; Morell, A.; Skvaril, F.: IgG2 deficiency in autoimmune cytopenias; in Hanson, Söderström, Oxelius, Monogr. Allergy, vol. 20, pp. 116-118 (Karger, Basel 1986).
15 Shackelford, P.G.; Polmar, S.H.; Mayus, J.L.; Johnson, W.L.; Corry, J.M.; Nahm, M.H.: Spectrum of IgG2 subclass deficiency in children with recurrent infections: prospective study. J. Pediat. *108:* 647-653 (1986).
16 Leickly, F.E.; Buckley, R.H.: Development of IgA and IgG2 subclass deficiency after sulfasalazine therapy. J. Pediat. *108:* 481-482 (1986).

A. Plebani, MD, Clinica Pediatrica, Università di Pavia,
P. le Golgi, 2, I-27100 Pavia (Italy)

Issues Concerning the Use of Intravenous Immunoglobulins for the Immunoprophylaxis of Cytomegalovirus Infections in Allogeneic Bone Marrow Transplant Recipients

David Emanuel

Bone Marrow Transplantation Service, Department of Pediatrics, Memorial Sloan-Kettering Cancer Center, New York City, New York, N.Y., USA

Cytomegalovirus (CMV) is a major cause of morbidity and is the commonest infectious cause of death in patients receiving allogeneic bone marrow transplants [1]. The primary cause of CMV infection in patients who are seropositive at the time of transplant appears to be the reactivation of latent virus, whereas seronegative patients probably acquire CMV infection from virus-containing blood products or bone marrow [1, 2]. Approaches to the prevention of CMV infection and related disease in recipients of both bone marrow and renal transplants have included the use of CMV-seronegative blood products and passive immunoprophylaxis with CMV immune plasma or globulin [3–9]. Most of these studies have reported that passive immunization with intravenous Ig containing CMV-specific antibodies can modify the severity of CMV infection and prevent interstitial pneumonia after bone marrow transplantation. Similarly, it has been shown that the use of CMV-seronegative blood products can prevent CMV infection in seronegative transplant recipients receiving marrow from a seronegative donor [3]. Based on the analyses of these studies, it has now become 'standard practice' in a number of transplant centers to provide passive CMV immunoprophylaxis with Ig to most patients. Whether the assumption that this approach is valid for all patients remains to be definitively determined by carefully controlled prospective clinical trials.

Comparison of data collected in previous CMV immunoprophylaxis trials is difficult as there are many variables in these studies. Primarily, the quantity and quality of products administered has been markedly different. This was because the availability of Ig preparations containing high titers of CMV-specific antibodies was limited. Also the criteria for selection of patients for participation in these studies has varied. A number of studies have only enrolled CMV-seronegative transplant recipients for passive CMV immunoprophylaxis on the grounds that (1) CMV-seropositive patients have a significantly lower risk of interstitial pneumonia, or (2) CMV infection is due to reactivation of latent virus in CMV-seropositive recipients and hence it is unlikely that passive immunoprophylaxis would be worthwhile in those patients [3–5, 8]. In addition, virological surveillance and diagnostic techniques in these studies have been markedly variable, again making comparisons difficult [4, 6].

Recently, however, a number of new intravenous Ig products have become available for use in the USA and Europe. By comparing the in vitro characteristics of specific lots of two Ig used successfully in previous clinical trials, with similar data from randomly selected lots of three currently available Ig, we hoped to define some baseline criteria for the selection of an Ig for use in a large prospective CMV immunoprophylaxis study planned for our patients. Each lot of product was assayed for CMV-specific immunoreactive antibody by enzyme-linked immunosorbent assay (ELISA) and for the titer of CMV-neutralizing antibodies as determined by a standard virus plaque-reduction assay [11, 12]. As we proceeded with this evaluation, we unexpectedly noted no direct or predictable correlation between the amount of CMV-specific IgG by ELISA and the in vitro functional activity as measured by virus neutralization. We noted significant differences between lots of the same product as well as marked variability between Ig from different manufacturers [13].

The characteristics and mode of production of the five intravenous Ig evaluated are outlined in table I. With the exception of the Minnesota CMV hyperimmune globulin, all are produced by classical Cohn cold ethanol fractionation followed by the various methods of purification as noted. The Minnesota globulin is prepared from citrated plasma followed by ion-exchange purification of the IgG fraction on QAE-50 Sephadex [6]. The three commercially available products in the USA, namely Sandoglobulin, Gammimune-N and Gammagard are produced from pooled venous plasma of from 2,000 to 8,000 normal US-based donors. Both Minnesota CMV Globulin and Cyto-

Table I. Characteristics of five intravenous Ig containing CMV-specific antibodies

Immune globulin (protein concentration)	Method of production
Gamimune-N (50 mg/ml) (Cutter)	Cohn fractionation and pH adjustment pH 4.25
Gammagard (50 mg/ml) (Hyland-Travenol)	Cohn fractionation and ion exchange pH 6.8
Minnesota CMV Globulin (50 mg/ml)	ion exchange pH 6.3
Sandoglobulin (30 mg/ml) (Sandoz)	Cohn fractionation, pepsin treatment and pH adjustment pH 6.6
Cytotect (110 mg/ml) (Biotest)	Cohn fractionation with β-propriolactone treatment

Table II. IgG subclasses in intravenous Ig and normal plasma (data supplied by manufacturers)

	IgG1, %	IgG2, %	IgG3, %	IgG4, %
Plasma	60	30	6	4
Gammagard (Hyland)	67	25	5	4
Gamimune-N (Cutter)	58	28	6	5
Sandogloblin (Sandoz)	60	30	7	3
Minnesota CMV	94	5	–	0.1
Cytotect (Biotest)	not available			

tect (Biotest) are produced from a much smaller prescreened pool of donors with high CMV antibody titers [6, 9].

The IgG subclass profiles of four of the five Ig and normal plasma are noted in table II. The subclass distribution of the three commercial products closely resemble normal human plasma. However, the Minnesota CMV globulin is almost entirely deficient in IgG3, the IgG subclass supposedly containing the bulk of antiherpes virus neutralizing activity [14]. Data on IgG subclass distribution in Cytotect (Biotest) was not available.

The titer of CMV-specific IgG was assayed in each lot of each product by ELISA as previously described [11]. We used a single lot of a commercially available glycine-extracted CMV Strain AD169 antigen preparation (Clark Laboratories, Jamestown, N.Y.) to insure standardization [13]. Each lot of each product was assayed at least

Table III. CMV antibody reactivity of different intravenous Ig

Immunoglobulin	Elisa titer[1]	Neutralization titer[1]	µg/ml of IgG required for 50% plaque reduction
Gamimune-N	1: 3,200	1: 500	100
Gammagard	1: 6,400	1:1,000	50
Minnesota CMV	1:64,000	1:1,000	50
Sandoglobulin	1: 1,600	1: 50	600
Cytotect	1:64,000	1:1,000	110

[1] Results represent the average of 3 experiments and a median of lots tested.

twice and to insure reproducibility of the ELISA, a standard CMV-IgG reference serum was assayed in parallel with all tests (Paul Ehrlich Institute CMV serum, 69.1 mg/0.5 ml, 30 PEI/ml, Paul Ehrlich Institute, Frankfurt, FRG). The titer of CMV-neutralizing antibodies in each lot of each preparation was assessed by a standard plaque reduction assay [12, 13]. The reciprocal of the highest dilution of the Ig that yielded a greater than 50% reduction in the number of virus plaques was taken as the neutralizing titer. In addition, the quantity of Ig required to reduce the number of virus plaques by 50% was calculated for each product tested. In addition, the ability of each lot of each product to neutralize 'wild' clinical isolates of CMV was evaluated. The results of all these experiments are summarized in tables III and IV.

All five products tested have high titers of CMV-IgG by ELISA. All five Ig were anticomplementary and thus unable to be assayed for CMV-IgG by complement fixation. As expected, the highest titers of CMV-IgG were found in the CMV hyperimmune preparations, with the three commercial Ig products having only slight lot-to-lot and product-to-product variation.

Although the hyperimmune CMV globulin products clearly had significantly higher CMV-IgG titers by ELISA when compared to the median titers of the standard γ-globulin products, this did not directly correlate with their having the higher titer of CMV-neutralizing antibodies. Both CMV-hyperimmune products had neutralizing-antibody titers of 1:1,000 as compared to Gammagard (1:1,000, median

Table IV. Quantitative neutralization of CMV clinical isolates and strain AD-169 by different intravenous human Ig

Immune globulins (lot No.)	CMV isolates 114 (38)[1]	123 (57)	421 (55)	588 (42)	595 (37)	642 (40)	2663 (50)	2830 (90)	average of 8 isolates %	AD-169 (250) %
Gamimune N (40PO5)	75[2]	76	95	79	60	61	83	80	76.1	96
Gammagard (850919)	79	88	81	85	59	60	82	86	77.5	96
Minnesota (18)	89	53	84	86	58	59	74	86	73.6	93
Sandoglobulin (53691260)	61	60	64	51	40	45	65	50	54.5	78
Biotest (441024)	70	67	75	74	69	56	70	67	68.5	84

[1] Number in parentheses indicates the PFU of virus used in assay.
[2] Results were given as percentage reduction of plaques compared to negative controls.

Table V. Relationship between the CMV-specific immunoreactive and functional activity of different lots of 5 intravenous Ig, as measured by ELISA and virus neutralization

Titer of CMV neutralizing antibodies	Titer of CMV-IgG by ELISA 800	1,600	3,200	6,400	12,800	64,000
0		S, S				
50						
100					GN	
200	S	S	GD, GD, GD			
500			GN, GN			
1,000			GD		GD, GD, GD, GD	M, M, B
2,000			GN		GD, GD, GD	
4,000			GD			

S = Sandoglobulin; GN = Gamimune-N; GD = Gammagard; M = Minnesota Hyperimmune Globulin; B = Biotest Hyperimmune Globulin.

of 12 lots) or Gammimune-N (1:500, median of 4 lots). By contrast, Sandoglobulin (1:50, median of 5 lots) had significantly lower neutralizing activity than the other products tested. A number of lots of both Gammagard and Gamimune-N had neutralizing-antibody titers equal to or greater than the two hyperimmune products tested, despite having significantly lower CMV-IgG titers by ELISA (table V). Of interest was the unexpected finding that 25% of all tested lots of Gammagard and Gamimune-N had neutralizing-antibody titers significantly below the median titer for that product, with no direct correlation with the CMV-IgG titer by ELISA in the same lot. Similarly, when the quantity of Ig required for virus neutralization was calculated for each product, using a quantitative plaque-reduction assay and allowing for differences in protein content and infusion concentrations, there were significant differences noted (table III). The amount of Ig required to neutralize the same titer of CMV ranged from 50 to 600 µg/ml. Of note is the finding that the two hyperimmune globulins required similar quantities of Ig for virus neutralization when compared to most lots of the three standard Ig tested.

The quantitative reduction in the number of viral plaques produced by each of the γ-globulin preparations when tested in a plaque reduction assay, was determined. Eight clinical isolates and one laboratory strain of H-CMV were used and results are outlined in table IV.

There were notable differences when each product was tested for the ability to neutralize wild clinical isolates of CMV. One of the three commercial intravenous Ig generally had a lower effective neutralization capacity when compared to the other products (table IV). Both 'hyperimmune' products were not more effective in neutralizing the clinical isolates of CMV when compared to the standard Ig.

These data show that in five intravenous Ig tested, there is no predictable relationship between the quantity of immunoreactive CMV-specific antibody by ELISA and in vitro functional activity as measured by virus neutralization. However, there is no data in humans of a direct correlation between an antibody's in vitro neutralization capacity and its possible effectiveness as a CMV prophylactic in vivo. It has been postulated in a murine CMV model that the beneficial clinical effect of antiserum containing CMV-neutralizing antibodies may be more related to the prevention of recurrent massive viral dissemination rather than by totally preventing low-grade organ infection [15]. This may mean that the ability to efficiently neutralize circulating or non-cell associated virus may be clinically important. Whether this murine data can in any way be extrapolated to the human is unknown. Unfortunately no animal model exists at present in which human CMV will grow, so the investigation of the mechanisms of CMV prophylaxis by antibodies will continue to be done by inference from in vitro data.

Both of the products shown to have previous clinical efficacy which were available for this study were in fact 'hyperimmune' products produced from plasma collected from donors selected for their high titer of CMV-specific antibodies by ELISA or complement fixation [6, 9]. Both products, despite having significantly higher amounts of CMV immunoreactive antibodies, were no more effective in neutralizing both clinical and laboratory isolates of CMV than were the standard Ig products. It is thus likely that there are subtle differences between those antibodies that are immunoreactive by ELISA and those that are functionally active in vitro by virus neutralization. If these data can be confirmed, they may have practical implications for the manufacturers of these products as well as to clinicians designing future clinical studies, e.g. it may be necessary for manufacturers to provide functional data on all lots of Ig they release, or for clinicians to be more aware that the quantity as well as quality of antibodies in these preparations is variable.

Bone marrow transplant recipients, like the normal population, appear to have a restricted immune reactivity to CMV, predominantly producing both CMV-specific IgG1 and IgG3 [16, 17]. IgG1 appears to be the predominant subclass in reactivated disease in CMV-seropositive patients, whereas both IgG1 and IgG3 were produced in primary CMV infections, with IgG3 appearing first [16]. In CMV-seropositive patients, however, CMV IgG3 may not always be present and may be an indicator of reactivated disease [17]. According to Wahren et al. [unpublished results], both CMV IgG1 and IgG3 appear to have CMV-neutralizing capacity, although Beck has previously reported that herpes virus-neutralizing activity primarily resides in the IgG3 subclass [14]. The Minnesota CMV Globulin used successfully in a previous CMV immunoprophylaxis trial [6] has no IgG3 but, as we have noted, still effectively neutralizes CMV in vitro (tables II–V). IgG1 accounts for greater than 90% of the IgG in this product. It is thus likely that IgG1 as well as IgG3 CMV-specific antibodies can effectively neutralize CMV in vitro. The role of IgG subclasses in CMV immunoprophylaxis is thus just one of a number of unresolved issues surrounding the use of intravenous Ig for the prevention of CMV infection and disease in allogeneic bone marrow transplant recipients. The exact role of Ig to alter the incidence and severity of reactivated infections in CMV-seropositive recipients has not been addressed, and as these patients account for a majority in most transplant centers, this is an important area of future study. The interaction of IgG subclasses with T-cell- and NK-cell-mediated immunity needs to be carefully studied. It is possible that the interaction of humoral with cell-mediated antiviral activity is the basis for the prophylactic and therapeutic effects of Ig noted in previous clinical trials. Until an animal model for human CMV is developed, evaluation of the in vivo efficacy of Ig to prevent or ameliorate human CMV infection in different patient groups will have to be defined in carefully designed and standardized prospective clinical trials.

References

1 Meyers, J.D.; Fluornoy, N.; Thomas, E.D.: Risk factors for cytomegalovirus infection after human marrow transplantation. J. infect. Dis. *153:* 478–488 (1986).
2 Hersman, J.; Meyers, J.D.; Thomas, E.D.; Buckner, C.D.; Clift, R.: The effect of granulocyte transfusions on the incidence of cytomegalovirus infection after allogeneic marrow transplatation. Ann. intern. Med. *96:* 149–152 (1982).
3 Bowden, R.A.; Sayers, M.; Fluornoy, N.; et al.: Cytomegalovirus immune globulin and seronegative blood products to prevent primary cytomegalovirus infection after marrow transplantation. New Engl. J. Med. *314:* 1006–1010 (1986).
4 Winston, D.J.; Pollard, R.B.; Ho, W.G.; et al.: Cytomegalovirus immune plasma in bone marrow transplant recipients. Ann. intern. Med. *97:* 11–18 (1982).
5 Meyers, J.D.; Lesczynski, J.; Zaia, J.A.; et al.: Prevention of cytomegalovirus infection by cytomegalovirus immune globulin after marrow transplantation. Ann. intern. Med. *98:* 442–446 (1983).
6 Condie, R.M.; O'Reilly, R.J.: Prevention of cytomegalovirus infection by prophylaxis with an intravenous, hyperimmune native, unmodified cytomegalovirus globulin; randomized trial in bone marrow transplant recipients. Am. J. Med. *76:* 134–141 (1984).
7 Syndman, D.R.; McIver, J.; Leszczynski, J.; et al.: A pilot trial of a novel CMV immune globulin in renal transplant recipients. Transplantation *38:* 553–557 (1984).
8 Winston, D.J.; Ho, W.; Lin, C.H.; et al.: Intravenous immune globulin for prevention of cytomegalovirus infection and interstitial pneumonia after bone marrow transplantation. Ann. intern. Med. *106:* 12–18 (1987).
9 Kubanek, B.; Ernst, P.; Ostendorf, P.; et al.: Preliminary data of controlled trial of intravenous immune globulin in the prevention of cytomegalovirus infection in bone marrow transplant recipients. Transplant. Proc. *17:* 468–469 (1985).

10 Neiman, P.E.; Reeves, W.; Ray, G.: A prospective analysis of interstitial pneumonia and opportunistic viral infection among recipients of allogeneic bone marrow grafts. J. infect. Dis. *136:* 754–767 (1987).
11 Middeldorp, J.M.; Jongsma, J.; Ter Haar, A.; Schirai, J.: The detection of immunoglobulin M and G antibodies against cytomegalovirus early and late antigens by enzyme-linked immunosorbent assay. J. clin. Microbiol. *20:* 763–771 (1984).
12 Wentworth, B.; French, L.: Plaque assay of cytomegalovirus strain of human origin. Proc. Soc. exp. Biol. Med. *135:* 253–258 (1970).
13 Chehimi, J.; Peppard, J.; Emanuel, D.: Selection of an intravenous immune globulin for the immunoprophylaxis of cytomegalovirus (CMV) infections: an in vitro comparison of currently available and previously effective immune globulins. J. Bone Marrow Trans. (in press).
14 Beck, O.E.: Distribution of virus antibody activity among human IgG subclasses. Clin. exp. Immunol. *43:* 626–632 (1981).
15 Rubin, R.H.; Wilson, E.J.; Barrett, L.V.; Medearis, D.N.: The protecive effect of hyperimmune anti-murine cytomegalovirus antiserum against lethal virus challenge: the case for passive-active immunization. Clin. Immunol. Immunopathol. *39:* 151–158 (196).
16 Linde, G.A.; Hammarström, L.; Persson, M.; Smith, C.I.E.; Sundqvist, V.A.; Wahren, B.: Virus-specific antibody activity of different subclasses of immunoglobulins G and A in cytomegalovirus infections. Infect. Immunity *42:* 237–244 (1983).
17 Wahren, B.; Linde, A.; Sundqvist, V.A.; Ljungman, P.; Lonnqvist, B.; Ringden,O.: IgG-subclass-specific CMV reactivity in bone marrow transplant recipients. Transplantation *38:* 479–483 (1984).

David Emanuel, MD, Bone Marrow Transplantation Service,
Department of Pediatrics, Memorial Sloan-Kettering Cancer Center,
New York City, New York, NY 10021 (USA)

Survival of Antigen-Specific Antibody Following Administration of Intravenous Immunoglobulin in Patients with Primary Immunodeficiency Diseases

Susanna H. Fischer[a], Hans D. Ochs[a], Ralph J. Wedgwood[a], Frantisek Skvaril[b], Andreas Morell[b], Harry R. Hill[c], Gerald Schiffmann[d], Lawrence Corey[a, 1]

[a] Department of Pediatrics, University of Washington School of Medicine, Seattle, Wash.; [b] Institute for Clinical Experimental Tumor Research, University of Bern, Bern, Switzerland; [c] Department of Pediatrics, University of Utah College of Medicine, Salt Lake City, Utah; [d] Downstate Medical Center, Brooklyn, N.Y., USA

Introduction

Metabolic properties of immunoglobulin isotypes and IgG subclasses were originally determined using ^{125}I- or ^{131}I-labeled myeloma proteins [1, 2]. The potential artefacts involved include protein damage during labeling and intrinsic abnormality of the myeloma protein itself. The availability of modified immunoglobulin preparations for intravenous use (IVIG) allows the infusion of large amounts of pooled normal, heterogeneous immunoglobulin consisting of polyclonal IgG antibodies to many specific antigens. Following administration of IVIG to patients with primary immune deficiency, half-life curves can be constructed for IgG and IgG subclasses and for clinically relevant antigen-specific antibodies. The dosage of IVIG required to achieve protective serum levels of specific antibodies throughout the interval between IVIG infusions depends on the survi-

---

[1] The authors wish to thank the staff of the Clinical Research Center at the University of Washington for its important contribution. The technical assistance of Mr. Samuel Heller, Ms. Joan Dragavon and Ms. Anne Cent and the secretarial assistance of Ms. Joan Palmer are gratefully acknowledged, as well as the support from Dr. R. Babington, Sandoz Pharmaceuticals.

Table I. Patient data

Patient	Sex	Diagnosis	Age years	Age at onset of symptoms years	Isohemagglutinin titer[1] (blood group)	Serum Ig concentrations at time of Dx IgG mg/dl	IgA mg/dl	IgM mg/dl	Peak Ab response to ΦX 174 1st	2nd	%IgG	Characteristics	Comments
A.C.G.	M	XLA	25	9/12	anti-A < 1:2 anti-B < 1:2 (0)	326	0	0	0	0	0	chronic pan sinusitis; chronic otitis; chronic restrictive lung dis; hx of arthritis	uncle of J.L.M.
J.L.M.	M	XLA	9	9/12	< 1:2 (A)	283	0	8	0.03	0.162	0	sinusitis; hx of otitis media	nephew of A.C.G.; affected younger sibling
J.A.R.	M	XLA	27	9/12	anti-A 1:2 (B)	435	0	6	0	0	0	chronic pansinusitis chronic restrictive and obstructive lung dis; hx of arthritis	has one affected nephew
J.M.S.	M	XLA	32	12	anti-B 1:2 (A)	153	6	0	0	0.26	0	chronic pansinusitis; chronic obstructive lung dis; hx of arthralgia; hx of *Giardia lamblia*	no positive family hx. Dx of XLA based on clinical characteristics
A.A.P.	M	CVI	31	10	anti-B 1:4 (A)	31	32	2	0.56	42.2	23	chronic pansinusitis chronic RUL	no positive family hx

Table I. (cont.)

J.J.C.	M	CVI	15	3	anti-A 1:64 (B)	220	0	12	0.40	328.0	1.7	infiltrate; chronic atopic dermatitis chronic sinusitis hx of *Giardia lamblia* infestation	no positive family hx; has balanced translocation of chromosomes 11 and 22
A.R.H.	F	CVI	58	30	anti-A 1:32 anti-B < 1:2 (0)	128	0	16	3.94	114.0	7	chronic pansinusitis chronic restrictive lung dis; Rt lobectomy	no positive family hx
S.M.S.	F	CVI	42	6	anti-A < 1:2 anti-A < 1:2 (0)	221	0	11	–	20.7	–	chronic pansinusitis chronic obstructive lung disease; Lt lobectomy	no positive family hx
C.S.D.	M	CVI	6	1	n.d.	260	0	126	6.33	11.6	0	chronic sinusitis hx of otitis media	no positive family hx
K.O.S.	M	CVI	36	5	anti-B 1:8 (A)	456	0	7	0.036	0.34	5.9	chronic pansinusitis; chronic laryngitis; chronic obstructive lung disease	has affected daughter
Normal control					anti-A 1:32–1:2,048 anti-B 1:8–1:512	650– 1,600	90– 425	50– 300	40– 150	500– 2,000	56 ± 24		

[1] Determined by hemagglutination detecting predominantly IgM antibody.

val time of the infused immunoglobulin. Because each of the four IgG subclasses has characteristic biological activities [3], we determined the survival of IgG subclasses and of a selection of antigen-specific antibodies following the infusion of a commercially available IVIG preparation (Sandoglobulin®, Sandoz) in 10 patients with humoral immunodeficiency.

Materials and Methods

Patients. Ten individuals with selective antibody deficiency were enrolled in the study (table I). Of the 10 patients, 4 had X-linked agammaglobulinemia (XLA) and were not able to make antibody to bacteriophage ΦX 174 [4]. The remaining 6 patients had common variable immune deficiency (CVID), and with the exception of patient A.A.P., failed to make significant amounts of IgG antibody to bacteriophage ΦX 174 after repeated immunization.

IVIG Infusions. The material used (Sandoglobulin) is prepared by submitting Cohn fraction II to mild acid treatment at pH 4 and the addition of 1:10,000 pepsin. Immediately before use the lyophilized material was reconstituted to a solution consisting of 6% IgG at a pH of 6.6. During the initial 3 months of IVIG therapy, each patient received 100 mg/kg/month of this material. After a 3-month 'washout' period the trough value prior to infusion had reached a 'baseline IgG level'. Thereafter, monthly infusions of 400 mg/kg were given resulting in a stepwise increase of the peak and trough IgG levels [5, 6]. After the 7th and 8th infusions, a steady state of both the peak and trough serum IgG levels, defined by similar levels after two consecutive infusions, was observed. Following the 8th IVIG infusion serum samples were collected for the survival studies immediately before, at 15 min following, and at days 1, 3, 5, 7, 10, 14, 18, 21, 24 and 28. Each serum sample was aliquoted and stored at –70 °C until processed.

Quantitation of Serum Immunoglobulin. Total serum IgG and IgG subclasses were determined by radial immunodiffusion using plates specific for IgG and IgG subclasses [6]. For analysis of the data, the immediate postinfusion (15 min) level was taken as 100% and subsequent levels converted to a percentage of this value.

Quantitation of Serum Antibodies. Antibody activity to streptococcal group A carbohydrate (A–CHO) was determined by enzyme-linked immunosorbent assay (ELISA). The antigen, A–CHO was extracted from streptococcus A strain J17A4 as described by Fuller [7]. The antigen was coupled to tyramine with cyanogen bromide and placed in microtiter plates (Dynatech, Plochingen, FRG); IgG1 and IgG2 anti-A-CHO antibodies were determined with subclass-specific antisera (Unipath, Bedford, England). Total IgG anti-A-CHO activity was determined using a goat antihuman IgG antisera (Tago, Burlingame, Calif.). The optical density values measured in each of the collected patient sera were converted to percent values of the immediate postinfusion sample.

Table II. Mean (10 patients) trough and peak levels (mg/dl), half-life data

	IgG	IgG1	IgG2	IgG3	IgG4
Preinfusion (trough 1)	541 ± 83	296 ± 42	233 ± 30	11 ± 5	11 ± 1
15 min after infusion (peak)	1,232 ± 129	703 ± 57	441 ± 35	56 ± 9	27 ± 3
Day 7	862 ± 90	437 ± 31	302 ± 22	21.6 ± 3	16.6 ± 3.5
Day 28 (trough 2)	578 ± 89	290 ± 56	214 ± 25	11 ± 3	10 ± 3
Half-life, days[1]	32.2	34.8	40.2	24.1	36.0

[1] Calculated as described in ref. [6].

Antibody to hepatitis B surface antigen (HBsAg) was determined by a commercially available radioimmunoassay (AUSAB Abbott Laboratory, Diagnostic Division, North Chicago, Ill.).

Antibody titers to coxsackie B types 1–4 were measured by a virus neutralization assay [8]. Antibody to pneumococcal polysaccharide types 1, 6a, and 7 were determined by a radioimmunoassay [9]. Antibody titers to rubella and cytomegalovirus (CMV) and to *Toxoplasma gondii* were measured by ELISA, using commercially available reagents (Whittaker A, Bioproducts, Watersville, Md.). Herpes simplex-specific antibodies were determined by a microneutralization assay.

Antibody titers to diphtheria and tetanus toxoid were determined by a standard hemagglutination assay and titers expressed as the reciprocal of serum dilution. A standard assay to measure phagocytosis and bacterial killing was used to determine the opsonic titers of the collected sera against *Klebsiella pneumoniae*. This complement-dependent assay was a modification of previously described procedures [10].

Results

The 4 XLA patients selected for the study, and 5 of 6 patients with CVID made either no antibody to bacteriophage ΦX 174 or a very small amount of IgG antiphage antibody. Thus, endogenous production of IgG antibody by study patients appears to be insignificant.

IgG Subclass Survival

The values for total IgG and IgG subclasses obtained at the preinfusion time (trough 1) and before the next infusion on day 28 (trough 2) are provided in table II. The two trough values are similar for total IgG and for each of the IgG subclasses. This suggests that the net catabolism of the infused IVIG must have approximated the actual

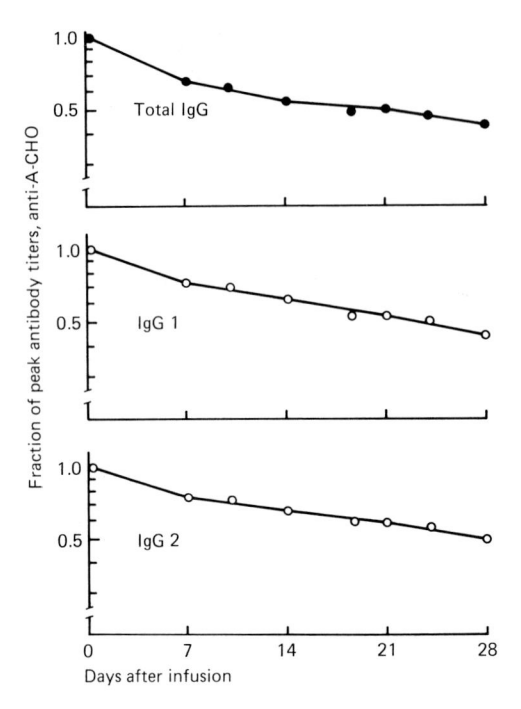

Fig. 1. The decline of antibody activity against A-CHO (IgG total, IgG1 and IgG2) after the 8th monthly IVIG dose of 400 mg/kg. Antibody titers (geometric mean of 10 patients) are shown for total anti-A-CHO IgG (●), IgG1 and IgG2 (○), expressed as percent of the immediate postinfusion sample calculated T½: 36.3 days (IgG); 27 days (IgG1); 35.6 days (IgG2).

monthly dosage of 400 mg/kg body weight per month. A lower rate of catabolism would have resulted in continuously increasing serum trough levels, a faster rate of catabolism in decreasing trough levels.

The peak levels obtained 15 min after infusion are approximately twice the preinfusion (trough) level for total IgG and for IgG1, IgG2, and IgG4. In contrast, the peak serum IgG3 level increased 5-fold. However, the decrement of IgG3 during the first week was extremely rapid; the value at 7 days was only twice baseline.

The half-lives for IgG and the IgG subclasses given in table II were calculated from the disappearance curves constructed from the individual values obtained at each time period of sample collection. The curves and the characteristics of the exponential equations have been published previously [6]. During the first week after infusion,

25–30% of the initially infused IgG1 and IgG4, 20% of the IgG2 and over 55% of the IgG3 had disappeared from the vascular space; presumably either catabolized or distributed extravascularly. Thereafter, the slopes of the curves (fractional catabolic rate) approximated –0.02 per day for IgG, IgG1, IgG2 and IgG4; and –0.03 per day for IgG3. The half-life values indicated in table II were derived from the disappearance curves between days 7 and 28. It appears that the infused IgG3 consisted of two populations of molecules; 50–55% of the infused IgG3 had a very short half-life and disappeared during the first week, the remainder showed a catabolic rate compatible with a half-life of 24 days.

Antigen Specific Antibody Disappearance

Antibody activity to A-CHO doubled after infusion of IVIG reaching a mean titer of 291 (± 52 SD) μg IgG/ml serum. The Sandoglobulin lot used for these studies had an IgG1:IgG2 anti-A-CHO antibody ratio of 3:7. The geometric mean of anti-A-CHO antibody activity is shown in figure 1 and expressed as percent of the OD determined in the samples obtained 15 min after termination of the infusion. Using a standard formula we determined the fractional catabolic rates for anti-A-CHO IgG (–0.019), IgG1 (–0.025) and for IgG2 (–0.019). The half-lives for anti-A-CHO antibody were accordingly 36 days for total IgG, 27 for IgG1 and 36 for IgG2 (fig. 1). The disappearance curves of antibody specific for HBsAg, CMV and three types of pneumococcal polysaccharides (PPS types 1, 6A and 7) are shown in figure 2. Titers were determined in sera collected on day 7, 14, 21 and 28. The curves of visual best fit follow a slope similar to the disappearance curve of total IgG determined simultaneously suggesting a half-life of 32 days.

In addition, antibody titers were determined to 11 common antigens including tetanus und diphtheria toxoid, *Klebsiella pneumoniae* (opsonizing antibody), *Toxoplasma gondii,* rubella, herpes simplex and coxsackie B types 1, 2, 3, 4, and 6 (fig. 3). The preparation of IVIG used in this study contained demonstrable antibody to all antigens except coxsackie B6. As expected, a rise of at least 2-fold in antibody titer to all antigens except coxsackie B6 was observed immediately after infusion. At day 7 the specific antibody titers were still above the preinfusion trough levels; at 28 days they were the same as the preinfusion levels and persistence beyond 7 days must be presumed.

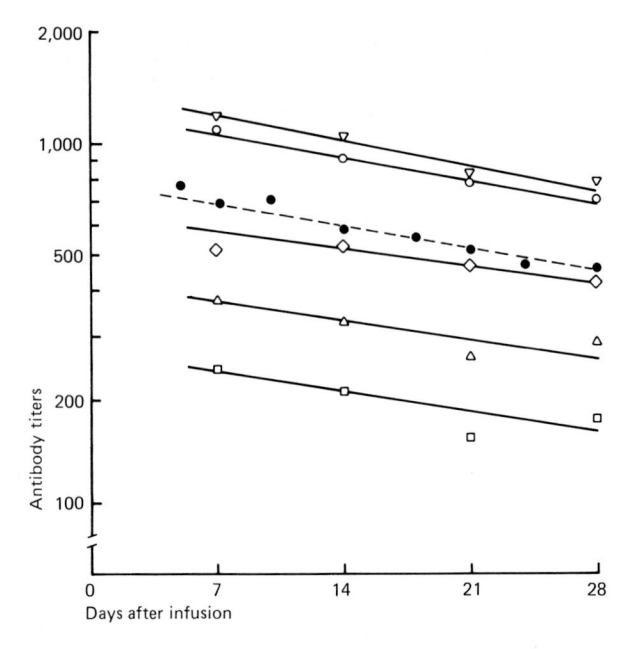

Fig. 2. The serum disappearance curves following the 8th monthly IVIG dose of 400 mg/kg are shown for specific antibodies to the following antigens: HBsAg (○) determined by RIA and expressed as cpm; CMV (◇) determined by ELISA and expressed as OD × 100; PPS type I (▽), type 6A (□), type 7 (△) determined by RIA and expressed as nanograms antibody N/ml. The slope of the disappearance curve for total IgG (●) representing a T½ of 32 days is shown for comparison.

Discussion

The availability of immunoglobulin preparations that are safe for intravenous use allow for effective therapy of patients with hypogammaglobulinemia. Normal or near normal serum IgG levels have been achieved in such patients [5, 11, 12]. Patients with severe antibody deficiency are excellent subjects for the measurement of half-lives of IgG, IgG subclasses and specific IgG antibodies, because their own production of IgG antibody is severely depressed or nonexistent.

The half-lives for total IgG, IgG subclasses and antigen-specific antibodies reported here are longer than those previously recorded in the literature [2]. This is particularly evident for IgG3 which, after rapid disappearance of half the infused amount during the first week, showed a slower than expected catabolic rate with a calculated half-

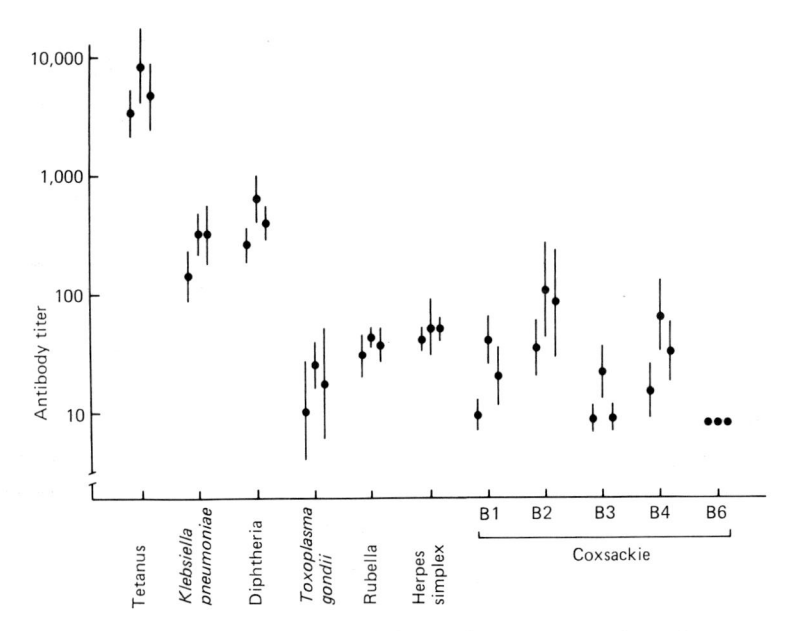

Fig. 3. Antibody titers to 12 different antigens, expressed as the geometric mean ± SD, were measured preinfusion; 15 min; and 7 days postinfusion of IVIG at a dose of 400 mg/kg. The IVIG lot used did not show any activity for coxsackie B6 and no antibody rise was observed after IVIG infusion.

life of 24 days. This contrasts sharply with previously reported IgG3 half-life of 6–8 days [2]. There are many possible reasons to explain the long half-lives observed in this study. Previously reported study techniques used radioactive tracers and a proportion of the immunoglobulin molecules may have been damaged during the labeling process. The myeloma proteins used for the half-life measurements may themselves have been intrinsically abnormal or altered during purification. Since IgG catabolism is concentration-dependent, it could be argued that the low levels of IgG3 7 days after infusion resulted in prolonged survival of the remaining IgG3. This mechanism is probably less likely for IgG1, IgG2 and IgG4 since the levels did not decline as markedly and the peak and trough values were significantly above 'baseline' values. Furthermore, previous half-life studies may have been performed in nonequilibrated patients and thus may not be comparable to this study.

Monthly infusion of large amounts of IVIG results in a most unphysiologic fluctuation between peak and trough serum IgG concentrations. Presumably, catabolism at the peak is more rapid than at the trough. These extremes can be avoided by more frequent infusions of smaller amounts of IVIG. Such a regimen can be facilitated by a program of self-administration of IVIG in the home. This mode of therapy is safe, effective and well accepted by patients; the IgG levels achieved are less fluctuant and within normal range [13, 14].

Summary

To measure the survival of IgG, IgG subclasses and antigen-specific antibody in immune-deficient patients, we infused 4 patients with X-linked agammaglobulinemia (XLA) and 6 patients with common variable immune deficiency (CVID) with modified immunoglobulin at a dose of 400 mg/kg per month until steady state was reached. Following the 8th monthly infusion, serial samples were obtained and analyzed for serum concentration of IgG, IgG subclasses and for specific antibody acivities against a battery of antigens. Half-lives for IgG and IgG subclasses were between 30 and 40 days except for IgG3 which appeared to consist of two populations of molecules, one showing a rapid decay, the other disappearing at a rate suggesting a half life of 22–24 days. Antigen-specific antibodies, including antibodies to HBsAg, cytomegalovirus, pneumococcal polysaccharides and streptococcal group A carbohydrate were similar to that for total IgG. These studies demonstrate that protective antibody titers to infective agents can be maintained for several weeks following high-dose intravenous immunoglobulin infusion.

References

1 Waldmann, T.A.; Strober, W.: Metabolism of immunoglobulins. Prog. Allergy, vol. 13, pp. 1–110 (Karger, Basel 1969).
2 Morell, A.; Terry, W.D.; Waldmann, T.A.: Metabolic properties of IgG subclasses in man. J. clin. Invest. *49:* 673–680 (1970).
3 Spiegelberg, H.L.; Fishkin, B.G.; Grey, H.M.: Catabolism of human γG-immunoglobulins of different heavy chain subclasses. I. Catabolism of γG-myeloma proteins in man. H. clin. Invest. *47:* 2323–2330 (1968).
4 Wedgwood, R.J.; Ochs, H.D.; Davis, S.D.: The recognition and classification of immunodeficiency diseases with bacteriophage ΦX 174; in Bergsma, Immunodeficiency in man and animals. Birth Defects, Orig. Article Ser., No. XI, pp. 331–338 (1975).
5 Ochs, H.D.; Fischer, S.H.; Wedgwood, R.J.; Wara, D.W.; Cowan, M.J.; Ammann, A.J.; Saxon, A.; Budinger, M.D.; Allred, R.U.; Rousell, R.H.: Comparison of high-

dose and low-dose intravenous immunoglobulin therapy in patients with primary immunodeficiency diseases. Proc. Symp. Intravenous Immune Globulin and the Compromised Host. Am. J. Med. 76: 78–82 (1984).
6   Ochs, H.D.; Morell, A.; Skvaril, F.; Fischer, S.H.; Wedgwood, R.J.: Survival of IgG subclasses following administration of intravenous gammaglobulin in patients with primary immunodeficiency diseases; in Morell, Nydegger, Clinical use of intravenous immunoglobulins, pp. 77–85 (Academic Press, London 1986).
7   Fuller, A.T.: Formamide method for the extraction of polysaccharides from hemolytic streptococci. Br. J. exp. Path. 19: 130–138 (1938).
8   Lennete, E.H.; Schmidt, N.J.: Diagnostic procedures for viral, rickettsial and chlamydial infections; 5th ed. (American Public Health Assn., Washington, DC 1979).
9   Robbins, J.B.; Austrian, R.; Cree, C.-J.; Rastogi, S.C.; Schiffmann, G.; Henrichsen, J.; Makela, P.H.; Broome, C.V.; Facklam, R.R.; Tiesjema, R.H.; Parke, J.C., Jr.: Considerations for formulating the second-generation pneumococcal capsular polysaccharide vaccine with emphasis on the cross-reactive types within groups. I. Infect. Dis. 148: 1136–1159 (1983).
10 Harper, T.E.; Christensen, R.D.; Rothstein, G.; Hill, H.R.: Effect of intravenous immunoglobulin G on neutrophil kinetics during experimental group B streptococcal infection in neonatal rats. Rev. Infect. Dis. 8: suppl. 4, pp. S401–408 (1986).
11 Morell, A.; Schnoz, M.; Barandun, S.: Build-up and maintenance of IgG serum concentrations with intravenous immunoglobulin in patients with primary humoral immunodeficiency. Vox Sang. 43: 212–219 (1982).
12 Roifman, C.M.; Lederman, H.M.; Lavi, S.; Stein, L.D.; Levison, H.; Gelfand, E.W.: Benefit of intravenous IgG replacement in hypogammaglobulinemic patients with chronic sinopulmonary disease. Am. J. Med. 79: 171–174 (1985).
13 Ochs, H.D.; Fischer, S.H.; Lee, M.L.; Delson, E.S.; Kingdon, H.S.; Wedgwood, R.J.: Intravenous immunoglobulin home treatment for patients with primary immunodeficiency diseases. Lancet i: 610–611 (1986) (letter).
14 Ashida, E.R.; Saxon, A.: Home intravenous immunoglobulin therapy by self-administration. J. clin. Immunol. 6: 306–309 (1986).

Hans D. Ochs, MD, Department of Pediatrics RD-20,
University of Washington, Seattle, WA 98195 (USA)
No reprints available.

New Biological Aspects of IgG Subclasses

Factors Influencing IgG Subclass Levels in Serum and Mucosal Secretions[1]

T. Söderström, R. Söderström, R. Andersson, J. Lindberg, L.Å. Hanson

Departments of Clinical Immunology, Internal Medicine and Infectious Diseases, University of Göteborg, Göteborg, Sweden

Introduction

Low IgG subclass levels have been associated with recurrent infections and other diseases, but may be seen also in healthy individuals. The subclass levels under which a deficiency may be of clinical relevance have not been settled. The striking variations in serum subclass levels among healthy persons during ontogeny suggest that the minimal level of a specific subclass required to withstand infections may vary depending on the functional capacity of the whole immune system. In this report, we present preliminary studies of factors affecting IgG subclass levels. In addition, we will discuss some aspects of IgG subclasses in relation to mucosal immunity.

Materials and Methods

The IgG subclass levels were measured by the Mancini technique [6] with subclass-specific monoclonal antibodies (clones JL5/2, GOM 1, Z 64, RJ4, Unipath, Bedford, England) as described [10]. Age-related normal ranges were used for comparison [7]. Antigen-specific antibodies were measured by enzyme-linked immunosorbent assay [3]. The immunohistochemical procedure for determination of IgG subclass specific pro-

---

[1] These studies were supported by grants by the Medical Research Council (No. 215), The Swedish Institute for Technical Development, the Ellen, Walter and Lenart Hesselman Foundation, KabiVitrum, Stockholm, Göteborg Medical Society, and Förenade Liv (Mutual Group Life Insurance Company, Stockholm, Sweden).

Table I. Distribution of IgG subclass deficiencies among infection prone patients low in single or multiple IgG subclasses

Subclass deficiency type	Number of adult patients males	females	Total %	Number of child patients males	females	Total %
IgG3	89	175	49.0	18	13	15.9
IgG1	29	60	16.5	21	5	13.3
IgG1+3	18	57	13.9	3	0	1.5
IgG2	10	29	7.2	52	39	46.7
IgG1+2	7	19	4.8	16	13	14.9
IgG1+2+3	4	22	4.8	5	1	3.1
IgG2+3	4	16	3.7	5	4	4.6

duction in mucosal tissue was previously described [2]. The methods employed for studies of the immune function of the patients [10] as well as the allotype determinations [3] were summarized previously. The various patient groups and specific methods will be briefly described in connection with the results.

Results

Age and Sex Variation

The distribution of IgG subclass deficiencies among 539 adults (> 16 years) and 195 children with low levels of one or several IgG subclasses investigated in our laboratory are shown in table I. Boys were 1.6 times more frequent than girls, and the difference was most pronounced among the IgG1-deficient children. 70% of the children with deficiency were diagnosed before they reached 6 years of age. The frequency order of deficiencies among children was IgG2 ≫ IgG3 > IgG1 + G2 > IgG1. Among the adults, females were 2.4 times more often found, and the order was IgG3 ≫ IgG1 > IgG1 + G3 > IgG2. The switch to female and IgG3 dominance seemed to occur at around 15–16 years of age.

Immunological Investigations

The immune status of 65 IgG subclass-deficient adult patients was investigated with flow cytometry analysis of B cells and T cell subpopulations using FITC-conjugated monoclonal antibodies (Leu-series,

Table II. Lymphocyte findings in IgG subclass-associated immunodeficiency

Subclass deficiency type	Number of patients	Percent of patients with decreased			
		T lymphocyte		B lymphocyte	
		CD4/CD8[1]	function[2]	number[3]	function[4]
IgG1	11	9.1	54.5	27.6	75.0
IgG2	9	22.2	55.6	11.1	71.0
IgG3	30	10.0	40.0	13.3	75.0
Combined	15	6.7	53.3	26.7	66.7

[1] Ratio between CD4/CD8 lower than 1.0.
[2] PHA or ConA stimulatory index lower than 0.8 compared to healthy control individuals.
[3] Less than 2% surface immunoglobulin-positive lymphocytes in peripheral blood.
[4] EBV- or PWM-stimulated protein A – plaque lower than 50% of healthy controls for IgG.

Becton Dickinson, Calif.). T cell function was studied with phytohemagglutinin (PHA) and concanavalin A (ConA) stimualted ^{3}H incorporation and B cell function with Epstein-Barr virus (EBV) and pokeweed mitogen (PWM)-stimulated Protein A plaque assay [9]. The results are shown in table II. As many as three quarters of the patients seemed to have demonstrable B- and/or T cell dysfunction.

Genetics

Several families with more than one member low in isolated subclasses were found. A pair of twins with IgG3 + IgG4 deficiency was investigated as well. In a collaborative part of the study patients with IgG3 deficiency were allotyped [3]. A strong correlation was demonstrated between the G3m(g) allotype and IgG3 deficiency in as much as persons heterozygous for G3m(g) were low and individuals homozygous for G3m(g) were very low in serum IgG3. These results suggest that allotyped-linked regulatory events might be associated with subclass deficiency, and that a gene dose effect may be seen.

Infections

Recurrent upper and lower respiratory tract infections were the most common diagnoses among the patients. Some of these indivi-

Table III. Progressive changes occurring in 8 patients with subclass deficiency

Initial deficiency	Subsequent deficiencies		
IgG1	IgG1 + 3		
	IgG1 + 2 + 3		
IgG2	IgG2 + 3	→	IgG2
	IgG3		
	IgG1 + 2 + 3		
IgG3	IgG1 + 3	→	IgG3
	IgG2 + 3		
	IgG1 + 2 + 3		

duals were sampled at the time of bacterial pneumonias, and they showed more pronounced deficiencies during acute illness. In addition, patients with long-standing infections, such as chronic Borrelia, herpes or cytomegalovirus infection were found as well as several young patients with myocarditis or pericarditis with IgG1 and/or IgG3 deficiency. In these cases, it was unclear whether the deficiency was present before the disease started. We also studied a boy with a history of varicellae at 5 months and severe herpes zoster ophthalmicus at 10 years of age. He was low in serum IgG2 and high in IgG4. A patient with congenital rubella infection was diagnosed as IgG3-deficient. No patients with parasitic infections were found. It has, in fact, been shown that patients with parasitic disease have significantly higher IgG4 levels than healthy control persons [5].

As part of a blind study of the effect of prophylactic γ-globulin administration, we have followed around 50 patients with subclass determination every 3 months. Five of these patients and 3 other patients who entered the study deficient in a single IgG subclass have added deficiencies in other subclasses, in some resulting in a hypogammaglobulinemia (table III). Since the patient code is not yet broken, we do not know if this has happened during immunoglobulin or saline treatment, and if the change was influenced by acute infections.

Treatment with Corticosteroids

Many patients with IgG subclass deficiencies show allergy-related symptoms like asthma or food hypersensitivity [10]. These patients have often been treated with steroids. To investigate the effect of corticosteroids on the IgG subclass levels, we have studied 7 patients given

Table IV. Effect of corticosteroid treatment prednisolone 40 mg/day for one week and then 25 mg/day on IgG subclass levels in 7 patients with giant cell arteritis

Time of sampling	Mean IgG subclass level, g/l			
	IgG1	IgG2	IgG3	IgG4
Before treatment	8.06	3.15	0.61	0.24
14 days after start of treatment	10.3	2.80	0.50	0.27

Prednisolon 30–40 mg/day during 1 week reduced to 15 mg/day because of giant cell arteritis. The subclass levels before treatment and 14 days after start of treatment are summarized in table IV. One patient developed IgG3 deficiency at 7 days, and one patient showed low IgG2 + 3 levels after 2 weeks. The mean subclass levels, however, showed no influence of the steroid treatment.

Effect of Surgery

Patients undergoing peripheral vascular surgery because of chronic leg ulcers were investigated for IgG subclass levels [10]. Following surgery there was a decrease in serum IgG, which affected all subclasses. After 2–3 weeks, a rebound effect causing slightly higher than starting levels was noted. Many patients were moderately IgG3-deficient already before surgery and some had low IgG1 or IgG2 levels. Three of these subclass-deficient patients developed severe postoperative infectious complications and even lower levels of the initially low subclass.

In a preliminary study of patients with surgery of the small intestine or colon because of inflammatory bowel disease, we noted effects on serum IgG subclasses. Removal of large parts of the small intestine in some patients resulted in low IgG2 levels lasting several months after the operation. Similarly, a period of IgG2 deficiency evolved in some patients following colectomy. One could speculate in at least two principal mechanisms resulting in IgG2 deficiency in these patients: (1) Removal of large masses of lymphoid tissue along the small intestine, where microbial antigens may have caused preferential IgG2 proliferation. (2) Removal of colon possibly causes a dramatic reduction in bacterial antigen stimulation of IgG2 production.

Chronic Active Hepatitis

Chronic active hepatitis is associated with increased serum immunoglobulin levels. Two alternative mechanisms have been proposed: impaired removal of antigen by the diseased liver or increased immunoreactivity [4]. We have studies 19 patients with chronic active hepatitis with serum IgG subclass levels determined at various stages of disease activity. Dramatic increases in serum Ig was observed during active disease. The levels often reached > 50 g/l and the antibodies were strikingly restricted to IgG1, sometimes combined with increased IgG3 levels. The restrictions to IgG1 and IgG3, often considered T-dependent subclasses, could suggest that locally produced lymphokines preferentially stimulating IgG1 production like IL-4 may be involved. Alternatively, processed microbial and dietary antigens may trigger the hyperreactive liver-associated lymphoid tissue differently as compared to the antigens present in the gut.

IgG Subclasses in the Mucosa

We have studied the local IgG subclass production in the nasal mucosa of IgG-subclass-deficient persons [2, 9]. Individuals with low serum IgG2 levels had few mucosal IgG2 producing lymphocytes. No correlation between serum IgG1 and IgG3 levels and mucosal lymphocytes making these isotypes could be found.

The salivary and nasal secretion response to the *Haemophilus influenzae* type b and tetanus toxoid antigens were studied following immunization of 21 IgG-subclass-deficient individuals with a polysaccharide-protein conjugate vaccine [1, 9]. No correlation was seen between the serum and secretory IgG subclass-specific responses. These studies suggest that the local environment may strongly influence the subclass-specific immune responses evoked by the antigen.

Individuals with Higher than Normal IgG Subclass Levels

The subclass-deficient individuals described above were found among patients investigated in our laboratory because of suspected immune dysfunction. We also looked at the distribution between subclasses in patients with increased subclass levels detected in the same patient material. As many as 259 children and 221 adults were found, which should be compared to the 195 children and 539 adults with subclass deficiency. Also in this group boys dominated among the

Table V. Factors suggested to influence IgG subclass levels

Genetic – gene deletions, allotype linkage
Age
Sex
Acute (and chronic?) infections
Stress – (vascular) surgery
Corticosteroid treatment
Surgical removal of lymphoid tissue – gut-associated lymphoid tissue
Colectomy – reduced antigenic stimulation
Chronic active hepatitis
Bone marrow transplantation
Protein-losing gastroenteropathy

children (1.2:1) and females among the adults (1.9:1). Among children, the frequency of high subclass levels distributed as follows: IgG1 ≫ IgG1 + G3 > IgG3 > IgG4 > IgG1 + G4 > other combinations > IgG2. Among the adult individuals, we found IgG1 > IgG3 > IgG2 > IgG1 + G3 > IgG4 and other combinations.

Concluding Remarks

We are obviously only beginning to understand the complex interactions leading to aberrations in IgG subclasses. Some of the many factors found to influence the serum IgG subclass levels are summarized in table V. Some of these items, like bone marrow transplantation and protein-losing syndromes have not been discussed. It is clear that subclass deficiency the way we define it at present is a good indication of underlying B and/or T cell dysfunction [8–10]. We do not know, however, if a high IgG subclass level functions equally well as an indicator. Since nature provides the newborn infant with high levels of all IgG subclasses one may assume that presence of a broad spectrum of antibodies may be beneficial in situations where the function of the immune system is not optimal.

References

1 Avanzini, M.A.; Söderström, T.; Schneerson, R.; Robbins, J.B.; Söderström, R.; Björkander, J.; Hanson, L.Å.: The heterogeneity of the antibody response in patients with IgG subclass deficiency is reflected on vaccination. Proc. 2nd Meet. European Group for Immunodeficiencies, 1986.

2 Brandtzaeg, P.; Kett, K.; Rognum, T.O.; Söderström, R.; Björkander, J.; Söderström, T.; Petruson, B.; Hanson, L.Å.: Distribution of mucosal IgA and IgG subclass-producing immunocytes and alterations in various disorders; in Hanson, Söderström, Oxelius, Immunoglobulin subclass deficiencies. Monogr. Allergy, vol. 20, 179–194 (Karger, Basel 1986).

3 Grubb, R.; Hallberg, T.; Hammarström, L.; Oxelius, V.-A.; Smith, C.I.E.; Söderström, R.; Söderström, T.: Correlation between deficiency of immunoglobulin subclass G3 and Gm allotype. Acta pathol. microbiol. scand., C, Immunol. 94: 187–191 (1986).

4 Lindberg, J.; Kaijser, B.; Lindholm, A.; Hermodsson, S.; Iwarson, S.: Humoral immunoreactivity in chronic active hepatitis: relation to HLA antigens. Int. Archs Allergy appl. Immun. 58: 75–81 (1979).

5 Magnusson, C.G.M.; Djurup, R.; Cesbron, J.T.; Johansson, S.G.O.: Automated assay of IgG4 in non-atopics, atopics and filariasis-infected patients using monoclonal antibody; in Hanson, Söderström, Oxelius, Immunoglobulin subclass deficiencies. Monogr. Allergy, vol. 20, p. 230 (Karger, Basel 1986).

6 Mancini, G.; Carbonara, A.O.; Heremans, J.F.: Immunochemical quantitation of antigens by single radial immunodiffusion. Immunochemistry 2: 235–254 (1965).

7 Oxelius, V.-A.: IgG subclass levels in infancy and childhood. Acta paediat. scand. 68: 23–27 (1979).

8 Quinti, J.; Papetti, C.; Festi, R.; Bonomo, R.; Aiuti, F.: IgG subclass deficiency in adults: a clinical and immunological study; in Hanson, Söderström, Oxelius, Immunoglobulin subclass deficiencies. Monogr. Allergy, vol. 20, pp. 143–148 (Karger, Basel 1986).

9 Söderström, T.; Söderström, R.; Avanzini, A.; Brandtzaeg, P.; Karlsson, G.; Hanson, L.Å.: Immunoglobulin G subclass deficiencies. Proc. 16th Meet. of the Collegium Internationale Allergologicum, 1987.

10 Söderström, T.; Söderström, R.; Bengtsson, U.; Björkander, J.; Hellstrand, J.; Holm, J.; Hanson, L.Å.: Clinical and immunological evaluation of patients low in single or multiple IgG subclasses; in Hanson, Söderström, Oxelius, Immunoglobulin subclass deficiencies. Monogr. Allergy, vol. 20, pp. 135–142 (Karger, Basel 1986).

Dr. T. Söderström, Department of Clinical Immunology,
Guldhedsgatan 10, S-413 46 Göteborg (Sweden)

Correlations of G2m(n) and Km(1) Allotypes with Subclass- and Light-Chain-Specific Antibody

Donna M. Ambrosino[a], Andreas Morell[b], Giuseppe Vassalli[b], Gerda G. de Lange[c], Frantisek Skvaril[b], George R. Siber[a, d]

[a] Laboratory of Infectious Disease, Dana-Farber Cancer Institute, Boston, Mass.;
[b] Institute for Clinical and Experimental Cancer Research, University of Berne, Berne, Switzerland; [c] Central Laboratory of the Netherlands, Red Cross Blood Transfusion Service, Amsterdam, The Netherlands; [d] Massachusetts Public Health Biologic Laboratories, Jamaica Plain, Mass., USA

Introduction

The major bacterial pathogens of childhood are polysaccharideencapsulated organisms. Antibodies to the capsular polysaccharides of these pathogens, *Haemophilus influenzae* type b (Hib), pneumococci, and meningococci are important in protection against infection [1–4]. Several observations suggest that the antibody response to polysaccharide antigens and susceptibility to these bacterial infections may be under genetic control. First, children who have recovered from meningitis have lower anti-Hib antibodies than age-matched siblings [5] and do not respond to immunizations as well as controls [6]. Second, siblings of patients with meningitis have lower antibody responses to a Hib-pertussis complex vaccine than control children [7]. Finally, certain ethnic populations, such as native Americans [8] and Alaskan Eskimos [9], have an extremely high incidence of infection by Hib and pneumococci. Although socioeconomic and epidemiologic factors may explain some of these observations, genetic factors are also likely to be important. We therefore have studied the relationship of immunoglobulin allotypes to polysaccharide antibody responses and disease susceptibility.

Human allotypes are genetic markers expressed as antigens on the constant regions of heavy or light chains of immunoglobulins. Human γ-chain and α-chain allotypes are designated Gm and Am, respectively. κ-Light chain allotypes are designated Km. The Gm and Am loci are located on chromosome 14 and the Km locus is located on chromosome 2 [10]. All allotypes are inherited in a Mendelian fashion and are co-dominant. Because the Km allotypes are expressed on light chains, they occur on molecules of all isotypes (IgG, IgM, IgA, IgD, and IgE). In contrast, the Gm allotypes are confined to IgG molecules and the Am allotypes are expressed only on IgA.

We have previously demonstrated that G2m(n) and Km(1), are correlated with polysaccharide-specific antibody responses in Caucasians [11, 12]. We will review these data and present new studies that confirm the original findings. In addition, we will define the subclass and light chain specificity of the relationship. This specificity offers an explanation for previous discrepancies in allotype correlations to polysaccharide antibody responses.

Methods

Study Population (Active Immunization)
58 male and 72 female Caucasian plasma donors with a mean age of 33 years were immunized with 0.5 ml 14-valent pneumococcal vaccine (Pneumovax, Lot 1912B, Merck, Sharp & Dohme, West Point, Pa.) and concurrently with 0.5 ml Hib vaccine (Lot 764-CF320; Merck, Sharp and Dohme) and 0.5 ml bivalent meningococcal vaccine (Menomune A/C, Connaught Laboratories, Swiftwater, Pa.), combined in the same syringe. Serum for Ig allotyping, Ig concentrations, and polysaccharide antibody assays obtained before and 4 weeks after immunization and stored at $-20\,°C$ until assay.

Study Population (Unimmunized)
Serum samples of 193 healthy young male adults (20-year-old Swiss recruits) were obtained from the Central Laboratory of the Swiss Red Cross Blood Transfusion Service and stored at $-70\,°C$ until assay.

Study Population (Disease Susceptibility)
98 children with Hib disease seen at Children's Hospital Medical Center, Boston, Mass., from 1977 to 1982 were studied. The case definition of Hib infection was outlined previously [24]. Controls were chosen from children with other febrile illnesses observed during the same period, matched to cases by age, sex, race, and neighborhood of resi-

dence using the postal code. Individuals with prior culture documented Hib, pneumococcal, or meningococcal infection were excluded.

Assays

Antibody to the capsular polysaccharide of Hib was measured by radioimmunoassay (RIA) [13], with tritiated capsular polysaccharide kindly provided by Dr. Porter Anderson (University of Rochester, Rochester, N.Y.). The assay was standardized with a standard serum (S. Klein) supplied by Dr. John Robbins (National Institutes of Health, Bethesda, Md.). Pneumococcal and meningococcal antibody was quantitated by RIA using radiolabelled pneumococcal type 3 antigen in Dr. G. Schiffman's laboratory [14] and meningococcal group C antigen in Dr. E. Gotschlich's laboratory [15].

IgG, IgM, and IgA antibody to the capsular polysaccharides of Hib, pneumococcus type 3 and meningococcus group C were quantitated by enzyme-linked immunosorbent assay (ELISA) using the respective antigens coupled to tyramine with cyanogen bromide as previously described [11]. Light-chain-specific anti-polysaccharide antibody was determined by an adaptation of this ELISA procedure using goat anti-human κ- and λ-alkaline phosphate conjugates (Tago, Burlingame, Calif.) as previously described [12]. Total κ- and λ-concentrations were determined by capturing immunoglobulin with goat anti-κ- and λ-IgG fractions (Atlantic Antibodies, Scarborough, Me.) [12]. The method of Zollinger and Boslego [16] was employed to estimate the concentrations of specific antibody in a human hyperimmune plasma pool as a reference for ELISA.

Serum concentration of IgG, IgM and IgA were measured by nephelometry [17]. Serum IgG subclass levels were determined with solid-phase competitive radioimmunoassays using sheep antisera to human IgG subclass proteins. These antisera were rendered specific by stepwise absorption with isolated IgG myeloma proteins. The World Health Organization serum pool 67/97 was used to establish the reference standard inhibition curves. Details of the reagents and the assay have been reported before [18, 19].

Antibodies to group-specific streptococcal A carbohydrate (A-CHO) were measured by ELISA [20]. For determinations of the subclasses of IgG antibodies to A-CHO monoclonal antibodies (moAg) to IgG subclasses (Unipath, Bedford, England) were used. The following clone numbers and dilutions of moAb were used: NL16 (anti-IgG1, 1:5,000) and GOM1 (anti-IgG2, 1:1,000). Results were expressed as OD values. Antibody concentrations of individual sera were compared with reference pool arbitrarily defined as 1000 U/ml and express in U/ml.

Antistreptolysin O activity in the sera was measured with a commercial hemolysis inhibition test (Behring Diagnostics, Marburg, FRG). Results were expressed as IU/ml. Immunoglobulin allotypes were determined by hemagglutinating inhibition in the laboratory of Dr. G. de Lange.

Each Gm marker carries the designation of the subclass on which it is detected. G1m(f) and G1m(a,z) or G1m(a,x,z) behave as allelic markers of IgG1. G3m(b) and G3m(g) are allelic markers of IgG3 molecules. IgG2 molecules are either positive or negative for G2m(n). The sum of Gm markers detected in a serum compose the Gm phenotype which can be grouped into haplotypes. Gm haplotypes most commonly found in Caucasians are Gm(f,n,b), Gm(f,b), Gm(z,a,g) and Gm(z,a,x,g).

Table I. Relationship between the G2m(n) allotype and anti-polysaccharide antibody concentrations before and after immunization

	Geometric mean antibody concentrations (p value)[1]			
	before immunization	before immunization	after immunization	after immuniztion
	antibody to G2m(n)+ (n=88)	antibody to G2m(n)− (n=42)	antibody to G2m(n)+ (n=88)	antibody to G2m(n)− (n=42)
H. influenzae type b (µg/ml)	2.17	1.70	35.0	21.3 (0.024)
N. meningitidis, (µg/ml)				
Group A	3.55	3.61	12.1	11.8
Group B	0.878	0.869	33.9	26.5
S. pneumoniae (ng protein N/ml)				
Type 1	1,010	874	2,100	1,660
3	152	116	1,930	1,260
6	211	144	723	445 (0.035)
7	438	177 (0.071)	2,040	955 (0.007)
8	555	434 (0.044)	1,530	1,030 (0.022)
9	72	55	476	288
12	1,760	985 (0.055)	3,440	2,150 (0.001)
14	501	293 (0.090)	1,690	1,010 (0.007)
18	700	361 (0.077)	2,540	1,460 (0.006)
19	167	100 (0.076)	1,050	334 (0.0001)
23	931	632 (0.011)	3,020	1,430 (0.001)
Geometric mean of types	520	423	1,870	1,220 (0.0005)

[1] A two-tailed t-test was used for normally distributed values and a Mann-Whitney test was used for nonnormally distributed values.

Statistical Methods

All statistical analyses were performed utilizing the PROPHET system, a national computer system sponsored by the Chemical/Biological Information Handling Program, National Institutes of Health. All statistical analyses such as correlations, multiple regression analyses and comparisons of means were performed on the logarithms of the concentrations.

Table II. Relationship between the G2m(n) allotype and class-specific postimmunization antibody concentrations to Hib, Pneumococcus type 14, and Meningococcus group C capsular polysaccharides

Antibody to	Geometric mean antibody concentrations, ELISA units/ml (p value)[1]	
	G2m(n)+ (n=88)	G2m(n)− (n=42)
H. influenzae type b		
IgG	12,950	5,735 (0.005)
IgM	1,425	1,201
IgA	1,408	1,425
S. pneumoniae type 14		
IgG	36,300	21,200 (0.014)
IgM	3,870	5,150
IgA	532	630
N. meningitidis group C		
IgG	5,140	2,430 (0.012)
IgM	1,690	1,890
IgA	557	630

[1] A two-tailed t-test was used for normally distributed values and a Mann-Whitney test was used for nonnormally distributed values.

For multiple linear regression analyses involving Ig allotypes, the presence of the presumptive haplotypes (f, n, b; f, b; z, a, g; or z, a, x, g) or allotype [Km(1), A2m(2)] was scored as 1 and the absence as 0. Significantly correlated variable were entered into the regression analysis one at a time, generally beginning with the variable with the highest correlation coefficient. Standard statistical tests were applied for comparisons of means and proportions, including the t-test for normal distributions with equal dispersions and the Mann-Whitney test for nonnormal distributions with equal dispersions.

Results

G2m(n) and Polysaccharide Antibody Response

We have previously shown that in 130 actively immunized Caucasian adults, G2m(n) allotype was significantly correlated with higher total binding postimmunization antibody levels to Hib and 8 of 11 pneumococcal types examined (p < 0.05) [11] (table I). We next examined the class-specific responses to three polysaccharides. The correlation of G2m(n) to increased antibody responses was confined to the IgG class (table II) for all three polysaccharides examined.

G2m(n) and Disease Susceptibility

To determine if the lack of G2m(n) was associated with increased susceptibility to infection, we compared the frequencies of various Ig allotypes in 98 children infected with Hib and 98 matched control as previously published [11]. Caucasian children with Hib infections other than epiglottitis were found to be significantly more likely to lack the G2m(n) allotype than controls (p < 0.05). G2m(n)-negative Caucasian children ≤ 18 months old had a 5.1-fold higher risk of nonepiglottic Hib infections than G2m(n)-positive children (p < 0.01).

We conclude that allotypic variants of the γ-2 heavy chain genes, or genes in linkage equilibrium with them, exert a regulatory influence on the Caucasian antibody response to a variety of immunologically distinct bacterial polysaccharide antigens. In addition, young Caucasian children of the low responder phenotype, i.e. those lacking the G2m(n) allotype, were found to be genetically predisposed to Hib and perhaps other bacterial infections.

Km(1) and Polysaccharide Antibody Response

Our results noted above demonstrated that G2m(n), an antigenic marker on the heavy chain of IgG2 subclass immunoglobulins, *was* correlated to the IgG antibody response to polysaccharides. We next examined the relationship of Km(1), a light chain marker, to the light-chain-specific response. We demonstrated that the 14 Km(1)-positive individuals had lower concentrations of κ-containing anti-polysaccharide antibody for Hib (p = 0.029) and *N. meningitidis* group C (p = 0.003) than the 115 Km(1) negatives (table III).

To determine if the Km(1) association was specific for antibody to polysaccharides we examined the relationship of Km(1) to total κ- and λ-antibody. The Km(1) positives had a lower geometric mean κ-antibody concentration of $12,800 \times 10^3$ ELISA units as compared with 14,500 ELISA units (p = 0.079) (table III). The presence of the Km(1) allotype did not significantly correlate with total λ-antibody concentrations.

Table III. Relationship between Km(1) allotype and light-chain-specific antibody concentrations after immunization with polysaccharide antigens

	Geometric mean antibody concentration (ELISA units) after immunization		p value[1]
	Km(1)+ (n = 14)	Km(1)— (n = 115)	
H. influenzae type b			
Kappa	5,320	11,600	0.029
Lambda	7,704	3,540	
N. meningitidis group C			
Kappa	8,280	16,200	0.003
Lambda	2,260	3,290	
S. pneumoniae type 3			
Kappa	3,980	3,750	
Lambda	5,950	7,830	
Total antibody ($\times 10^3$)			
Kappa	12,800	14,500	0.079
Lambda	7,300	7,800	

[1] A two-tailed t-test was used for normally distributed values and a Mann-Whitney test for nonnormally distributed values.

G2m(n) and Subclass-Specific Antibody to Group A Streptococcae Carbohydrate (A-CHO)

To confirm our G2m(n) finding and further define the relationship to subclass-specific antibody, we decided to study a different population and assay subclass-specific antibody. We hypothesized that the correlation of G2m(n) to increased IgG antibody concentrations would be confined to the IgG2 subclass. We chose to examine antibody to the group-specific carbohydrate of group A streptococci (A-CHO). Due to universal exposure, most normal adults have measurable quantities of antibodies to this carbohydrate antigen. We determined the serum concentrations of specific IgG, IgM, IgG1 and IgG2 subclass antibody in 193 normal adult Swiss males. IgG and IgM anti-A-CHO could be detected in all sera. At serum dilutions of 1:50 and 1:100, IgG1 anti-A-CHO was found in 123 (63%) sera and IgG2 anti-A-CHO in 107 (55%) sera.

Table IV. Relationship between G2m(n) allotype and total immunoglobulin concentrations in 193 adults

	Geometric mean concentration, mg/100 ml (p value)	
	G2m(n)+ (n = 131)	G2m(n)— (n = 62)
IgG	1,282	1,297
IgM	117	135 (0.0001)
IgA	198	186
IgG1	759	867 (0.0001)
IgG2	317	214 (0.0001)
IgG3	76	71
IgG4	44	31 (0.009)

By a multiple linear regression analysis, the G2m(n) was positively correlated with IgG2 anti-A-CHO levels (p = 0.007). Interestingly, G2m(n) was negatively correlated with IgG1 anti-A-CHO levels (p < 0.0001). As a consequence, the two opposite relationships cancelled out the correlations between Gam(n) and IgG anti-A-CHO (r = +0.071, n.s.). Furthermore, this correlation was not specific for antibody to carbohydrates. Gam(n) was correlated with increased total IgG2 subclass concentrations (p < 0.0001) and decreased total IgG1 subclass concentrations (p = 0.022). The relationship of G2m(n) to total and specific antibody concentrations is shown in tables IV and V.

Finally, it was noted that G2m(n)-positive individuals had higher IgG4 concentrations and lower total IgM as well as IgM anti-A-CHO concentrations compared to G2m(n) negatives. Serum antistreptolysin concentrations were not significantly different in these two groups (table V).

Discussion

We have previously reported that the G2m(n) and Km(1) allotypes are correlated with the antibody response to polysaccharides in adult Caucasians [11, 12]. We noted that the G2m(n) allotype, a marker expressed on γ-chains, was only associated with regulation of the IgG isotype. This association was of clinical significance in that children

Table V. Relationship between G2m(n) allotype and antibody concentrations to group A Streptococcus in 193 adults

	Geometric mean concentration (p value)	
	G2m(n)+ (n = 131)	G2m(n)− (n = 62)
Anti-A-CHO antibody		
IgG, µg/ml	124	105
IgG1, OD values	0.141	0.283 (0.0001)
IgG2, OD values	0.188	0.114 (0.007)
IgM, µg/ml	47	60 (0.032)
Antistreptolysin O, IU/ml	111	114

lacking the G2m(n) allotype were at significantly increased risk of infection [11]. The Km(1) allotype was shown to correlate with decreased antibody response to certain polysaccharides. The association was restricted to the specific antibody type expressing the allotype. Km(1) individuals had a decreased concentration of antibody containing κ-light chains. Although not reaching significance, the Km(1) negatives also had lower total κ-antibody. This then suggested that the allotype association was not restricted to polysaccharides.

These two studies suggested that allotype associated regulation would not be specific for polysaccharides, but rather specific for the total subclass or total light chains expressing the marker. To confirm our findings and further define the subclass-specific nature of the G2m(n) association, we examined the total subclass concentrations and the subclass-specific antibody to A-CHO in 193 Caucasian adults. The G2m(n) allotype was significantly correlated with increased total IgG-2 concentrations ($p < 0.0001$) and specific IgG-2 anti-A-CHO concentrations ($p = 0.007$). Interestingly, G2m(n) allotype was also correlated with a decreased total IgG-1 concentration ($p = 0.0001$) and decreased specific IgG-1 anti-A-CHO ($p = 0.0001$). Thus, if only IgG had been determined, not subclass-specific antibody, the correlation to G2m(n) allotype would be missed (tables IV and V).

This subclass specificity of allotype correlations may explain the apparent discrepancies between laboratories. Granoff et al. [21] have not found any association between G2m(n) allotype and the IgG antibody response to either Hib polysaccharide *B. pertussis* vaccine or to Hib PS vaccine in white children. However, IgG2 subclass-specific antibody was not measured. In fact, young children responding to polysaccharide vaccine may produce substantial amounts of IgG1 antibody and this may be exaggerated by immunization with complexed vaccines [22]. Thus, if only IgG antibody is measured, no G2m(n) allotype association would be detected.

Regarding Km(1) correlations, we have noted a decreased antibody response in whites with Km(1) allotype. In contrast, Granoff et al. [23] have reported an increased response to Hib polysaccharide vaccine and a decreased risk of developing Hib meningitis in black children. Again, the differences may relate to the specific light chains (κ or λ) composing the response. Light-chain-specific antibody was not determined. Alternatively, the racial differences between our Km(1) studies may explain the discrepancies. The Km(1) locus in blacks may be linked to different regulatory genes than in whites. Such linkage differences are problematic for extending allotype observations to different ethnic populations. In a recent study, G2m(n) was reported not to be associated with Hib disease susceptibility in North America [14]. However, only 5% of total population expressed the G2m(n) allotype. To duplicate our G2m(n) finding in white children in this population would have required a far larger sample size.

In summary, we find allotype-associated regulation to be restricted to the heavy or light chain expressing the allotype. Secondly, we suggest that allotype-associated regulation is not antigen-specific. Antibody to antigens, such as polysaccharides, may be correlated with specific allotypes, such as G2m(n), because the antibody response is preferentially IgG2 [25]. Allotype-associated regulation of antibody response may have clinical significance in such situations.

References

1   Schneerson, R.; Rodrigues, L.P.; Parke, J.C.; Robbins, J.B.: Immunity to disease caused by *Haemophilus influenzae* type b. II. Specificity and some biologic characteristics of 'natural' infection acquired, and immunization induced antibodies to the capsular polysaccharide of *Haemophilus influenzae* type b. J. Immun. *107:* 1081–1089 (1971).
2   Peltola, H.; Kayhty, H.; Sivonen, A.; Makela, P.H.: *Haemophilus influenzae* type b capsular polysaccharide vaccine in children: a doubleblind field study of

100,000 vaccines 3 months to 5 years of age in Finland. Pediactrics *60:* 730–737 (1977).
3   Austrian, R.: Some observations on the pneumococcus and on the current status of pneumococcal disease and its prevention. Rev. infect. Dis. *3:* S1–17 (1981).
4   Artenstein, M.S.; Gold, R.; Zimmerly, J.G.; Wyle, F.A.; Schneider, H.; Harkins, C.: Prevention of meningococcal disease of group C polysaccharide vaccine. New Engl. J. Med. *282:* 417–420 (1970).
5   Whisnant, J.K.; Rogentine, G.N.; Gralnick, M.A.; Schlesselman, J.J.; Robbins, J.B.: Host factors and antibody response in *Haemophilus influenzae* type b meningitis and epiglottitis. J. infect. Dis. *133:* 448–455 (1976).
6   Norden, C.W.; Michaels, R.H.; Melish, M.: Effects of previous infection on antibody response of children to vaccination with capsular polysaccharide of *Haemophilus influenzae* type b. J. infect. Dis. *132:* 69–74 (1975).
7   Granoff, D.M.; Squires, J.E.; Munson, R.S.; Suarez, B.: Siblings of patients with *Haemophilus meningitis* have impaired anticapsular antibody reponse to Haemophilus vaccine. J. Pediat. *103:* 185–191 (1983).
8   Lozonsky, G.A.; Santosham, M.; Sehgal, V.; Zwahlen, A.; Moxon, E.R.: *Haemophilus influenzae* disease in the White Mountain Apaches. Pediat. Infect. Dis. *3:* 539–547 (1984).
9   Ward, J.I.; Margolis, H.S.; Lum, M.K.W.; Fraser, D.W.; Bender, T.R.: *Haemophilus influenzae* disease in Alaskan Eskimos: characteristics of a population with an unusual incidence of invasive disease. Lancet *i:* 1281–1285 (1981).
10 Loghem, E. van: Genetic studies on human immunoglobulins; in Weir, Handbook of experimental immunology, vol 1 (Blackwell, Oxford 1978).
11 Ambrosino, D.M.; Schiffman, G.; Gotschlich, E.C.; Schur, P.H.; Rosenberg, G.A.; DeLange, G.G.; Loghem, E. van; Siber, G.R.: Correlation between G2m(n) immunoglobulin allotype and human antibody response and susceptibility to polysaccharide encapsulated bacteria. J. clin. Invest. *75:* 1935–1942 (1985).
12 Ambrosino, D.M.; Barrus, V.A.; deLange, G.G.; Siber, G.R.: Correlations of the Km(1) immunoglobulin allotype with anti-polysaccharide antibodies in Caucasian adults. J. clin. Invest. *78:* 361–365 (1986).
13 O'Reilly, R.J.; Anderson, P.; Ingram, D.L.; Peter G.; Smith, D.H.: Circulating polyribophosphate in *Haemophilus influenzae* type b meningitis: correlation with clinician course and antibody response. J. clin. Invest. *56:* 1012–1022 (1975).
14 Schiffman, G.; Douglas, R.M.; Bonner, M.J.; Robbins, M.; Austrian, R.: A radioimmunoassay for immunologic phenomena in pneumococcal disease and for the antibody response to pneumococcal vaccines. I. Method for the radioimmunoassay for anticapsular antibodies and comparison with other techniques. J. immunol. Methods *33:* 133–144 (1980).
15 Gotschlich, E.; Rey, M.; Triau, R.; Sparks, K.J.: Quantitative determination of the human immune response to immunization with meningococcal vaccines. J. clin. Invest. *51:* 89–96 (1972).
16 Zollinger, W.D.; Boslego, J.W.: A general approach to standardization of the solid-phase radioimmunoassay for quantitation of class-specific antibodies. J. immunol. Methods *46:* 129–140 (1981).
17 Alper, C.A.: Plasma protein measurements as a diagnostic aid. New Engl. J. Med. *291:* 287–290 (1974).

18 Morell, A.; Skvaril, F.; Steinberg, A.G.; Loghem, E. van; Terry, W.D.: Correlations between the concentrations of the four subclasses of IgG and Gm allotypes in normal human sera. J. Immun. *108:* 195–206 (1972).

19 Morell, A.; Loghem, E. van; Nef, M.; Theilkas, L.; Skvaril, F.: Determination of IgG subclasses and Gm allotypes in culture supernatants of pokeweed mitogen-stimulated human blood lymphocytes. J. Immun. *127:* 1099–1102 (1981).

20 Morell, A.; Vassalli, G.; Lange, G.G., de; Skvaril, F.; Ambrosino, D.M.; Siber, G.R.: Class and subclass composition of natural antibodies to group A streptococcal carbohydrate. Correlations with serum immunoglobulin concentrations and allotypes (in press).

21 Granoff, D.M.; Shackleford, P.G.; Pandey, J.P.; Boies, E.G.: Antibody responses to *Haemophilus influenzae* type b polysaccharide vaccines in relation to Km(1) and G2m(23) immunoglobulin allotypes. J. infect. Dis. *154:* 257–264 (1986).

22 Insel, R.A.: B cell developmental pathway responses to polysaccharides. Pediat. Res. *20:* 295A (1986).

23 Granoff, D.M.; Pandey, J.; Boies, E.G.; Squires, J.E.; Munson, R.S.; Suarez, B.: Response to vaccines and risk of Haemophilus type b disease in children with the Km(1) immunoglobulin allotype. J. clin. Invest. *74:* 1708–1714 (1984).

24 Petersen, G.M.; Silimperid, D.R.; Rotter, J.I.; et al.: Genetic factors in *Haemophilus influenzae* type b disease susceptibility and antibody acquisition. J. Pediat. *110:* 228–233 (1987).

25 Yount, W.J.; Dorner, M.M.; Kunkel, H.G.; Kabat, E.A.: Studies on human antibodies. VI. Selecting variations in subgroup composition and genetic markers. J. exp. Med. *127:* 633–646 (1968).

Donna M. Ambrosino, MD, Laboratory of Infectious Disease,
Dana-Farber Cancer Institute, Boston, MA 02115 (USA)

Further Immunologic Evaluation of Children Who Develop Haemophilus Disease Despite Previous Vaccination with Type b Polysaccharide Vaccine[1]

Dan M. Granoff, Katherine E. Sheetz, Moon H. Nahm, Joseph V. Madassery, Penelope G. Shackelford[2]

Edward Mallinckrodt Department of Pediatrics, and the Department of Pathology, Washington University School of Medicine, St. Louis, Mo., USA

Introduction

Haemophilus influenzae type b polysaccharide vaccine was licensed in the USA in April 1985. In the USA, the vaccine is currently recommended for all children from 24 to 59 months of age [1]. Because this vaccine is not 100% effective, some 'vaccine failures', i.e. cases of type b Haemophilus disease occurring in previously vaccinated children, are expected [2]. We have reported that most vaccine failure children have normal serum immunoglobin concentrations, including IgG2 [3]. However, for reasons that remain unexplained, these children produce abnormally low levels of serum anticapsular antibody in response to both vaccination and to type b Haemophilus disease.

In a study recently presented at the Society for Pediatric Research (USA), Insel et al. [4] also reported finding impaired serum anticapsular antibody responses to immunization and infection in another

---

[1] This work was supported by US Public Service grants R01 AI 17962, AI 19350, AI 19676 from the National Institutes of Health, and RR-36 from the General Clinical Research Branch, and 1902 from the Tobacco Research Council.

[2] Michael T. Osterholm, Minnesota Department of Health; Trudy V. Murphy, University of Texas, Southwestern, Dallas; and Robert S. Daum, Tulane University School of Medicine, New Orleans, provided many of the serum samples from the patients in this study. Kathleen Lottenbach, Venita Boelloeni, and Sharon Bader provided excellent technical assistance.

group of 44 vaccine failure children. In contrast to the patient group we studied, these authors found that approximately 40% of their patients had deficient serum concentrations of one or more immunoglobulin isotypes, particularly IgA, IgG and/or IgG2. The reasons for the discordant results in the two studies could not be explained.

The primary purpose of the present study was to determine the frequency of immunoglobulin deficiency in an expanded group of vaccine failure patients. We also provide further data on the anticapsular antibody responses of the patients following immunization and recovery from type b Haemophilus disease.

Methods

Vaccine Failure Patients. Serum samples from 92 patients with onset of invasive Haemophilus disease three weeks or more after vaccination with type b polysaccharide vaccine were sent to us by physicians in 28 states, the District of Columbia, and two provinces in Canada. This group includes 46 patients who were previously reported [3]. Twenty-five of the 92 cases (27%) were detected as part of active surveillance for Haemophilus disease in Dallas County, Texas, and Minnesota [5], or in Connecticut [Shapiro, unpublished]. Seven other cases were cared for at Cardinal Glennon Hospital, St. Louis, or at St. Louis Children's Hospital. The remaining cases were reported by physicians in other areas who wanted to determine serum antibody responses to type b polysaccharide, or who learned that we were interested in evaluating such cases. *Haemophilus influenzae* was isolated from blood or CSF from 91 patients. In the remaining patient with typical epiglottitis, culture specimens were not obtained but type b antigen was detected in serum and urine by both latex agglutination and countercurrent immunoelectrophoresis.

Control Subjects. Serum samples were available from 25 patients who had been hospitalized previously in St. Louis with invasive *Haemophilus influenzae* type b disease, and who had not been vaccinated with Haemophilus vaccine. This control group is identical to the one described in detail previously [3]. In addition to the unimmunized patient control group, 67 healthy children from St. Louis who had been participants in vaccine trials served as a second group of controls for evaluation of serum IgG2 concentrations. The 67 included 28 children who had served as controls for IgG2 levels in our previous study [3]. The healthy control subjects were selected to match as closely as possible the ages of the vaccine failure patients (±3 months).

Laboratory Methods. Serum IgG, IgA and IgM concentrations were measured by nephelometry (ICS, Beckman, Brea, Calif.). In 23 patients, more than 1 specimen was tested. In our analysis, the values from the most recently obtained samples were used. The median interval between onset of hospitalization for Haemophilus disease and obtaining the serum to measure Ig concentrations was 80 days (range 0–423). Serum IgG2 concentrations were measured using a particle concentration fluorescence immunoassay [6], and a murine monoclonal anti-IgG2 antibody [GOM 1, ICN Immunobiologicals, Lisle, Ill.] [7]. The assay was found to be IgG2 subclass-specific and reproducible (interassay coefficient of variation ~ 10%). Because we previously measured serum IgG2 concentrations in vaccine failure patients using an IgG2 assay based on a heterologous antiserum, we compared the new assay with the old assay. The geometric mean of the IgG2 concentrations in 28 replicate sera measured with the new assay was about half of that measured with the old assay. The sensitivity of the new assay was approximately 380 µg/ml of serum IgG2.

Despite the lower sensitivity and overall lower values obtained with the monoclonal antibody, because it has been characterized in many laboratories, and is distributed commercially on a worldwide basis, its potential advantages would appear to outweigh the possible disadvantages of its relatively low affinity. In the present study, IgG2 was measured in sera from 70 vaccine failure patients and 63 healthy control children. Approximately equal numbers of specimens from controls and patients were coded and assayed together on the same day.

Serum antibody concentrations to type b polysaccharide were measured by a radioactive antigen-binding assay performed as described by Kuo et al. [8] except that ^{125}I-polysaccharide was used as the antigen instead of ^{3}H-polysaccharide. Acute (0–3 days), convalescent (10–93 days) and 'late' convalescent sera (>93 days) from individual subjects were assayed in parallel. The US Office of Biologics postimmunization adult serum pool was the reference standard.

Statistical Methods. Statistical analysis was performed using SAS and RS1 software on a VAX 11/785 computer (Digital Equipment Co.). For calculation of the geometric mean, values below the limit of the assay were assigned values of 50% of the limit (i.e. 0.035 µg/ml for anticapsular antibody, and 190 µg/ml for IgG2).

Results

Clinical. Table I summarizes selected clinical information on the 92 vaccine failure patients: 54 (58.7%) were male; 76 (82.6%) were white, 8 (8.7%) were black, and 8 (8.7%) were of mixed races or were American Indian, Hispanic, or Asian. At the time of vaccination, 6 patients (6.5%) were known to have host factors which might have predisposed them to developing invasive bacterial disease. These patients included one each with sickle cell disease, Shwachman syndrome, recent chelation therapy for an elevated blood lead concentration, and Down's syndrome. Two children had central nervous system shunts which may have predisposed them to developing bacterial meningitis. One of these 2 children had been born prematurely and had a history of bronchopulmonary dysplasia and recurrent pneumonia. None of

Table I. Characteristics of the 92 vaccine failure patients

Number (%)		
Male	54	(58.7)
White	76	(82.6)
Age (Months)		
Immunization		
Mean ± SD	27.7 ± 6.3	
Range	(18–47)	
Hospitalization		
Mean	33.4 ± 8.1	
(Range)	(20–64)	
Number (%) with		
Meningitis	59	(64.1)
Epiglottitis	16	(17.4)
Other	17	(18.5)

the 92 children had a history of prior invasive bacterial disease. Two of the patients had a sibling with a recent history of invasive type b Haemophilus disease.

The mean age ± SD of the vaccine failure patients at the time of immunization was 27.7 ± 6.3 months (range 18–47 months, table I): 15 (16%) were immunized between 18 and 23 months of age, 66 (72%) were immunized between 24 and 35 months of age, and 11 children (12%) were immunized between 36 and 47 months of age. Two children were immunized twice, at 19 months and 24 months, and at 18 and 24 months, respectively. Both developed disease after the second immunization. In our analysis, these children were each counted once, and the dates of the second immunizations were used. The median interval between immunization and onset of hospitalization was 123 days (range 20–670 days). The mean age at the time of hospitalization was 33.4 months (range 20–64 months, table I).

Meningitis was the principal diagnosis in 59 children (64%), epiglottitis in 16 (17%) and other invasive diseases in 17 (19%). One child developed a second episode of type b Haemophilus disease (cellulitis) 7 months after recovery from his first episode (pneumonia).

Immune Evaluation

Immunoglobulins. Table II summarizes the prevalance of low (>2 SD below the mean for age), or borderline serum immunoglobulin

Table II. Serum immunoglobulin concentrations in 92 vaccine failure patients

	Number (%) with		
	Low values*	Borderline values**	Low or borderline values
IgM, IgG or IgA[+]	5 (5.4)	5 (5.4)	10 (10.9)
IgM	1 (1.1)	1 (1.1)	2 (2.2)
IgA	4 (4.3)	4 (4.3)	8 (8.7)
IgG	2 (2.2)	1 (1.1)	3 (3.3)

* > 2 SD below mean for normal children of similar age.
** 2 SD below mean for normal children of similar age.
[+] Some children had low or bordeline levels of more than one isotype.

Table III. Serum IgG2 concentrations of the vaccine failure patients

Subjects	Number tested	Mean age months	Serum IgG2, µg/ml		
			geometric mean	n	< 380[1] (%)
Vaccine failures	70	34.8	644	11	(15.7)
Healthy controls	63	32.2	781	8	(12.7)
Probability			0.13		> 0.5

[1] Lower limit of assay

concentrations (~2 SD below the mean for age) in the vaccine failure children. Two children had low or borderline IgM values, 8 had low or borderline IgA values, and three had low or borderline IgG values. Because more than one isotype was low or borderline in some children, a total of 10 of the 92 children (10.9%) had low or borderline concentrations of IgM, IgA, or IgG. Note however, that only 5 of the 92 patients (5.4%) had concentrations below the normal range for age.

Table III summarizes the serum IgG2 concentrations of the vaccine failure patients and healthy control children. The geometric mean IgG2 concentration of the vaccine failure group was lower than that of the healthy age-matched control children but the difference was not statistically significant (p = 0.13). Eleven of 70 vaccine failure subjects

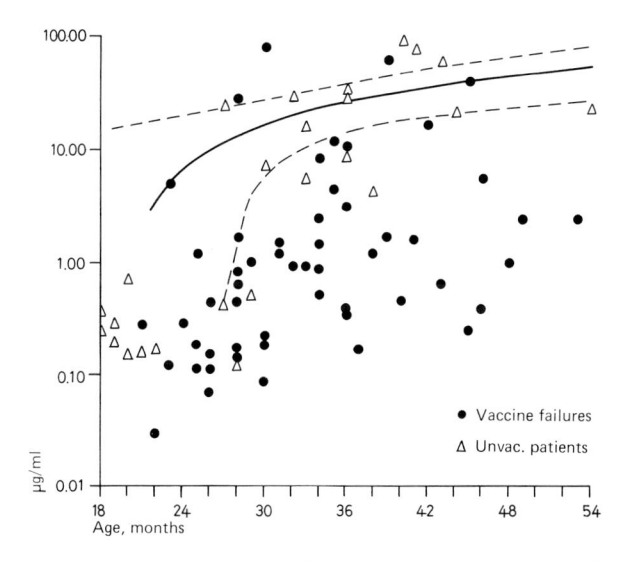

Fig. 1. Total *Haemophilus influenzae* type b anticapsular antibody concentration in convalescent sera obtained 10–93 days after hospitalization, as measured by a radioantigen binding assay [8]. The solid line shows the best fit for the antibody responses of the children who had not been previously vaccinated. The dashed lines show the 95% confidence intervals.

tested (15.7%) had serum IgG2 concentrations <380 µg/ml (the lower limit of the assay) compared with 8 of 63 controls (12.7%, p>0.5). Two of the 11 vaccine failure subjects with serum IgG2 levels <380 µg/ml also had low serum concentrations of IgA (77 and 184 µg/ml).

Antibody to Type b Polysaccharide. Serum samples were obtained during the first 3 days of hospitalization from 36 vaccine failure patients and 17 unimmunized control patients. There was no significant difference between the geometric mean concentrations of antibody to type b polysaccharide in acute-phase sera from the two groups (0.27 and 0.44 µg/ml, p>0.10). The geometric mean of the antibody concentration to type b polysaccharide in the 55 vaccine failure patients tested increased significantly to 0.83 µg/ml in convalescent serum obtained 10–93 days after hospital admission (p < 0.03). This value was significantly lower than that in convalescent sera of the 25 unimmunized control patients (0.83 vs. 4.07 µg/ml, p = 0.0002, by analysis of covariance with age as a covariate). In 33 vaccine failure patients, there was no significant further increase in antibody in 'late' convalescent sera obtained 95-423 days after onset of disease (median = 190 days) (geometric mean antibody = 0.84 µg/ml).

Figure 1 shows the individual anticapsular antibody concentrations in convalescent sera obtained from vaccine failure and control patients 10-93 days after onset of hospitalization. Most vaccinated and unvaccinated patients who developed disease between 18 and 30 months of age had convalescent antibody concentrations <1.0 µg/ml. In contrast, all control patients >30 months of age who had not been previously vaccinated developed high concentrations of antibody (>4.0 µg/ml) whereas almost half of the 32 vaccine failure children tested in this age group had concentrations ≤1.0 µg/ml.

The vaccine failure patients with borderline or low serum Ig concentrations included high- and low-antibody responders to the type b capsule. Nine of the 11 vaccine failure patients with serum IgG2 concentrations <380 µg/ml had convalescent or 'late' convalescent sera available for measurement of antibody to type b polysaccharide. Of the 7 who were older than 30 months of age at the time of disease, one, who also was deficient in IgA, had 42.5 µg/ml of serum anticapsular antibody. Two others had anticapsular antibody levels of 2.45 and 2.5 µg/ml, and 4 had levels <0.5 µg/ml. One of the 2 children with low serum IgG2 levels who was <30 months of age at the time of disease had an antibody level of 0.18 µg/ml, and the other child, who also had low serum levels of IgM, IgA and total IgG, had an anticapsular antibody level of 0.84 µg/ml.

Six of the 8 vaccine failure patients with normal serum concentrations of IgG2, and low or borderline serum concentrations of IgM, IgA or IgG had anticapsular antibody levels measured in convalescent sera. One child with low serum IgA had 2.45 µg/ml of anticapsular antibody, and 3 children with borderline serum IgA levels had anticapsular antibody levels of 0.57, 1.7 and 2.2 µg/ml; one child with low serum IgG and borderline IgA had 12.5 µg/ml of antibody, and one child with borderline serum IgM had an anticapsular antibody level of 0.17 µg/ml. Thus, of 15 children tested with low or borderline serum concentrations of IgM, IgA, IgG or IgG2, 6 had high anticapsular antibody responses to disease (>2.0 µg/ml), 2 had intermediate responses (0.8-1.9 µg/ml), and 7 had low responses (<0.8 µg/ml).

Response to Reimmunization. Two patients were reimmunized with type b polysaccharide vaccine approximately one year after recovery

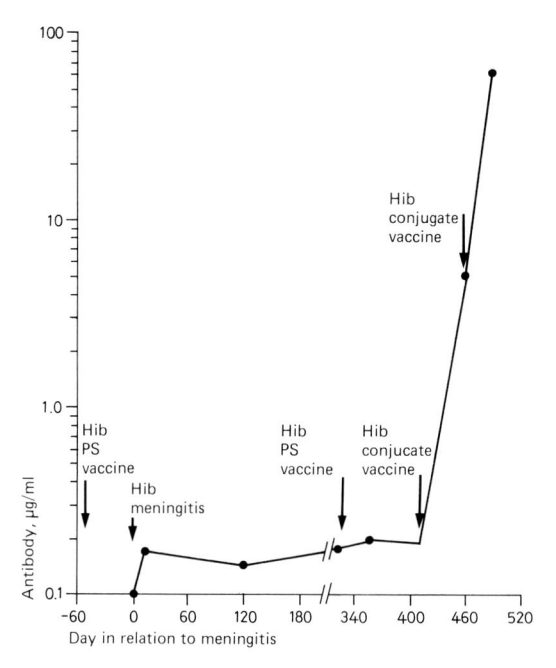

Fig. 2. Serum anticapsular antibody concentrations in a patient who developed type b Haemophilus meningitis despite previous immunization with tye b polysaccharide vaccine. The patient was reimmunized with conventional type b polysaccharide vaccine approximately one year after onset of disease and failed to respond. He was subsequently give two injections, separated by 2 months, of type b oligosaccharide-CRM conjugate vaccine prepared by Porter Anderson (University of Rochester).

from Haemophilus disease. One subject was 58 months of age at the time of reimmunization, and had normal serum immunoglobulin concentrations, including IgG2 (1,807 µg/ml). His IgM concentration was 473 µg/ml, a value just above the lower limit of normal for age (440 µg/ml). The other subject was 45 months of age, and had normal total serum immunoglobulin concentrations. His IgG2 level, measured in a sample obtained at 36 months of age, was 341 µg/ml. Neither child responded to reimmunization (anticapsular antibody concentrations of <0.3 µg/ml in postimmunization sera). The first subject was then reimmunized with two i.m. injections, separated by two months, of type b oligosaccharide-CRM conjugate vaccine (C12, kindly provided by Dr. Porter Anderson, University of Rochester, N.Y.) [9]. As shown in figure 2, this child had high antibody responses (serum concentrations of 5.0 and 62.5 µg/ml of total antibody after the first and second injections, respectively) to immunization with the conjugate vaccine. The second post-immunization sample contained 32 µg/ml of IgG anticapsular antibody as measured by enzyme-linked immunosorbent assay [10].

Discussion

This report extends our previous observations on the immunologic status of children who developed invasive Haemophilus disease despite previous vaccination with type b polysaccharide vaccine. At the time of vaccination, 16% of the patients were 18–23 months of age and, therefore, might be expected to have lower antibody responses to vaccine than the older children [2]. Six children (6.5%), including one immunized at 23 months of age, had conditions such as sickle cell disease or Down's syndrome which might have predisposed them to developing bacteremic disease or meningitis. We identified 5 additional children, including 2 immunized at <24 months age age, with low concentrations of serum IgM, IgA or IgG, a frequency of 5.4%. This frequency is similar to the 6.5% frequency in the subgroup of 46 patients reported in our first study [3]. Five others of the 92 children (5.4%) had borderline serum concentrations of IgM, IgA or IgG, with values just above the lower limit of normal for age. These results differ markedly from those reported by Insel et al. [4] who found low serum concentrations of IgA in 34% of the 44 vaccine failure patients they studied, and low IgG values in 25%.

The reasons for the discrepant results between the two studies are not apparent. We measured the concentrations of IgM, IgA and IgG by a standard nephelometry method which has a high degree of precision. We also repeated the IgA determinations by radial immunodiffusion (Kallestad, Austin, Tex.) in a subset of 10 serum samples. These samples were selected based on availability, and having IgA values as determined by nephelometry that were just above or below the lower limit of normal for age. There was a high degree of concordance in the respective results by the two methods, and none of the samples with values within the normal range by nephelometry where abnormal when remeasured by radial immunodiffusion.

One difference between our study and Insel's is that approximately half of the serum samples we assayed for Ig concentrations were obtained within 80 days from onset of the patient's illness, whereas Insel only assayed samples obtained in 'late' convalescence [Insel, personal communication]. Interestingly, all of the 5 patients in our study identified as having low serum concentrations of IgM, IgA or IgG were tested at intervals >80 days from onset of disease. However, even if we only included patients with sera available from more than 80 days, the frequency of *low* concentrations of serum IgM, IgA, or IgG in our sample would be only 11.4%, substantially lower than the 35–40% frequency reported in Insel's study.

Two other possible explanations for the discrepant results between the two studies are that we may have used different definitions for the lower limit of normal, or there may have been differences in patient referral patterns. With respect to the latter, it is noteworthy that, to date, we have obtained serum samples from 85% of the patients reported to us. These patients include nearly all those identified in several geographic areas in the USA where active, prospective surveillance is employed for detecting cases of type b Haemophilus disease. In contrast, Insel and his co-workers obtained samples from a vaccine manufacturer or the US Centers for Disease Control, and the cases they studied represent only a small proportion of the total number of reported cases. Therefore, it is possible that their sample may be biased as a result of selective reporting and/or referring serum from more severe cases, or from children with underlying diseases.

In the present study, 15.7% of the 70 vaccine failure patients tested had serum concentrations of IgG2 <380 µg/ml (the lower limit of our current assay), whereas in our first study where a heterologous antiserum was employed to measure IgG2, no child had a serum IgG2 concentration >2 SD below normal [3]. However, the results of both studies are consistent in that in the present study, the frequency of serum IgG2 <380 µg/ml in the vaccine failure patients was not significantly different from that found in a group of healthy control children (15.7 vs 12.7%, p>0.5). However, with our current assay, we cannot exclude the possibility that vaccine failure children with levels <380 µg/ml have lower IgG2 values than the healthy control children with levels <380 µg/ml. Therefore, these sera are being investigated further.

Our data indicate that many vaccine failure patients have impaired serum anticapsular antibody responses to immunization with type b polysaccharide vaccine and to type b Haemophilus disease (fig. 1). The majority of these children have normal serum concentrations of Ig, including IgG2 and, we have previously reported, they also have normal serum antibody concentrations to tetanus toxoid protein [3]. The biologic basis for the impaired antibody responses to type b polysaccharide is unknown.

We have previously found that certain Gm immunoglobulin phenotypes were associated with altered relative risk of Haemophilus vaccine failure [3]. This finding suggested that failure to respond to immunization may relate, in part, to genetic factors. Another possible explanation for the poor antibody responses is that prior vaccination with the type b vaccine might induce immune tolerance in some susceptible children. However, tolerance would be expected to be antigen-specific. In a separate study, we immunized 32 vaccine failure patients and 20 healthy control children with pneumococcal vaccine. We found lower IgG antibody responses to type 23, but not to type 3 pneumococcal polysaccharide, in the patients [authors' unpublished data]. Thus, some of the Haemophilus vaccine failure patients have deficient antibody responses to heterologous polysaccharides.

Conceivably, our selection of patients who developed disease despite prior vaccination with type b polysaccharide vaccine may simply have detected many healthy children with low anticapsular antibody responses which are representative of the lower part of the bell-shaped, normal distribution of vaccine responses for any given age group [11]. However, two of the vaccine failure patients were reimmunizd with type b polysaccharide vaccine approximately one year after recovery from Haemophilus disease, and both failed to respond with serum anticapsular antibody. The ages of these children at the time of reimmunization were 45 and 58 months, ages when nearly all normal children respond [11]. Interestingly, one of the two showed high antibody responses to subsequent immunization with a type b oligosaccharide-protein conjugate vaccine (fig. 2). Insel et al. [4] also noted that a number of vaccine failure patients showed poor antibody responses to reimmunization with isolated type b polysaccharide vaccine but responded to immunization with a conjugate vaccine. Therefore, it is likely that many of these patients have a defect in antibody response to isolated type b polysaccharide vaccine but, in some, the unresponsiveness can be circumvented by use of the new conjugate vaccines.

In summary, patients with vaccine failure probably represent a heterogenous group. A small proportion will have easily identifiable predisposing factors such as sickle cell disease, Down's syndrome, hypogammaglobulinemia or other conditions known to impair serum antibody responses to polysaccharide vaccines, or to increase susceptibility to diseases caused by encapsulated bacteria. An additional group, also probably small in number, will have isolated IgG2 deficiency. However, identification of these patients remains problematic because of interassay differences and difficulties in defining the lower limit of normal serum IgG2 concentrations in children of different ages. Clearly, more work is needed to define the role of IgG2 deficiency in children who fail to respond to polysaccharide vaccines, and in susceptibility to Haemophilus disease. Another, perhaps sizable proportion of the vaccine failure children, may have no underlying disease, and their low serum anticapsular antibody responses will be representative of the lower range of normal. However, it is likely that many of the vaccine failure children, despite having normal serum Ig concentrations, will prove to have either a selective impairment of antibody responses to the type b polysaccharide, or a broader impairment of serum antibody responses to include the type b polysaccharide and certain heterologous polysaccharides. Whatever the biologic basis for the impaired antibody responses of these children, it is likely that much information can be learned about normal and abnormal immune responses to polysaccharides by careful investigation of this heretofore unrecognized patient group.

References

1. American Academy of Pediatrics, Committee on Infectious Diseases: Haemophilus type b polysaccharide vaccine. Pediatrics 76: 322–324 (1985).
2. Granoff, D.M.; Cates, K.L.: *Haemophilus influenzae* type by polysaccharide vaccines (Medical Progress). J. Pediat. 107: 330–336 (1985).
3. Granoff, D.M.; Shackelford, P.G.; Suarez, B.K.; et al.: *Haemophilus influenzae* type b disease in children vaccinated with type b polysaccharide vaccine. New England J. Med. 315: 1584–1590 (1986).
4. Insel, R.A.; Gellin, B.; Broome, C.; Smith, D.: IgG2 subclass deficiency presenting as *H. influenzae* b disease after immunization with Hib vaccine. Pediat. Res. 21: 312A (1987).
5. Murphy, T.V.; Osterholm, M.T.; Pierson, L.M.; et al.: Prospective surveillance of *Haemophilus influenzae* type b disease in Dallas County, Texas and Minnesota. Pediatrics 79: 173–180 (1987).

6 Mayus, J.; Macke, K.; Shackelford, P.G.; et al.: Human IgG subclass assays using a novel assay method. J. immunol. Methods *88:* 65–73 (1986).
7 Jeffries, R.; Reimer, C.; Skvaril, F.; et al.: Evaluation of monoclonal antibodies having specificity for human IgG sub-classes: results of an IUIS/WHO Collaborative study. Immunol. Lett. *10:* 223–252 (1985).
8 Kuo, J.S.-C.; Monji, N.; Schwalbe, R.S.; McCow, D.W.: A radioactive antigen-binding assay for the measurement of antibody to *Haemophilus influenzae* type b capsular polysaccharide. J. immunol. Methods *43:* 35–47 (1981).
9 Anderson, P.W.; Pichichero, M.E.; Insel, R.A.; et al.: Vaccines consisting of periodate-cleaved oligosaccharides from the capsule of *Haemophilus influenzae* type b coupled to a protein carrier: structural and temporal requirements for priming in the human infant. J. Immun. *137:* 1181–1186 (1986).
10 Shackelford, P.G.; Granoff, D.M.; Nelson, S.J.; et al.: Subclass distribution of human antibodies to *Haemophilus influenzae* type b capsular polysaccharide. J. Immun. *138:* 587–592 (1987).
11 Granoff, D.M.; Munson, R.S., Jr.: Prospects for prevention of *Haemophilus influenzae* type b disease by immunization. J. infect. Dis. *153:* 448–461 (1986).

Dan M. Granoff, MD, St. Louis Children's Hospital,
400 South Kingshighway Blvd., St. Louis, MO 63110 (USA)

IgG Subclass Composition of the Antibody Response of Healthy Adults, and Normal or IgG2-Deficient Children to Immunization with *H. influenzae* type b Polysaccharide Vaccine or Hib PS-Protein Conjugate Vaccines[1]

Penelope G. Shackelford, Dan M. Granoff

Edward Mallinckrodt Department of Pediatrics, Washington University School of Medicine, St. Louis, Mo., USA

Introduction

Healthy children less than 2 years of age respond poorly to many polysaccharide antigens, including the capsular polysaccharide of *Haemophilus influenzae* type b (Hib PS) [1]. This inability to produce type specific anticapsular antibody is thought to be a major factor in susceptibility of young children to invasive Hib infection. Reports of the relative restriction of antipolysaccharide antibodies to the IgG2 subclass [2, 3], and the late maturation of IgG2 in normal children [4], prompted us to study the IgG subclass distribution of anti-Hib PS antibodies. Our hypothesis was that restriction of the anti-Hib PS antibody response to IgG2 might explain the inability of healthy young children to respond to this antigen. To assess further the relation of serum IgG2 concentration to the response to polysaccharide antigens, we also measured the anti-Hib PS antibody responses of children with recurrent infection who had low serum concentrations of IgG2.

---

[1] This work was supported by US Public Service grants R01 AI 19350, AI 17962, AI 19676 from the National Institutes of Health, and RR-36 from the General Clinical Research Branch.

Methods

Antibody Assays. Total antibody to Hib PS was measured using a radioactive antigen binding assay (RABA) with ^{125}I-labelled antigen [5]. The assay was quantitated using the US Office of Biologics serum reference pool as a standard.

Enzyme-linked immunosorbent assays (ELISA) were used to measure IgG, IgG1, and IgG2 antibodies to Hib PS [6]. Hib PS conjugated to poly-l-lysine was used to coat microtiter plates. Test sera were titrated in the plate and binding was detected with biotinylated conjugates of secondary antibodies. The anti-IgG reagent was a commercially available affinity-purified goat antiserum (Tago, Burlingame, Calif.). The anti-IgG1 reagent was a murine monoclonal (HG 11) developed at Washington University, St. Louis [7]. The anti-IgG2 reagent was a murine monoclonal (HP 6014) purchased from ICN, Immunobiologics (Lisle, Ill.). Since HP 6014 was available in ascites, its binding was detected using a biotinylated goat antimouse antiserum (6650, Tago, Burlingham, Calif.) which had been absorbed to remove reactivity with human IgG. These assays were quantitated using affinity purified IgG1 and IgG2 fractions prepared from a postvaccination serum pool [6]. The anti-Hib PS antibody concentrations of these fractions were assigned using the RABA.

Measurement of Serum IgG Subclass Concentrations. Serum concentrations of IgG subclasses were measured using two types of solid-phase competitive inhibition assays. In one assay, polyvinyl microtiter plates were coated with subclass-specific antibodies and serum samples were titrated as inhibitors of the binding of ^{125}I-labelled myeloma protein to these antibodies [7]. In the other assay [8], latex particles were coated with the purified subclass specific antibodies and were loaded into special multiwell plates (PANDEX). Test sera were added as inhibitors of the binding of fluorescein-conjugated myeloma proteins to the antibody-coated latex particles. The plates were washed and the fluorescence measured in a special 'screen machine'. In both of these competitive inhibition assays, purified myeloma proteins and the World Health Organization standard reference serum (67/97) were used as standards.

The subclass-specific reagents used in these assays were the murine monoclonal antibody specific for IgG1 (HG 11), a monkey antiserum specific for IgG2 [7], and murine monoclonals specific for IgG3 (C3-8 provided by Dr. M.E. Conley) and for IgG4 (provided by Dr. D. Capra).

Vaccines and Subjects. Thirty-five healthy adults were immunized s.c. with 25 μg of conventional Hib PS vaccine prepared by Praxis Biologics (Rochester, N.Y.). Eighty-two healthy children from 18 to 83 months of age were vaccinated i.m. with 5 μg of conventional Hib PS vaccine prepared by Porter Anderson, University of Rochester [5].

Fifteen healthy adults were immunized i.m. with 20 μg of Hib PS covalently linked to diphtheria toxoid (Hib PS-D) (Connaught, Lot 3344), and 15 additional adults were immunized i.m. with 20 μg of Hib PS vaccine (Connaught). Sera from the first eight vaccinees in each group were arbitrarily selected for study of IgG subclass-specific responses [6].

Hib PS conjugated with a partially purified outer membrane protein from group B *Neisseria meningitidis* (Hib PS-OMP) (Lot 1003/C-L680, Merck Sharp & Dohme Re-

Table I. Measurement of IgG1, IgG2 and IgG in affinity-purified anti-Hib PS antibody

Subject No.	Vaccine	Immunoglobulin[1], µg/ml			% IgG1 anti-Hib PS antibody[2]	IgG2/IgG1 ratio	
		IgG1	IgG2	IgG		serum	anti-Hib PS antibody
2105	Hib PS-D	15.5	10.3	27.3	57	0.28	0.66
2106	Hib PS-D	8.8	7.8	28.0	31	0.36	0.88
2116	Hib PS-D	17.7	8.1	22.9	77	0.23	0.46
2124	Hib PS-D	20.2	14.6	35.0	58	1.12	0.72
2114	Hib PS	21.6	12.0	30.0	72	0.28	0.55
2119	Hib PS	11.2	6.0	18.6	60	0.10	0.54

Reprinted by permission from ref. [6].
[1] IgG1, IgG2 and total IgG affinity purified anti-Hib PS antibodies were measured by solid-phase inhibition radioimmunoassay.
[2] Calculated from IgG1/IgG × 100 in affinity-purified antibody

search Laboratories, West Point, Pa.) was given to 6 adults and 40 children in a dose containing 7 µg of Hib PS and 43 µg of OMP. Children 2–6 months of age received 2 injections separated by one month; children 7–17 months of age usually received one injection, although a few children with < 2 µg/ml of anti-Hib PS antibody following immunization were given a second injection of vaccine [9]. Thirty children immunized between 2 and 17 months of age were boosted 10–15 months later with Hib PS vaccine (Praxis), and 10 additional children were boosted with Hib PS-OMP vaccine [10].

Results

Initial Studies. We recently reported the IgG subclass distribution of anti-Hib PS antibody in healthy adults immunized with conventional Hib PS vaccine or Hib PS-D conjugate vaccine [6]. Table I summarizes the results of direct measurement of IgG, IgG1, and IgG2 in affinity-purified preparations of anti-Hib PS antibody. These antibodies were purified by absorption of post-immunization sera with Hib PS-Sepharose 4B followed by elution of the antibody with 3.5 M $MgCl_2$. As shown, the proportion of IgG1 in the IgG anti-Hib PS antibody ranged from 31 to 77%, and there were no apparent differences

Table II. Effect of absorption of IgG1 on IgG anti-Hib PS antibody

Subject No.	Vaccine	Total μg of anti-Hib PS antibody[1]		% IgG1 anti-Hib PS
		before abs.	after abs. of IgG1	
2105	Hib PS-D	9.2	5.7	38
2106	Hib PS-D	5.3	3.2	40
2114	Hib PS	4.1	2.2	46
Serum pool[2]	Hib PS	6.3	2.4	62

Reprinted by permission from ref. [6].
[1] Measured by radioactive antigen binding assay.
[2] Serum pool prepared from 7 adults immunized with Hib PS vaccine.

between subjects immunized with Hib PS or Hib PS-D. It should be noted that although IgG1 predominated in these affinity-purified preparations (i.e. contributed more than 50% of Hib PS), in most cases there was relative enrichment of IgG2 in the affinity-purified antibody compared to that in total serum IgG. In other words, although IgG1 predominated, there was evidence for preferential expression of IgG2 in anti-Hib PS antibody.

Because recovery of bound antibody from the affinity columns ranged from 23 to 61%, we were concerned that we may have preferentially eluted lower affinity antibodies. If the subclass composition of the antibodies varies in relation to affinity, then the composition of our affinity-purified antibodies would be skewed. Thus, we next assessed the subclass distribution of anti-Hib PS antibodies by a second method that was not affected by polysaccharide antigen-binding activity. Anti-IgG1 affinity columns were prepared and used to absorb IgG1 from purified IgG fractions of serum [6]. The contribution of IgG1 to anti-Hib PS antibody was then determined by subtraction. As shown in table II, 38–62% of the IgG anti-Hib PS antibody was removed by absorption of IgG1, confirming that IgG1 is important in the IgG responses to this polysaccharide. Finally, in collaboration with Moon Nahm at Washington University, we used isolectric focusing to visualize directly the contribution of IgG1 and IgG2 to the clonal repertoire of the IgG response [6]. Figure 1 shows the focusing patterns ob-

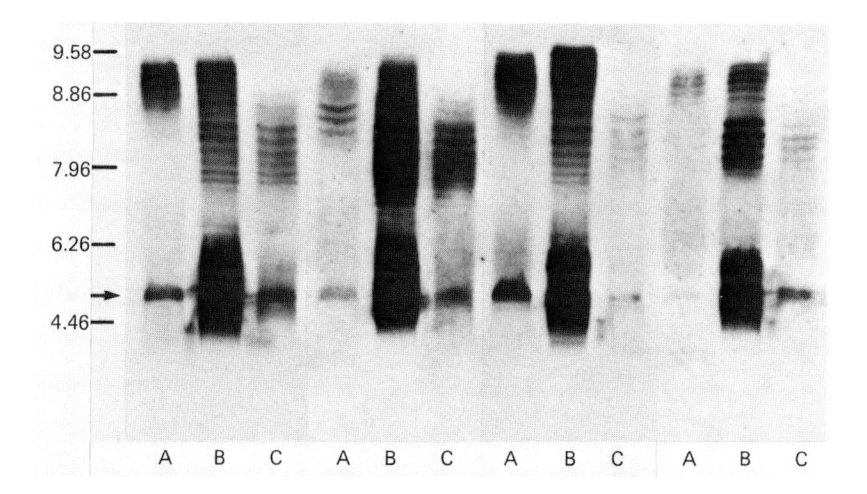

Fig. 1. IEF to visualize anti-Hib PS antibodies in serum and in IgG1 and IgG2 affinity-purified fractions from 4 subjects. A lanes show the clonal patterns of IgG1 fractions. B lanes show the clonal patterns of whole sera, and C lanes show the clonal patterns of IgG2 fractions. The heavy staining in the acidic regions (pH 4–6) is IgM anti-Hib PS as shown by disappearance after absorption of IgM (data not shown). Heavy staining in the application site (arrow) is probably denatured and aggregated anti-Hib PS antibody. Gels prepared in collaboration with Moon Nahm, Washington University, St. Louis. Reprinted by permission from ref. [6].

tained with sera from 4 representative immunized adults. Clearly, both IgG1 and IgG2 contribute to the spectrotypic pattern of anti-Hib PS antibody.

ELISA. The methods described above are not practical for assaying subclasses in large numbers of samples, particularly from children in whom frequently only small volumes are available for study. ELISA were therefore developed for measurement of IgG, IgG1, and IgG2 anti-Hib PS antibodies [6].

Response to Hib PS Vaccine. Using an ELISA, we measured the subclass composition of anti-Hib PS antibody in serum from 30 adults and 82 children immunized with Hib PS vaccine (table III). The adults in this sample are different individuals than those immunized in our first study [6] described above. Also, in the second study, our analysis was restricted to IgG 'responder subjects', that is individuals who had

Table III. Subclass composition of Hib PS antibodies in IgG responder adults and children immunized with Hib PS

Isotype	Anticapsular antibody (geometric mean), µg/ml		
	adults (n = 30)	children (n = 37)[1]	p value
IgG	30.9	10.0	<0.001
IgG1	9.1	5.8	n.s.
IgG2	7.9	1.7	<0.001

[1] 16–83 months of age (mean = 49 months).

> 1.9 µg/ml of IgG anti-Hib PS antibody in postimmunization serum. This level was chosen arbitrarily to avoid the error inherent in measuring IgG subclass composition of specific antibody in lower titer samples. Thirty-seven of 82 children (mean age, 49 months) and 30 of 35 adults hat IgG anti-Hib PS concentrations > 1.9 µg/ml. As expected, the IgG anti-Hib PS antibody response of the adults was greater than that of the responder children (geometric means of 30.9 vs 10.0 µg/ml, p < 0.001). The IgG2 responses of the adults were 4-fold greater than those of the responder children (geometric means of 7.9 vs 1.7 µg/ml, p < 0.001). Interestingly, the IgG1 responses of the two groups were not significantly different (9.1 vs 5.8 µg/ml, p > 0.10). The higher IgG2 responses of the adults resulted in a lower geometric mean ratio of IgG1/IgG2 in the adults than in the children (1.2 vs 3.5, p < 0.001).

Response to Hib PS-OMP Conjugate Vaccine. Immunization of 6 adults with Hib PS-OMP conjugate vaccine produced IgG, IgG1, and IgG2 responses similar to those described above for adults immunized with Hib PS vaccine; the geometric mean IgG1/IgG2 ratio of the adults given the conjugate vaccine was 1.2. When 11 children, 2–17 months of age (mean age, 10 months), were immunized with Hib PS-OMP vaccine, a geometric mean IgG response of 6.3 µg/ml was observed. In contrast to the adults vaccinated with conventional or conjugate vaccine, the IgG responses of the infants to conjugate vaccine consisted almost entirely of IgG1 (4.5 µg/ml) with relatively little IgG2 present (geometric mean 0.3 µg/ml). The resulting geometric mean IgG1/IgG2 ratio was 14.5.

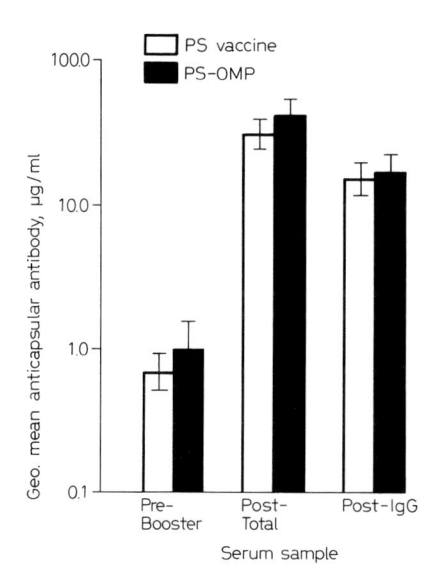

Fig. 2. Anticapsular antibody responses of children (14–31 months of age) to booster immunization with conventional Hib PS vaccine and Hib PS-OMP conjugate vaccine 10–14 months after priming in infancy with Hib PS-OMP vaccine.

In view of the T-cell-dependent (TD) characteristics of Hib PS-protein conjugate vaccines [11] and the striking predominance of IgG1 in the primary responses of the infants, we were interested to determine the subclass composition of the antibody responses of subjects boosted later with either Hib PS vaccine or Hib PS-OMP vaccine [10]. Children 14 to 31 months of age were given either conventional Hib PS vaccine (n = 30) or conjugate vaccine (n = 10) approximately 1 year after immunization with conjugate vaccine. Figure 2 summarizes the antibody responses of the two groups. Both groups of children responded with total and IgG anti-Hib PS antibody responses of similar magnitudes as those measured in adults immunized with Hib PS for the first time, and there were no significant differences in the antibody responses of the two groups of children boosted with either vaccine. In each group, IgG1 antibody accounted for the majority of the IgG response, although the geometric mean IgG2 anti-Hib PS antibody levels achieved after Hib PS vaccine (3.9 µg/ml) or after Hib PS-OMP vaccine (4.2 µg/ml) represent a 30-fold increase over the respective prebooster geometric mean IgG2 antibody levels. Following the boos-

Table IV. IgG subclass distribution of anti-Hib PS antibody response of white adults in relation of the G2m(23) allotype[a]

IgG1/IgG2 anticapsular antibody	Number tested	Number G2m(23) positive[b]	%[c]
≤ 0.5	20	17	85
0.5–4.9	44	29	66
≥ 5.0	15	6	40

[a] Adults were immunized with Hib PS vaccine (see text).
[b] Allotype status determined by Janardan Pandey, Medical University of South Carolina, Charleston.
[c] $\chi^2 = 7.7$ (d.f. = 2, p = 0.02).

ter, the geometric mean ratio of IgG1/IgG2 anticapsular antibody for children given Hib PS-OMP was higher than that of the children given Hib PS (5.1 vs 2.9), but the difference was not statistically significant (p = 0.2).

Subclass Response in Relation to the G2m(23) Allotype. We have observed marked heterogeneity in the subclass composition of the anti-Hib PS responses of healthy adults immunized with conventional Hib PS vaccine or Hib PS protein conjugate vaccines. To test for possible genetic factors which might influence the isotype responses of individuals immunized with conventional Hib PS vaccine, in collaboration with Janardan Pandey at the Medical University of South Carolina, we studied the relation of the subclass distribution of anti-Hib PS antibody to the G2m(23) allotype. This allotype is a genetic marker on IgG2 and was previously designated G2m(n). In a previous study, G2m(23)-positive adults immunized with Hib PS vaccine were found to have higher IgG responses than those who were negative for this allotype [12]. In our study, subjects were divided into groups based on those with a predominance of IgG1 in their anticapsular antibody response (IgG1/IgG2 ratios > 5.0), those with a predominance of IgG2 (ratio < 0.5), and those in the intermediate range (ratios > 0.5 and < 5). The individuals studied included 35 subjects immunized with Hib PS vaccine prepared by Praxis Biologics, and 44 additional subjects who received either Praxis vaccine along with 23 valent pneumococcal vaccine and meningococcal A, C, Y, W-135 vaccine (n = 21), or Hib PS vaccine prepared by Porter Anderson [5] along with meningococcal A, C vaccine (n = 23). The data from the 3 groups were combined. As shown in table IV, there was an over-representation of G2m(23)-positive individuals among those responding with predominantly IgG2 antibody, and an under-representation of those with this allotype in the group with predominant IgG1 responses (p = 0.02). Subjects in the intermediate range had a proportion of G2m(23) positive individual which was similar to that in the general population (66%). Thus, it appears that the G2m(23) allotype is a marker for a preferential IgG2 responses in adults immunized with conventional Hib PS vaccine.

Responses to IgG2 Deficient Children. Finally, to understand better the relationship between low serum concentrations of IgG2 and responses to polysaccharide antigens, we measured the antibody responses of 13 IgG2-deficient (G2D) children who were immunized with Hib PS. With one exception, these children presented with recurrent or severe infections including recurrent sinopulmonary infection (7 patients), recurrent sinusitis (3 patients), recurrent Hib infection (1 patient), and severe pneumococcal meningitis (1 patient). The exception was a child who was a healthy sibling of the G2D patient with pneumococcal meningitis. Eleven children had serum IgG2 concentrations more than 3 SD below the geometric mean for age, and the 2 remaining children had IgG2 values between 2 to 3 SD below the mean. Only 3 of the children had abnormal concentrations of one or more total serum immunoglobulins: one had low levels of both IgG and IgA, and one each had low levels of IgG or IgA.

The 13 G2D children were immunized s.c. with 25 μg of Hib PS vaccine (Praxis). Their mean age at immunization was 53.9 months (range 24–162 months). The responses of this group were compared to those of 51 control children immunized at a mean age of 49.5 months. Although the ages of G2D and control subjects did not differ significantly, statistical evaluation of the responses was performed using analysis of covariance with age as a covariate. The total (by RABA) and IgG anti-Hib PS responses of the G2D children were significantly less than those of the control children (table V). Not surprisingly, the IgG2 antibody responses of G2D children were almost undetectable (geometric mean, 0.08 μg/ml), and were significantly less than those of the controls (geometric mean, 0.5 μg/ml, p < 0.001). However, the geo-

Table V. Antibody responses of IgG2-deficient children immunized with Hib PS vaccine

Subjects(n)	Anticapsular antibody (geometric mean), µg/ml			
	total	IgG	IgG1	IgG2
G2D (13)	1.2	0.7	0.5	0.08
Control (51)	9.2	2.7	2.3	0.50
p(2-tail)	<0.001	<0.01	<0.01	<0.001

metric mean IgG1 response of the G2D children also was significantly less than that of the healthy control children (0.5 vs 2.3 µg/ml, $p < 0.01$).

Notably there was marked heterogeneity in the responses of the G2D patients; 5 of 13 showed normal antibody responses, i.e. they produced > 2.0 µg/ml total antibody to Hib PS vaccine in postimmunization sera. There was no apparent correlation between total serum IgG2 concentrations and response to Hib PS within this group. In preliminary studies of the ability of these children to respond to other PS antigens, 3 of the 5 Hib PS 'responders' also showed normal antibody responses to pneumococcal types 3 and 23 polysaccharides.

Discussion

Immunization of healthy adults with Hib PS vaccine evokes an IgG antibody response composed of either IgG1, IgG2 or both. The majority of adults show a predominance of IgG1 (IgG1/IgG2 > 1.0). However, the proportion of IgG2 in anti-Hib PS antibody represents a slight IgG2 preference when compared to the relative concentrations of total IgG1 and IgG2 in serum. Children 18–83 months of age who respond to Hib PS vaccine show a higher proportion of IgG1 antibody than adults (geometric mean IgG1/IgG2 of 3.5 vs 1.2, $p < 0.001$).

When anti-Hib PS antibody responses are evoked in infants less than 17 months of age by immunization with a PS-protein conjugate vaccine (Hib PS-OMP), an almost exclusive IgG1 response is seen (geometric mean IgG1/IgG2 = 14.5) Evidence has been presented that conjugation of Hib PS to a protein carrier confers TD characteristics to the PS [11]. However, in the studies reported here, it is impossible to determine if the predominant IgG1 response to the conjugate vaccine in infants was caused by the effects of T cell regulation or by the young age at the time of immunization since children < 17 months of age produce little or no antibody response to conventional Hib PS vaccine. In other studies, the subclass distribution of anti-Hib PS antibody in adults immunized with Hib PS-D [6], or Hib PS-OMP was similar to that of adults immunized with Hib PS. However, in contrast to the infants immunized with the conjugate vaccine, it is likely that most, if not all, of the adults have been previously exposed to type b polysaccharide or to cross-reacting antigens.

The antibody responses of the children primed in infancy with Hib PS-OMP conjugate vaccine and boosted with either Hib PS vaccine or Hib PS-OMP conjugate vaccine were striking (fig. 2). Although the booster responses of the primed children were predominantly IgG1, there was also evidence of substantial increases in IgG2 antibody. Thus, priming with a TD form of Hib PS (Hib PS-OMP) in infancy, does not suppress IgG2 antibody expression at a later age with subsequent exposure to Hib PS.

In summary, the IgG subclass composition of the antibody response to Hib PS appears to depend upon the age of the individual at the time of exposure and, perhaps, to a lesser extent, on the form of the antigen. In addition, the association of the G2m(23) allotypic marker with relatively higher IgG2 than IgG1 responses in white adults, immunized with Hib PS vaccine, suggests that genetic factors also may affect the IgG subclass response. It is also possible that the route of antigenic exposure may affect the characteristics of the response, although studies to date in this area are limited [13].

Finally, our data confirm previous reports that G2D children have deficient serum antibody responses to immunization with Hib PS. However, our data indicate that there is clear heterogeneity in the responses of this group that is unrelated to the degree of serum IgG2 deficiency, and that some of the G2D children show normal responses to Hib PS vaccine. Also, the low IgG responses of the G2D children were not necessarily related directly to the low serum IgG2 levels, since in most subjects with low responses, the IgG1 as well as IgG2 responses were abnormal. Thus, a low serum IgG2 concentration appears to be a marker of impaired IgG responses to this polysaccharide, rather than a cause of the low response.

Future studies are needed to determine the reasons why healthy infants and older G2D children with recurrent infection fail to respond to Hib PS. Examination of B cell populations and assessment of IgG subclass expression on the surface of B cells and in plasma cells, as well as regulation IgG subclass secretion in vitro, are needed. It will also be of interest to determine if unique B cell subpopulations have been activated by TD forms of Hib PS or rather, if the same B cells are driven to alternate subclass expression by T cell effects.

References

1. Robbins, J.B.: Vaccines for the prevention of encapsulated bacterial diseases: current status, prospects for the future. Immunochemistry *15:* 839–854 (1978).
2. Yount, W.J.; Dorner, M.M.; Kunkel, H.G.; Kabat, E.A.: Studies on human antibodies. VI. Selective variations in subgroup composition and gentic markers. J. exp. Med. *127:* 633–648 (1968).
3. Riesen, W.F.; Skvaril, F.; Braun, D.G.: Natural infection of man with group A streptococci. Levels, restriction in class, subclass, and type; and clonal appearance of polysaccharide group-specific antibodies. Scand. J. Immunol. *5:* 383–390 (1976).
4. Schur, P.H.; Rosen, F.; Norman, M.E.: Immunoglobulin subclasses in normal children. Pediat. Res. *13:* 181–183 (1979).
5. Granoff, D.M.; Shackelford, P.G.; Pandey, J.P.; Boies, E.G.: Antibody responses to *Haemophilus influenzae* type b polysaccharide vaccine in relation to the Km(1) and G2m(23) immunoglobulin allotypes. J. infect. Dis. *154:* 257–264 (1986).
6. Shackelford, P.G.; Granoff, D.M.; Nelson, S.J.; Scott, M.G.; Smith, D.S.; Nahm, M.H.: Subclass distribution of human antibodies to *Haemophilus influenzae* type b capsular polysaccharide. J. Immun. *138:* 587–592 (1987).
7. Scott, M.G.; Nahm, M.H.: Mitogen induced human IgG subclass expression. J. Immun. *133:* 2454–2460 (1984).
8. Mayus, J.; Macke, K.; Shackelford, P.G.; Kim, J.; Nahm, M.H.: Human IgG subclass assays using a novel assay method. J. immunol. Methods *88:* 65–73 (1986).
9. Einhorn, M.S.; Weinberg, G.A.; Anderson, E.L.; Granoff, P.D.; Granoff, D.M.: Immunogenicity in infants of *Haemophilus influenzae* type b polysaccharide in a conjugate vaccine with *Neisseria meningitidis* outer-membrane protein. Lancet *ii:* 299–302 (1986).
10. Weinberg, G.A.; Einhorn, M.S.; Lenoir, A.A.; Granoff, P.D.; Granoff, D.M.: Immunologic priming to capsular polysaccharide in infants immunized with *Haemophilus influenzae* type b polysaccharide – *Neisseria meningitidis* outer membrane protein conjugate vaccine. J. Pediat. *111:* 22–27 (1987).
11. Schneerson, R.; Barrera, O.; Sutton, A.; Robbins, J.B.: Preparation, characterization and immunogenicity of *Haemophilus influenzae* type b polysaccharide – protein conjugates. J. exp. Med. *152:* 361–376 (1980).

12 Ambrosino, D.; Shiffman, M.G.; Gotschlich, E.G.; Schur, R.H.; Rosenberg, G.A.; DeLange, G.G.; VanLoghem, E.; Siber, G.R.: Correlation between G2m(n) immunoglobulin allotype and human antibody response and susceptibility to polysaccharide encapsulated bacteria. J. clin. Invest. *75:* 1935–1942 (1985).
13 Rosales, S.V.; LaScolea, L.J.; Ogra, P.L.: Development of respiratory mucosal tolerance during *Haemophilus influenzae* type b infection in infancy. J. Immun. *132:* 1517–1521 (1984).

Penelope G. Shackelford, MD, St. Louis Children's Hospital,
400 South Kingshighway Blvd, St. Louis, MO 63110 (USA)

Development of IgG Antipolyribosylribitolphosphate Antibodies in the Course of *H. influenzae* Type b Meningitis in Infants below 2 Years of Age

Ger T. Rijkers[a], John J. Roord[b], Marlies C. Struyvé[a], Jan T. Poolman[c], Ben J.M. Zegers[a]

[a] Department of Immunology, and [b] Infectiology, Universtiy Hospital for Children and Youth 'Het Wilhelmina Kinderziekenhuis', Utrecht; [c] National Institute for Public Health and Environmental Hygiene, Bilthoven, The Netherlands

Introduction

Haemophilus influenzae type b (Hib) is an encapsulated gram-negative bacterium and is the major causative agent of endemic meningitis in children [Sell and Wright, 1982]. Antibodies against the capsular polysaccharide, a linear polymer of ribosylribitolphosphate (PRP), confer protection against Hib diseases [Peltola et al., 1984]. The antibody response to polysaccharide antigens has a number of characteristics which distinguishes these responses from antibody responses to protein antigens. Capsular polysaccharides are type 2 T-cell-independent (Tl-2) antigens [Rijkers and Mosier, 1985] while the response to protein antigens is strictly T-cell-dependent. Antipolysaccharide antibodies in man are mainly of the μ and γ2 isotype [Freijd et al., 1984; Bird et al., 1984] antiprotein antibodies are predominantly γ1 [Stevens et al., 1983]. In general, the in vivo onset of antipolysaccharide responsiveness is relatively late: children below 18–24 months of age do not produce antibodies upon immunization with polysaccharide vaccines [Peltola et al., 1977; Cowan et al., 1978]. Group A meningococcal polysaccharides, however, can induce an antibody response early in life [Käyhty et al., 1981]. We recently have obtained data indicating that polysaccharide-specific B cells are present already at the neonatal age [Rijkers et al., in preparation]. Since these B cells obviously are not triggered by polysaccharide-containing vaccines, we were interested whether in vivo exposure to Hib would lead to induction of anti-PRP antibodies. The data presented show that Hib infection may elicit IgG type anti-PRP antibodies in children below the age of 18 months.

Material and Methods

Patients and Controls

Bacterial isolates were recovered from cerebrospinal fluid taken from patients who were admitted to our hospital with clinical signs of meningitis and were identified by standard bacteriological methods. The capsular type of *Haemophilus influenzae* was determined by a slide agglutination technique using antisera against capsular types of *Haemophilus influenzae* (Wellcome, Beckenham, England) or by latex coagglutination [van Alphen et al., 1983]. Children with the age of 6–60 months visiting the outpatient clinic with a medical history free from systemic infections and without an increased susceptibility to infections comprised the control group. Blood was collected from patients at admittance and during reconvalescence and from controls. Sera were stored at –70 °C until use.

Hib Antibody Assay

Flexible polyvinylchloride flat bottom 96 well enzyme-linked immunosorbent assay (ELISA) plates (Flow, Irvine, UK) were coated with 5 µg/ml tyramine conjugated Hib PRP [Robbins et al., 1973] overnight at room temperature. Individual wells were sequentially incubated with 0.1% bovine serum albumin in PBS-0.05% Tween (30 min, room temperature) serial dilutions of serum samples (3 h at 37 °C), peroxidase-conjugated rabbit antihuman IgG or antihuman IgM (Tago, 2 at 37 °C) and orthophenylenediamine (0.2 mg/ml). After 20–30 min, the reaction was stopped by addition of 1 N H_2SO_4 and absorbance read at 498 nm on an ELISA reader. An anti-Hib PRP hyperimmune serum (containing 40 µg/ml antibody [Robbins et al., 1973], Office of Biologics, US Food and Drug Administration) was used as a standard in all assays and was assigned 100 U/ml IgM anti-PRP and 100 U/ml IgG anti-PRP. Specificity of the assay was demonstrated by preincubation of the standard serum with 10 µg/ml PRP, a procedure which resulted in a >90% reduction in optical density. Preincubation with an irrelevant antigen (type 4 pneumococcal polysaccharide) was without any effect (data not shown).

Results

In sera from healthy children below the age of 2 years no significant levels of IgM anti-PRP are detectable. Thereafter, a gradual increase in IgM titers is observed but IgG anti-PRP remains low (fig. 1). These data reflect the relative late onset of antipolysaccharide responsiveness in ontogeny.

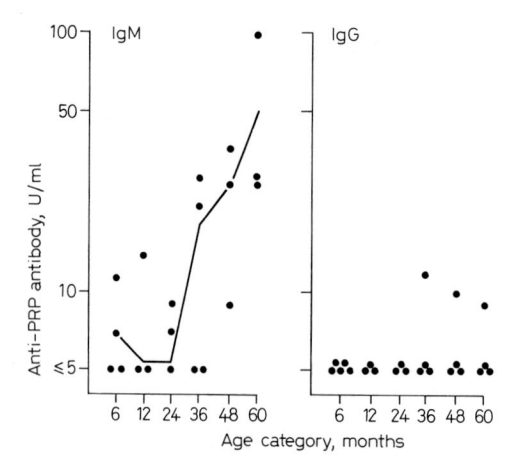

Fig. 1. Development of anti-PRP antibody in healthy children. Children are divided in age categories: 0–6 months (6), 6–12 months (12), 12–24 months (24), 24–36 months (36), 36–48 months (48), and 48–60 months (60). IgM (left panel) and IgG (right panel) anti-PRP are expressed in arbitrary units (see Methods).

A substantial anti-PRP response was observed in children during the course of Hib meningitis, including those below the age of 2 years (patients 1–4 in fig. 2). Both IgM and IgG type anti-PRP was demonstrable and, in those cases in which the development of anti-PRP could be followed in time, maximum titers were obtained at 15–30 days after onset of clinical symptoms of Hib infection. It should be noted that in patients 6 and 7 (3–4 years old), in whom neither IgM nor IgG anti-PRP could be detected, Hib meningitis had a fatal outcome.

Retrospectively, we have analyzed sera from patients who had suffered from Hib meningitis before the age of 2 years old. Elevated IgM and IgG anti-PRP titers could be demonstrated up to 18 months following the onset of Hib meningitis (data not shown). The presence of IgM anti-PRP for such prolonged periods is suggestive for persistence of PRP antigen in these, clinically healthy, children.

Discussion

The available repertoire of the human immune system is restricted early in life as compared to the adult situation [Pabst and Kreth, 1980].

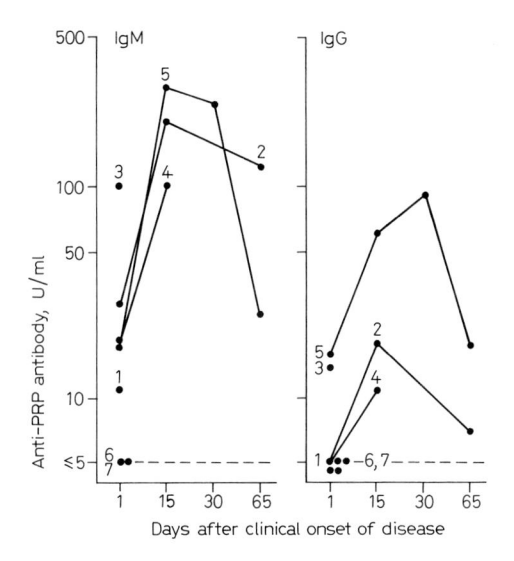

Fig. 2. Anti-PRP antibodies during Hib meningitis in children. Numbers indicate individual patients: 1 = 6 months old; 2 = 16 months; 3 = 12 months; 4 = 13 months; 5 = 29 months; 6 = 36 months; 7 = 39 months. Broken line indicates upper limit of healthy age-matched controls. IgM (left panel) and IgG (right panel) anti-PRP are expressed in arbitrary units (see Methods).

The most prominent restriction is the incapability of young children to mount an adequate antipolysaccharide antibody response. This delay in antibody responsiveness is a 'physiological phenomenon' for type 2 T-cell-independent antigens, a category of antigens to which polysaccharides belong [Mosier and Subbarao, 1982; Rijkers and Mosier, 1985]. Vaccination studies with PRP-containing vaccines have invariably shown that children below 18–24 months of age fail to produce anti-PRP antibodies [Anderson et al., 1972; Peltola et al., 1977; Pincus et al., 1982]. Vaccination with PRP combined with pertussis toxin [Coulehan et al., 1983; Lepow et al., 1984] or vaccination with PRP-protein conjugate vaccines [Anderson et al., 1985, 1986; Eskola et al., 1985] does elicit anti-PRP antibodies in high titers and at a younger age as compared to vaccination with native PRP. The latter observations indicate that the form in which PRP is presented to the immune system determines whether PRP-specific B cells are triggered. Our data demonstrate that children below the age of 2 years clearly develop anti-

PRP antibodies during the course of Hib meningitis. In the light of the above reasoning it is tempting to speculate that PRP present in vivo in the capsule of Hib bacteria is recognized by cells of the immune system in association with other capsular constituents (of which outer membrane proteins are an attractive candidate).

Originally, it has been reported that children below 2 years of age with meningitis caused by Hib do not develop anti-PRP antibodies [Norden et al., 1972]. Later on it was shown, using sensitive radioimmunoassays, that a proportion of those children can develop low titers of anti-PRP antibodies during the course of meningitis; 1.5 years of age seems to be a 'turning point' [O'Reilly et al., 1975; Käyhty et al., 1981]. The data presented in figure 2 confirm that young children (i.e. below the age of 18 months) can produce anti-PRP antibodies, including antibodies of the IgG class.

IgG antipolysaccharide antibodies predominantly reside in the IgG2 subclass. A recent study, however, showed that following PRP vaccination a substantial fraction of IgG anti-PRP in adults is of the IgG1 subclass [Shackelford et al., 1987]. IgG1 and IgG2 have been demonstrated to possess equivalent functional activities in terms of complement-mediated bactericidal and opsonic activity in vitro and protection against experimental Hib bacteremia in infant rats [Weinberg et al., 1986]. It would be of interest to be informed about the subclass distribution of IgG anti-PRP produced during the course of natural Hib infection in young children. To that end we are currently setting up ELISA techniques for quantitation of the subclass distribution of antipolysaccharide-specific antibodies in order to address this issue.

References

Alphen, van L.; Riemens, T.; Poolman, J.; Hopman, C.; Zanen, H.C.: Homogeneity of cell envelope protein subtypes, lipopolysaccharide serotypes, and biotypes among *Haemophilus influenzae* type b from patients with meningitis in the Netherlands. J. infect. Dis. *148:* 75–81 (1983).

Anderson, P.; Peter, G.; Johnston, R.B.J.; Wetterlow, L.H.; Smith, D.H.: Immunization of humans with polyribophosphate, the capsular antigen of *Haemophilus influenzae* type b. J. clin. Invest. *51:* 39–44 (1972).

Anderson, P.; Pichichero, M.E.; Insel, R.A.: Immunization of 2-month-old infants with protein coupled oligosaccharides derived from the capsule of *Haemophilus influenzae* type b. J. Pediat. *107:* 346–351 (1985).

Anderson, P.; Pichichero, M.E.; Insel, R.A.; Betts, R.; Eby, R.; Smith, D.H.: Vaccines consisting of periodate-cleaved oligosaccharides from the capsule of *Haemophilus influenzae* type b coupled to a protein carrier: structural and temporal requirements for priming in the human infant. J. Immun. *137:* 1181–1186 (1986).

Bird, P.; Lowe, J.; Stokes, R.P.; Bird, A.G.; Ling, N.R.; Jefferies, R.: The separation of human IgG into subclass fractions by immunoaffinity chromatography and assessment of specific antibody activity. J. immunol. Methods *71:* 97–105 (1984).

Coulehan, J.L.; Hallowell, C.; Michaels, R.H.; Welty, T.K.; Lui, N.; Kuo, J.S.: Immunogenicity of a *Haemophilus influenzae* type b vaccine in combination with diphtheria-pertussis-tetanus vaccine in infants. J. infect. Dis. *148:* 530–534 (1983).

Cowan, M.J.; Ammann, A.J.; Wara, D.W.; Howie, V.M.; Schultz, L.; Doyle, N.; Kaplan, M.: Pneumococcal polysaccharide immunization in infants and children. Pediatrics *62:* 721–727 (1978).

Eskola, J.; Käyhty, H.; Peltola, H.; Karanko, V.; Mäkelä, P.H.; Samuelson, J.; Gordon, L.K.: Antibody levels achieved in infants by course of *Haemophilus influenzae* type B polysaccharide/diphtheria toxoid conjugate vaccine. Lancet *i:* 1184–1186 (1985).

Freijd, A.; Hammarström, L.; Persson, M.A.A.; Smith, C.I.E.: Plasma anti-pneumococcal antibody activity of the IgG class and subclasses in otitis prone children. Clin. exp. Immunol. *56:* 233–238 (1984).

Käyhty, H.; Jousimies-Somer, H.; Peltola, H.; Mäkelä, P.H.: Antibody response to capsular polysaccharides of groups A and C *Neisseria meningitidis* and *Haemophilus influenzae* type b during bacteremic disease. J. infect. Dis. *143:* 32–41 (1981).

Lepow, M.L.; Peter, G.; Glode, M.P.; Daum, R.S.; Calnen, G.; Knight, K.M.; Mayer, D.; Kuo, J.S.; Lui, N.S.: Response of infants to *Haemophilus influenzae* type b polysaccharide and diphtheria-tetanus pertussis vaccines in combination. J. infect. Dis. *149:* 950–955 (1984).

Mosier, D.E.; Subbarao, B.: Thymus-independent antigens: complexity of B lymphocyte activation revealed. Immunol. Today *3:* 217–222 (1982).

Norden, C.W.; Melish, M.; Overall, J.C., Jr.; Baum, J.: Immunologic responses to *Haemophilus influenzae* meningitis. J. Pediat. *80:* 209–214 (1972).

O'Reilly, R.; Anderson, P.; Ingram, D.L.; Peter, G.; Smith, D.H.: Circulating polyribophosphate in *Haemophilus influenzae*, type b meningitis. Correlation with clinical course and antibody response. J. clin. Invest. *56:* 1012–1022 (1975).

Pabst, H.F.; Kreth, H.W.: Ontogeny of the immune response as a basis of childhood disease. J. Pediat. *97:* 519–534 (1980).

Peltola, H.; Käyhty, H.; Sivonen, A.; Mäkelä, H.: *Haemophilus influenza* type b capsular polysaccharide vaccine in children: a double-blind field study of 100,000 vaccinees 3 months to 5 years of age in Finland. Pediatrics *60:* 730–737 (1977).

Peltola, H.; Käyhty, H.; Virtanen, M.; Mäkelä, P.H.: Prevention of *Haemophilus influenzae* type b bacteremic infections with the capsular polysaccharide vaccine. New Engl. J. Med. *310:* 1561–1566 (1984).

Pincus, D.J.; Morrison, D.; Andrews, C.; Lawrence, E.; Sell, S.H.; Wright, P.F.: Age-related response to two *Haemophilus influenza* type b vaccines. J. Pediat. *100:* 197–201 (1982).

Rijkers, G.T.; Mosier, D.E.: Pneumococcal polysaccharides induce antibody formation by human B lymphocytes in vitro. J. Immun. *135:* 1–4 (1985).

Robbins, J.B.; Parke, J.C.; Schneerson, R.; Whisnant, J.K.: Quantitative measurement of 'natural' and immunisation-induced *Haemophilus influenza* type b capsular polysaccharide antibodies. Pediat. Res. *7:* 103–110 (1973).

Sell, S.H.; Wright, P.F. (eds): *Haemophilus influenzae:* epidemiology, immunology and prevention of disease (Elsevier, Biomedical Press, New York 1982).

Shackelford, P.G.; Granoff, D.M.; Nelson, S.J.; Scott, M.G.; Smith, D.S.; Nahm, M.H.: Subclass distribution of human antibodies to *Haemophilus influenza* type b capsular polysaccharide. J. Immun. *138:* 587–592 (1987).

Stevens, R.; Dichete, D.; Keld, B.; Heiner, D.: IgG1 is the predominant subclass of in vivo and in vitro produced anti-tetanus toxoid antibodies and also serves as the membrane IgG molecule for delivering inhibitory signals to anti-tetanus toxoid antibody-producing B cells. J. clin. Immunol. *3:* 65–73 (1983).

Weinberg, G.A.; Granoff, D.M.; Nahm, M.H.; Shackelford, P.G.: Functional activity of different IgG subclass antibodies against type b capsular polysaccharide of *Haemophilus influenzae.* J. Immun. *136:* 4232–4236 (1986).

Ger T. Rijkers, PhD, Department of Immunology, University Hospital for Children and Youth 'Het Wilhelmina Kinderziekenhuis', PO Box 18009, NL-3501 CA Utrecht (The Netherlands)

Subject Index

Acquired immunedeficiency syndrome
 children, γ-globulin therapy 191
 congenital, immunoglobulin G antibody response 133
 hypergammaglobulinemia 92
 hypogammaglobulinemia 92
 T helper cell 83
Agammaglobulinemia 5, 229, see also Hypogammaglobulinemia
 X-linked 160
Agglutination inhibition 12
Anti-D
 antibodies, interaction with Fc receptors 76
 therapy 75
Anti-Sm antibodies 50
 electrophoretic mobility 51
Antibiotics, immunotherapy 171, 190
Antibody(ies)
 anti-DNA 51
 anti-RNP 51
 anti-Sm 50, 51
 anti-SS-B 51
 antinuclear 50
 antipolysaccharide 18
 autoantibodies, see Autoantibodies
 monoclonal, see Monoclonal antibodies
 polysaccharide antigens 69
 protein antigens 69
Antibody-dependent cellular
 cytotoxicity 75
 anti-D antibody 76
Antigen(s)
 HLA class II 113
 polysaccharide 69, 282
 protein 69, 282
 T cell 106, 282
 types 105
Antisera 2, 61
L-Asparaginase, anaphylactic reaction 38
Assays 61–72, see also specific assays
 comparison 68
 method, selection 67
 polyclonal antisera, production 61
Asthma 172, 239
Ataxia telangiectasia
 bone marrow transplantation 123
 immunodeficiency 113
Autoantibodies
 anti-Sm 50
 systemic lupus erythematosus 41
Autoimmune disease 164

B cell
 activation 106–109
  T cell-dependent 106–108
  T cell-independent 108, 109
 malignant 8
 polysaccharide-specific 282
 precursors 51
Bee venom 33, 34
Bone marrow transplantation 242
 ataxia telangiectasia 123
 cytomegalovirus infection 222
 immunodeficiency 114, 123
 immunoglobulin A 123
 immunoglobulin G 118, 242
  herpes virus reactivation 30
 T cell function 123
Bronchiectasis 180, 196
 immunoglobulin subclass 2 deficiency 164
 immunotherapy 172
Bronchitis, chronic, immunotherapy 172
Bronchodilators 172
Bronchopulmonary dysplasia 191, 258

Cancer 8
Capsular polysaccharides, see also Haemophilus influenzae type b
 adult immunization 132
 immunoglobulin subclass 2 response 133
Casein 36
Chelation therapy 258
Chemotherapy, immunoglobulin M deficiency 122
Chest pain 168
Children, see also Infants, Neonate
 Haemophilus influenzae type b vaccine failures 256–268
 immunoglobulin G deficiency 97, 168
  defined 194
  immunoglobulin A deficiency 194

Subject Index

immunotherapy 168–176, 194–203
Coeliac disease 36
Cold virus 8
Common varied immunodeficiency 113, 160, 228
Complement activation, immunoglobulin subclass 2 22
Corticosteroids 172, 239, 240
Coxsackie B virus 231
Cytomegalovirus 27
   infection 239
      cause 216
         passive immunoprophylaxis 217
         prevention 216
         transplant recipients 216
Cytotect 218, 219

DiGeorge's syndrome 113
Diphtheria toxin 231
Down's syndrome 258
Dysgammaglobulinemia 103

Echovirus encephalitis 214
Electrophoresis 1
   immunoglobulin G 3
Encephalitis
   echovirus 214
   herpes simplex, diagnosis 30
Endometritis 138
Enzyme immunoassays 12
Enzyme-linked immunosorbent assay 14, 62–65, 130
   advantage 67
   vs radial immunodiffusion 67
Epilepsy 204–215
Epstein-Barr virus 27, 93

Fc receptor 22
Food allergy 36, 239

G2m(23) allotype 276
Gamimune-N 218, 219
Gammagard 218, 219
Gastrointestinal infections 18
Gliadin 36
γ-Globulin
   fractions 1

therapy 168–176, *see also* Immunotherapy
   recurrent infection 100
Glomerulonephritis 117, 124
Graft-versus-host disease 114
   chronic 120
   immunodeficiency 123

Haemophilus influenzae 18
   conjugate vaccines, immunoglobulin G 130
   type b 109, 115, 128
      antibody 261, 262, 282
         assay 273
         immunoglobulin subclass 2 269, 277
         meningitis 286
         radioimmunoassay 246
      capsular polysaccharide 128, 188, 246
      conjugate vaccine 128, 130, 274–276, 285
      immunoglobulin subclass 2 269, 277
      meningitis 253, 286
      response to reimmunization 262
      vaccine 256
         failures 256, 259, 260
Hemophilia 52
Hepatitis 241
Hepatitis B virus 27
Herpes infection 239
Herpes simplex virus 27, 231
Herpes zoster ophthalmicus 239
Histamine release 6
HLA class antigens 113
Hypergammaglobulinemia
   acquired immunodeficiency disease 86
   immunodeficiency virus infection 83
Hypogammaglobulinemia 103, 195
   acquired 177
   acquired immunodeficiency syndrome 86
   congenital 177
   mycoplasma infection 184
   sinopulmonary infection 178

Immunization 98
   immunoglobulin G deficiency 99
Immunodeficiency 7, *see also*
   Immunoglobulin G, deficiency
   ataxia telangiectasia 113
   bone marrow transplantation 114

Subject Index

clinical characteristics 162
common varied 113, 160, 228
DiGeorge's syndrome 113
humoral 228
immunoglobulin G 82, 113–134
primary 113
Purtilo's syndrome 113
severe combined 113
T cell function 78
Immunodeficiency virus infection
hypergammaglobulinemia 83
immunoglobulin A 83
immunoglobulin G 83
Immunoelectrophoresis 1
immunoglobulin G 2
Immunoglobulin(s)
α-chain allotypes 245
γ-chain allotypes 245
cytomegalovirus-specific antibodies 218
exogenous, production 217
homogenous 78
Immunoglobulin A 1
deficiency
bone marrow transplantation 114, 123
immunoglobulin G antibody response 103, 133
selective 113
gastrointestinal infections 18
immunodeficiency virus infection 83
Immunoglobulin D 4
Immunoglobulin G
age dependency 34
agglutination inhibition 12
allotypy 2, 245
antibodies, isoelectric points 132
antiglomerular basement membrane nephritis 114
L-asparaginase therapy 39
assays 62–69, see also Assays
bone marrow transplantation 30, 118, 242
corticosteroids 239, 240
cytomegalovirus immunoprophylaxis 222
deficiency
asthma 239
autoimmune disease 164
bacterial capsular saccharides 103
bone marrow transplantation 114

bronchiectasis 164
bronchopulmonary dysplasia 191
chest pain 168
children 97, 168, 194–203, see also Children, immunoglobulin G deficiency
chronic Borrelia 239
cytomegalovirus infection 239
epilepsy 204
food hypersensitivity 239
genetics 238
herpes infection 239
herpes zoster ophthalmicus 239
immunization 99
maturation 214
myocarditis 239
pericarditis 239
recurrent infections 195, 238, 239
stress 242
surgery 240
electrophoresis 3
Fab region, antigen-binding specificity 74
Fc region, effector function 74
food allergy 36
G2m(n) allotype 252
graft-versus-host disease 123
Haemophilus influenzae
conjugate vaccines 130
type b 115
vaccine failures 260
half-life 230
heavy chain 2
hepatitis, chronic active 241
herpes simplex encephalitis, diagnosis 30
idiopathic membranous nephropathy 114
immunity transfer from mother to fetus 75
immunodeficiency disease 82
immunodeficiency virus infection 83
immunoelectrophoresis 2
immunotherapy, see Immunotherapy
indicator of therapeutic efficacy 34
interrelationships among subclasses 189, 190
Km(1) allotype 252
light chain 2
low birth weight infant 158

Subject Index

metabolic properties 225
monoclonal antibodies 8, 59
myeloma proteins 2
natural killer cell-mediated immunity 223
neutralizing efficacy of subclasses 31
placental transfer 151
polyclonal antibodies 59
polyclonal antisera 61
prednisolone 240
production, T cell antigens 109
protein quantitation 12–14
publications 6, 7
regulation 7
replacement therapy, see Immunotherapy
rheumatoid factor 41
septicemia 143–145
serum levels
  factors affecting 236
  normal 188
streptococci, group B 142, 149
subclasses 1, 3
  percentage composition 33
T cell 51, 52
Immunoglobulin G subclass 1
anti-D therapy 75
anti-SS-B 48
antibodies 133
anticapsular polysaccharide 18, 189
L-asparaginase therapy 39
bee venom 35
deficiency 189
dominant antiviral subclass 27
food allergy 37
half-life 74
herpes virus 30
low birth weight infant 158
protein antigens 69
ribosylribitolphosphate 23
Immunoglobulin G subclass 2 19
antibody response, age 132
antigenic marker 250
clonotypes 134
complement activation 22
deficiency 18, 100, 113, 124, 150, 164, 187, 210, 239, 270
Fc receptors 22

G2m(23) allotype 276
glomerulonephritis 117, 124
Haemophilus influenzae type b antibody 269
half-life 74
immunoglobulin A deficiency 103
low birth weight infant 158
polysaccharide antigens 69
ribosylribitolphosphate 23
streptococci antigen, group B 151, 152
Immunoglobulin G subclass 3 21
anti-D therapy 75
anti-SS-B 48
antiviral 27
L-asparaginase therapy 39
cytomegalovirus infection 30
deficiency 99, 239
half-life 74
marker for viral infections 29
mumps virus 28
protein antigens 69
rotaviruses 27
serum level 187
Immunoglobulin subclass 4
bee venom 33, 35
coagulation factors 52
deficiency 113, 187, 239
food allergy 37
half-life 74
hemophilia 52
herpes simplex virus 27
histamine release 6
rheumatoid factor 42, 52
serum level 187
vascular permeability 42
Immunoglobulin M 1
deficiency
  bone marrow transplantation 114
  chemotherapy 122
streptococci antigen, group B 142
T cell antigens 109
Immunotherapy 34, 100, 160–186
acquired immunodeficiency syndrome, children 191
agammaglobulinemia, X-linked 160
antibiotics 171, 190
antibody production 196

asthma 172
bronchiectasis 172, 180
bronchodilators 172
chest symptoms 168–176
children 168–176, 191, 194–203
chronic bronchitis 172
common varied immunodeficiency 160
concomitant therapies 172
corticosteroids 172
dosage 177, 184
echovirus encephalitis 214
efficacy 164, 172, 180, 195, 210
   hypogammaglobulinemia 232
epilepsy 204
γ-globulin 'cripples' 175
high-dose vs low-dose 184
hydrocortisone premedication 183
immunoglobulin G subclass 4
   deficiency 190
indications 164
intramuscular 160
   efficacy 164, 195
   vs intravenous replacement 178, 190
   limitations 177
intravenous 160, 204
   anaphylactoid reaction 161
   coxsackie B virus 231
   cytomegalovirus antibody
     reactivity 219
   diphtheria toxin antibody 231
   dosage 177
   group A streptococcal antibodies 231
   herpes simplex 231
   immunoglobulin G subclasses 218
   vs intramuscular 178, 190
   Klebsiella pneumoniae antibody 231
   production 218
   rubella 231
   tetanus antibody 231
   Toxoplasma gondii antibody 231
liver function 184
lupus erythematosus, systemic 195
meningococcal sepsis 191
pneumonia, recurrent 172
pulmonary function testing 180, 183
route of administration 160
seizures 205

serum immunoglobulin G level 179, 180
side-effects 173, 183, 198
   immunoglobulin G aggregation 161
staphylococcal infection 190
subcutaneous 196
Infants, low birth weight
   cell-mediated immunity 156, 157
   immunoglobulin G 158
   morbidity data 156
Infections, *see also* specific pathogens, e.g.
   Cytomegalovirus, *Haemophilus influenzae*
   immunodeficiency virus 83
   recurrent 97–102

Klebsiella pneumoniae 231

Leukemia
   acute lymphocytic 79
   chronic lymphocytic 104
Lupus erythematosus, systemic 195
   autoantibodies 41
Lymphadenopathy syndrome 113
   lymphoid interstitial pneumonitis 114

Meningitis
   antibody production 286
   group B streptococci 138
   Haemophilus influenzae type b 205
   pneumococcal 277
Meningococcal sepsis 191
Minnesota CMV globulin 218, 219
Monoclonal antibodies 18, 130
   immunoglobulin G subclasses 8, 59
Monoclonal gammopathies 78
Mumps virus, envelope antigens 28
Myeloma proteins, similarity to
   immunoglobulin 1
Myocarditis 2, 39

Neisseria meningitidis 18, 250
Neonatal cord serum 133
Neonate, pneumonia, group D
   streptococci 139
Nephelometry 12
Nephritis 114
Nephropathy, idiopathic
   membranous 114

Subject Index

Otitis media 100
  recurrent 97
    immunotherapy 107
Ovalbumin 36

Pericarditis 195, 239
Placental transfer 151
Pneumonia 97, 100
  group B streptococci, neonatal 138
  recurrent, immunotherapy 172
Polyribosylribitolphosphate 99, 132
Prednisolone 240
Purtilo's syndrome 113

Radioimmunoassay 62
  immunoglobulin G 12
Radio-immunodiffusion 14, 62
  vs enzyme-linked immunosorbent assay 67
  immunoglobulin G 12
Radio-immunoelectrophoresis 14
Radio-immunoprecipitation 14
Rheumatoid arthritis, vasculitis 42
Rheumatoid factor
  immune complex formation 42
  immunoglobulin G 41, 51
Ribosylribitolphosphate 23
Rocket immunoelectrophoresis 12
Rotaviruses 27
Rubella virus 27, 231

Sandoglobulin 218, 219
  humoral immunodeficiency 228
Seizures 205
Septicemia, group B streptococci 138
  predisposing factors 138, 139
Severe combined immunodeficiency 113
Shwachman syndrome 258
Sickle cell anemia 258
Sinopulmonary infection 277
Sinusitis 100, 277
Sjögren's syndrome 41
Solid phase immunoassay 14
Splenomegaly 104
SS-B
  antibodies 41
  viral RNA 41

Staphylococcus aureus 190
Streptococcus, group A
  antibodies, quantitation 228
  antigenic structure 140, 141
  endometritis 138
  immunoglobulin G 142
  immunoglobulin M 142
  meningitis 13
  opsonization, in vitro 141
  osteomyelitis 138
  pneumonia 138
  septicemia 138
    infants 143, 144
  type Ia antigen 149
Stress 242
Surgery 240

T cell
  antibody production 51
  antigens
    B cell activation 106–109
    immunoglobulin G 109
    immunoglobulin M 109
  B cell precursors 51
  bone marrow transplantation 123
  function, impaired 78
  immunoglobulin G 51, 52
T cell-independent antigens 282
Tetanus 231
Thrombocytopenia purpura 214
Turbidimetry 12

Ultracentrifugation 1
Ureaplasma urealyticum 184

Vaccination
  Haemophilus influenzae, see *Haemophilus influenzae*
  perinatal group B streptococcal sepsis 153
Varicella zoster virus 30
Vasculitis 42
Virus vaccine 98
  immunoglobulin G deficiency 99

Wiskott-Aldrich syndrome 79
  immunoglobulin G antibody response 133